Digestive Wellness

5TH EDITION

Strengthen the Immune System and
Prevent Disease Through Healthy Digestion

Elizabeth Lipski, PhD, CNS, FACN, IFMCP

New York   Chicago   San Francisco   Athens   London   Madrid
Mexico City   Milan   New Delhi   Singapore   Sydney   Toronto

1 2 3 4 5 6 7 8 9   QVS   24 23 22 21 20 19

ISBN   978-1-260-01939-1
MHID   1-260-01939-X

e-ISBN   978-1-260-01940-7
e-MHID   1-260-01940-3

Interior design by Sue Hartman

McGraw-Hill books are available at special quantity discounts to use as premiums and sales promotions or for use in corporate training programs. To contact a representative, please visit the Contact Us pages at www.mhprofessional.com.

Praise for *Digestive Wellness*

"Dr. Lipski is whip-smart and has years of experiences as a clinician and teacher. She comes from a strong evidence-based background, and also embraces traditional models of medicine, what we called 'nature-cure' in my training. Most importantly, Liz is a heart-centered teacher whose warmth comes through in whatever medium you experience her. You'll want to learn from Liz, as will your patients."

Kara Fitzgerald, ND, IFMCP
Author of *The Methylation Diet and Lifestyle* and
FxMed Podcast series.

"Liz Lipski's fifth edition of *Digestive Wellness* is a must-have guide for the millions of Americans with gut-related illness. She continues to translate scientific advances into practical health solutions using natural approaches."

Gerard Mullin, MD
Johns Hopkins School of Medicine
Senior Editor of *Integrative Gastroenterology*,
Oxford University Press

"Whilst a mystery to many, that the gut should hold the key to health and illness, Dr. Lipski puts it front and center in this masterpiece of connections and evidence. If you really want to understand how health is co-dependent on your digestive function, read this book!"

Michael Ash, DO, ND, BSc, RNT
Managing Director, NutriLink

"The health of our microbiome is now known to be at the center of chronic health challenges, digestive and otherwise. Dr. Liz Lipski is a beacon of hope and clarity when it comes to providing in-depth education and insights around GI health, microbial interactions and interventions, and techniques for effectively using food as medicine both personally and professionally. *Digestive Wellness* is a masterwork of the most up to date science and clinical pearls for the most important system in our body. I keep this invaluable resource at the top of my bookshelf and recommend that the clinicians I teach do so as well."

Andrea Nakayama, MSHNFM, FLNP, CNC, CNE
Founder of the Functional Nutrition Alliance

"Liz Lipski's revised edition of *Digestive Wellness* details everything you need to know about the gut. If any health problems plague you, you'll find solutions in this book because they all lead back to your digestive tract. This book is a must-read for literally everyone, but it should be required reading in all medical schools."

Donna Gates
Author of *Body Ecology*

"Liz Lipski's most recent edition of *Digestive Wellness* is even better than its previous guide to the mysteries of the pay down the tunnel that begins at our lips."

Sidney Baker, MD, Sag Harbor, NY

"Liz Lipski does it again with her new fifth edition of *Digestive Wellness*. She is a sought-after health expert and speaker, always bringing a wealth of practical wisdom to her students and as an author. I know many people will greatly benefit from the wisdom she shares on healing the digestive system."

Jill C. Carnahan, MD, ABIHM, ABoIM, IFMCP

This book is dedicated to Barbara Lipski (my sister), Allison Holms (my daugher-in-law), and to the many other brave and generous living donors and families of the bereaved who have donated organs so that others may live.

CONTENTS

Why Is Your Gut Making You Sick?

Doctors are trained to identify diseases by where they are located. If you have asthma, it's considered a lung problem; if you have rheumatoid arthritis, it must be a joint problem; if you have acne, doctors see it as a skin problem; if you are overweight, you must have a metabolism problem; if you have allergies, immune imbalance is blamed. Doctors who understand health this way are both right and wrong. Sometimes the causes of your symptoms do have some relationship to their location, but that's far from the whole story.

As we come to understand disease in the twenty-first century, our old ways of defining illness based on symptoms and location in the body are not very useful. Instead, by understanding the origins of disease and the way in which the body operates as one whole, integrated ecosystem we now know that symptoms appearing in one area of the body may be caused by imbalances in an entirely different system. Everything is connected. The center of that connection is the gut. Nowhere are those connections made clearer, and nowhere will you find a better owner's manual for your gut and how to keep it healthy, than in Dr. Lipski's updated edition of *Digestive Wellness*, which I have used successfully in my practice for more than a decade.

If your skin is bad or you have allergies, can't seem to lose weight, suffer from an autoimmune disease, struggle with fibromyalgia, or have recurring headaches, the real reason may be that your *gut is unhealthy*. This may be true even if you have *never* had any digestive complaints.

There are many other possible imbalances in your body's operating system that may drive illness as well. These include problems with hormones, immune function, detoxification, energy production, and more. But very often the gut may be at the root of your chronic symptoms.

SYMPTOMS THROUGHOUT THE BODY ARE RESOLVED BY TREATING THE GUT

Many today *do* have digestive problems, including reflux or heartburn, irritable bowel syndrome, bloating, constipation, diarrhea, and colitis. In fact, belly problems account for more than 200 million doctor's visits and billions in healthcare costs annually. But gut problems cause disease far beyond the gut. In medical school I learned that patients with colitis could also have inflamed joints and eyes, and that patients with liver failure could be cured of delirium by taking antibiotics that killed the toxin-producing bacteria in their gut. Could it be that when things are not quite right down below it affects the health of our entire body, including many diseases we haven't linked before to imbalances in the digestive system?

The answer is a resounding yes. Normalizing gut function is one of the most important things I do for patients, and it's so simple. The "side effects" of treating the gut are quite extraordinary. My patients find relief from allergies, acne, arthritis, headaches, autoimmune disease, depression, attention deficit, and more—often after years or decades of suffering. Here are a few examples of the results I have achieved by addressing imbalances in the function and flora of the gut:

- A 58-year-old woman with many years of worsening allergies, asthma, and sinusitis who was on frequent antibiotics and didn't respond to any of the usual therapies was cured by eliminating a worm she harbored in her gut called Strongyloides.
- A 52-year-old woman who had suffered with daily headaches and frequent migraines for years found relief by clearing out the overgrowth of bad bugs in her small intestine with a new nonabsorbed antibiotic called Xifaxan.
- A six-year-old girl with severe behavioral problems including violence, disruptive behavior in school, and depression was treated for bacterial yeast overgrowth, and in less than 10 days her behavioral issues and depression were resolved.
- A three-year-old boy with autism started talking after treating a parasite called giardia in his gut.

These are not miracle cures, but common results that occur when you normalize gut function and flora through improved diet, increased fiber intake, daily probiotic supplementation, enzyme therapy, the use of nutrients that repair the gut lining, and the direct treatment of bad bugs in the gut with herbs or medication.

A number of recent studies have made all these seemingly strange reversals in symptoms understandable.

RESEARCH LINKING GUT FLORA AND INFLAMMATION TO CHRONIC ILLNESS

Scientists compared gut flora or bacteria from children in Florence, Italy, who ate a diet high in meat, fat, and sugar to children from a West African village in Burkina Faso who ate beans, whole grains, vegetables, and nuts. The bugs in the guts of the African children were healthier, more diverse, better at regulating inflammation and infection, and better at extracting energy from fiber. The bugs in the guts of the Italian children produced by-products that create inflammation; promote allergy, asthma, and autoimmunity; and lead to obesity.

Why is this important?

In the West our increased use of vaccinations and antibiotics, along with enhancements in hygiene, have led to health improvements for many. Yet these same factors have dramatically changed the ecosystem of bugs in our gut, and this has a broad impact on health that is still largely unrecognized. Our diet has changed significantly in the past 10,000 years, and even more in the past 100 years with the industrialization of our food supply. This highly processed, high-sugar, high-fat, low-fiber diet has dramatically altered the bacteria that historically grew in our digestive tracts, and the change has not been good. Many other modern inventions including antibiotics (both those prescribed to us and those in our food supply), acid blockers, anti-inflammatory medication, aspirin, steroids, and chronic stress all injure the gut, alter our gut flora, and lead to systemic inflammation and chronic disease. Is your gut contributing to your chronic disease or symptoms? It is very likely it is.

Think of your gut as one big ecosystem. It contains 500 species of bacteria that amount to three pounds of your total weight. There are more than 100 trillion microbial cells. There is 100 times more bacterial DNA than human DNA in your body. A whole new field of research has emerged on the human "microbiome" and how it interacts to create health or disease and even weight gain or weight loss. These bugs control digestion, metabolism, inflammation, and your risk of cancer. These bugs produce vitamins, beneficial nutrients, and molecules that sustain your body and your ecosystem through a symbiotic relationship with you. The gut microbiome, probiotics and prebiotics are well-covered here in *Digestive Wellness*.

When the balance of bacteria in your gut is optimal, this DNA works for you to great effect. For example, some good bacteria produce short-chain fatty acids. These healthy fats reduce inflammation and modulate your immune system. Bad bugs, on the other hand, produce fats that promote allergy and asthma, eczema, and inflammation throughout your body.

Another recent study found that the bacterial fingerprint of gut flora of autistic children differs dramatically from healthy children. Simply by looking at the by-products of their intestinal bacteria (which are excreted in the urine—a test I do regularly in my practice called organic acids testing), researchers could distinguish between autistic and normal children.

Think about this: Problems with gut flora are linked to autism. Can bacteria in the gut actually affect the brain? They can. Toxins, metabolic by-products, and inflammatory molecules produced by these unfriendly bacteria can all adversely impact the brain. I explore the links between gut function and brain function in much greater detail in my book, *The UltraMind Solution* and you'll also find much about that here in *Digestive Wellness*.

Autoimmune diseases are also linked to changes in gut flora. A recent study showed that children who use antibiotics for acne may alter normal flora, and this, in turn, can trigger changes that lead to autoimmune disease such as inflammatory bowel disease or colitis.

The connections between gut flora and system-wide health don't stop there. A recent study in the *New England Journal of Medicine* found that you could cure or prevent delirium and brain fog in patients with liver failure by giving them an anti-biotic. Toxins from bacteria were scrambling their brains. Remove the bacteria that produce the toxins, and their symptoms clear up practically overnight.

Other similar studies have found that clearing out overgrowth of bad bugs with a nonabsorbed antibiotic can be an effective treatment for restless leg syndrome and fibromyalgia.

Even obesity has been linked to changes in our gut ecosystem that are the result of a high-fat, processed, inflammatory diet. This has been termed "microobesity." Bad bugs produce toxins called lipopolysaccardies (LPS) that trigger inflammation and insulin resistance or prediabetes, and thus promote weight gain.[7] You'll find a chapter in *Digestive Wellness* that discusses the role of obestity, insulin resistance and diabetes in more detail.

It seems remarkable, but the little critters living inside of you have been linked to everything from autism to obesity, from allergies to autoimmunity, from fibro-myalgia to restless leg syndrome, from delirium to eczema to asthma. In fact, more links between chronic illness and gut bacteria are discovered every day.

These bacteria thrive on what you feed them. If you feed them whole, fresh, real foods, good bugs will grow. If you feed them junk, bad bugs will grow. And when the population of bugs changes, the bad bugs begin to produce nasty toxins. Instead of *symbiosis*—a mutually beneficial relationship between you and your bugs—you create *dysbiosis*—a harmful interaction between bugs and host.

The ecosystem in your gut must be healthy for you to be healthy. When unfriendly bacteria grow in there, the friendly bacteria are pushed out and a toxic environment develops. This toxic environment affects your body and your metabolism in surprising ways.

If you have a chronic illness, even if you don't have digestive symptoms, you might want to consider what is living inside your gut. *Digestive Wellness* is the user's manual for the most important organ in the body, which connects to every other system in the body. A healthy gut is the center of a healthy life. Tending to the garden within can be the answer to many seemingly unrelated health problems.

Mark Hyman, MD

Endnotes

Bass, N. M. Bass, K. D. Mullen, K. D., A. Sanyal, A., et al. (2010). "Rifaximin treatment in hepatic encephalopathy," *New England Journal of Medicine*. 362(12): 1071–81.

Cani, P. D., J. Amar, J., M. A. Iglesias, M. A., et al., (2007). "Metabolic endotoxemia initiates Initiates obesity and insulin resistance.," *Diabetes*. 56(7): 1761–72.

De Filippo, C. De Filippo, D. Cavalieri, D., M. Di Paola, M., et al. (2010). "Impact of diet in shaping gut microbiota revealed by a comparative study in children from Europe and rural Africa,". *Proceedings from the Natl Natlional Academy of Sciience USA*. 107(33): 14691–96.

Margolis, D. J. Margolis, M. Fanelli, M., O. Hoffstad, O., and J. D. Lewis. (2010). "Potential association between the oral tetracycline class of antimicrobials used Used to treat acne and inflammatory bowel disease," *American Journal of Gastroenterology*. 105(12):2610–6. Epub 2010 Aug 10.

Pimentel, M. Pimentel, D. Wallace, D., D. Hallegua, D., et al. (2004). "A link Link between irritable Irritable bowel Bowel syndrome Syndrome and fibromyalgia may be related to findings on lactulose breath testing," *Annals of Rheumatic Disease*. 63, no. 4: 450–52.

Sandin, A. Sandin, L. Bråbäck, L., E. Norin, E., and B. Björkstén. (2009). "Faecal short chain fatty acid pattern and allergy in early childhood," *Acta Paediatrica*. 98, no. 5: 823–27.

Weinstock, L.B., S. E. Fern, S.E., and S. P. Duntley. (2008). "Restless legs syndrome in patients with irritable bowel syndrome: response to small intestinal bacterial overgrowth therapy," *Digestive Diseases and Science*, 53(5): 1252–56.

Yap, I. K. Yap, M. Angley, M., K. A. Veselkov, K.A., et al. (2010). "Urinary metabolic phenotyping differentiates children with autism from their unaffected siblings Siblings and age-matched controls," *Journal of Proteome Research*. 9(6): 2996–3004.

ACKNOWLEDGMENTS

Digestive Wellness takes a functional medicine approach to digestive and systemic health issues. It's foundation rests on the ideas of many people whose minds have helped inform my own—people like Jeffrey Bland, PhD, Sidney Baker, MD, Leo Galland, MD, Russel Jaffe, MD, PhD, Daniel Hardt, ND, Sally Fallon, MS, Patrick Hanaway, MD, Gerard Mullin, MD, Paula Bartholomy, DSc, the faculty at the Institute for Functional Medicine, and many researchers, colleagues, and clients who have taught me so much.

I am grateful to McGraw-Hill for all of their behind-the-scenes work on this edition. Specifically, I want to thank Christopher Brown, my publisher, for giving me this opportunity to thoroughly update *Digestive Wellness*. I appreciate your support and flexibility in this creative process. It felt like Daina Penikas, my production editor at McGraw-Hill, was by my side. I'd also like to thank Ishan Chaudhary, the project manager for this book, and his team of editors for their careful eyes in reviewing every word of this book several times. I specifically want to acknowledge Julie Angel for her insights, edits, and questions. Finally, I am grateful to Ever Olano for creating the detailed index.

And to my husband, Chris Dennen. Your unwaivering love and support allow me to spread my creative wings and fly.

PREFACE TO THE 5TH EDITION

Welcome to the fifth edition of *Digestive Wellness*. The original idea for this book grew from the emergence of an idea: What if imbalances in the digestive system caused not only digestive symptoms, complaints, and disease, but also symptoms, imbalances, and disease throughout the body? And what if by balancing our digestion, we could have more energy, think more clearly, experience less pain, and have better quality of life?

It's estimated that scientific knowledge doubles every two to three years. I've read that data is now doubling within months. That means, conservatively, that there is at least 60 times as much known now as when *Digestive Wellness* was first published in 1995. There was little that was known then, and I primarily wrote the book because I was curious and wanted to learn more. It was the first book to talk about leaky gut, dysbiosis, and the systemic effects of imbalanced digestion.

What we once thought of as a simple system becomes more complex with each advance of knowledge.

Yet the basic principles of great health—whole natural food, rest, satisfying work, communicative relationships, and movement—haven't changed. This book takes the science and melds it with the practical. I've spent the past four decades working with clients; teaching; learning from colleagues, students, and experts; and delving into the research to see how to interpret the research into a more basic question: How can we help people to actually feel better and optimize their health?

Research and information on how digestion affects overall health have mushroomed. What I thought would be a simple update of the fourth edition turned into an enormous rewrite. Daily, I am exposed to new research on gut barrier function, the microbiome both in and out of balance, the gut-brain connection, the mind-body connection, probiotics from supplements and food, autoimmune disease, and the mechanisms of how all of this works and interacts. In recent years, we have been finding out more about the role of the microbiome in kidney health and disease, bone health, cancer prevention and treatment, Alzheimer's disease, and loss of cognitive function.

We've also had seven more years to learn about the mechanisms of how natural, whole foods enhance digestive and overall health and reduce inflammation. Research on gut-healing diets, like the FODMAP diet, Specific Carbohydrate Diet, and other elimination diets can reduce inflammation and rapidly produce relief. This book also offers clues to help you determine which plan may match your needs or those of your patients.

The right diet in the right person can make changes in just a week or two. Just this week, I spoke with a woman who has been suffering for years from mental health and digestive issues. After two weeks on the FODMAP diet, her mental and digestive issues are resolving.

We've learned more about prebiotics from food and supplements, which are the fertilizer for the microbiome; and we have an expanded view of how they also play an important role in systemic health.

We've seen a revolution in lab testing since the fourth edition. We can easily do genomic and microbiome testing from the comfort of our own homes. Well-established labs have grown, merged, and developed new tests. Newer labs have stretched the boundaries of testing to refine earlier testing. We've gone from the 2.0 versions of tests to the 4.0 versions. Conventional laboratories have adopted what used to be considered "fringe" tests into their regular line of products, so that many of them are easier to obtain. Insurance companies (and often Medicare) are more regularly reimbursing for tests that were considered experimental less than a decade ago.

What also astounded me is the increase in diagnoses of so many of the conditions discussed in *Digestive Wellness*. People are more ill than before. The incidence of eczema in infants remains constant, at 10 to 20 percent, but in adults, the rates have risen from 0.5 to 1 percent to 1 to 3 percent (a doubling or tripling). The number of known autoimmune conditions jumped from 80 to 100. Celiac disease keeps rising. People with chronic fatigue syndrome went from 500,000 to between 836,000 to 2.5 million. And so it goes for nearly every condition listed. Part of this is due to much better diagnostics, and part is because the 21st-century way of living is incongruous with excellent health.

Our way of life is slowly killing us. We don't sleep as much as we need; we eat highly processed foods; we move our bodies less; we are lonelier; and we have less leisure time. According to the Environmental Working Group, the average American woman is exposed to 160 chemicals daily, and the average man 80 chemicals.

The more I learn, the more I believe that to a great extent, healing from digestive issues and systemic inflammation is in our own hands. Nutrition and lifestyle changes are your number one therapy. While it is fun to grab for shiny items like genomic and fancy testing, we must begin with the basics. Most people will get better this way. It won't be enough for some people, though, so then we can dive more deeply and do advanced testing, as well as explore how emotional and physical trauma keep people stuck.

If you are looking for an eight-week plan or a quick solution, you'll be disappointed. *Digestive Wellness* is a detailed guide into looking for root issues and solutions to optimize your health over the long term. While you may be remarkably better in two, four, six, or eight weeks, that's not the point. The point is long-term, positive health change.

It's easy to talk about making change and hard to actually make these changes. When you don't feel well, your body is sending an alarm: Something is not right here!!! It's an opportunity for us to listen. As we implement these changes and our lives look different a year or two from now, we also will find improved health and well-being. So, as difficult as it is to stop and listen to the messages our body gives us, the rewards can be great. Do what you can, peel away the layers bit by bit, and with time, your health and life will have shifted radically.

Over the last 24 years, people have sent me fan letters, stopped me in grocery stores, and written emails telling me how this book changed or even saved their lives. This book will empower you. No one knows how you feel or what works and doesn't feel right better than you do. If you don't find the solutions here, working with a team of health professionals may speed up your quest for optimal health. If you get stuck, find a new team member. You are the executive director of your own care. Teams will look different, but consider about working with a physician; specialists such as gastroenterologists, neurologists, infectious disease doctors, and rheumatologists if needed; nutrition professionals such as a Registered Dietitian (RD) or a Certified Nutrition Specialist (CNS); a health or lifestyle coach; someone who does structural work like a physical therapist, chiropractor, or massage therapist; someone who does energetic work like an acupuncturist, cranial sacral therapist, or homeopath; and a therapist on mental/spiritual issues to give you a rounded approach.

Prof. Liz Lipski, PhD, CNS, FACN, IFMCP, BCHN, LDN

WHAT'S NEW IN THIS EDITION

My understanding of how to assess digestive imbalances and disease has grown and continues to change nearly every day. One of the places where I have learned the most is by being on a team at the Institute for Functional Medicine. A group of us discussed what was known, what was believed, what seemed to work, and what we saw in our practices. From this consensus, Patrick Hanaway, MD, Gerard E. Mullin, MD, Tom Sult, MD, Dan Lukaczer, ND, and I developed a 2½-day course that we have taught to thousands of clinicians around the world. For me, the main shift was in how we assess digestive imbalances and diseases. We call this the DIGIN model.

The DIGIN model allows us to look at the underlying mechanisms to assess and come up with a plan for restoring health. These areas are:

- D: Digestion and absorption
- I: Intestinal permeability
- G: Gut microbiome
- I: Inflammation and immune
- N: Nervous system

A DIAGNOSIS IS NOT A CURE—IT'S A STARTING POINT

Two people can have the same diagnosis but different treatments. And they can have different diagnoses and the same treatment. People with the same diagnosis may have different reasons for it. Recently, I've worked with four people who all had been diagnosed with irritable bowel syndrome (IBS). We discovered that each of them had a different issue, and yet the same diagnosis. The first person had a low-grade infection, called small intestinal bacterial overgrowth (SIBO). The second had food sensitivities to dairy and gluten-containing grains. The third had a parasitic infection. And the fourth realized that rest, stress management, and exercise were the key to her bowel issues.

On the other hand, it's also possible for people with various diagnoses to have the same underlying issues. As you'll read later on, people with IBS, fibromyalgia, restless leg syndrome, and interstitial cystitis may all have SIBO as the underlying cause. When treated with antibiotic or antimicrobial herbs and low-carbohydrate and prebiotic foods they improve.

HOW TO USE THIS BOOK: 21ST-CENTURY MEDICINE: FUNCTIONAL MEDICINE

In *Digestive Wellness*, you'll find a Functional Medicine approach seen through the lens of a nutritionist. What is Functional Medicine ? The original idea was developed by Jeffrey Bland, PhD, and David Jones, MD, and continues to be refined and expanded by the thousands of health professionals who use it every day. Functional Medicine, as evolved through the Institute for Functional Medicine, incorporates all of what is considered to be the best medical practices, while also embracing a wide philosophy of health and healing. It looks to find root causes of disease and to find ways to remove them. It offers clinicians a system for quickly assessing and evaluating underlying antecedents and triggers of disease. Functional Medicine cuts across all disciplines and includes all types of clinicians—medical doctors, osteopaths, naturopathic physicians, chiropractors, acupuncturists, nutritionists, nurses, physical therapists, psychologists, massage therapists, and more. It blends the best of science with the art and care of the person to find a personalized, patient-centered approach toward well-being.

In Functional Medicine, finding the underlying triggers of illness and listening to the person's story are key. For example, I recently had a client whose main complaints were stomach pain, diarrhea, fatigue, and a feeling that she was failing. She'd been to many doctors with no relief, and she'd tried many approaches. After a single conversation, it became apparent to me that she had detoxification issues. Her health issues all began about a year after she moved into a brand-new home that was out-gassing (releasing into the environment) toxic chemicals. Treating her digestive issues and fatigue would have been the norm. Yet finding a way to gently detoxify her achieved the best results. On the other hand, I recently worked with a client whose main complaints were depression and fatigue. Although she didn't express issues with digestion at first, supporting her digestive system and switching to an elimination diet were key to her improved mental health and overall well-being.

Functional Medicine embraces person-centered therapies rather than setting protocols. It recognizes and honors the biochemical uniqueness of each person. Throughout this book, use your own story and initial triggers of disease to guide you. Recognize that one size does not fit all, and try what makes sense.

Begin with the recommendations on diet and lifestyle. If you aren't eating well, sleeping, moving, or spending time to relax and renew, begin with small changes in lifestyle.

USING THIS BOOK AND ITS ORGANIZATION

Here's what you'll find in the new *Digestive Wellness*:

Digestive Wellness is divided into five parts. In Part I, we walk through the digestive system. This grounds you in a basic understanding of the system, which makes the rest of the book easier to "digest."

Part II delves into what I consider to be the heart of the book, the DIGIN model. The DIGIN essentials work for many health conditions, and once these are balanced and corrected, health emerges. The features of DIGIN are as follows:

- **Digestion/Absorption (Chapter 3):** We move through fundamentals, such as how you can know whether you are digesting and absorbing your food. If you aren't, how can you balance that?
- **Intestinal Permeability (Chapter 4):** Increased intestinal permeability, also called leaky gut, is explained along with what issues and symptoms it's related to and how to heal from it.
- **Gut Microbiome (Chapters 5–7):** Next, we move into the gut microbiome and look at healthy gut ecology, biofilms, prebiotics, and probiotics.
- **Immune/Inflammation (Chapter 8-9):** We then move into the role of the immune system and inflammation in the gut including food sensitivities, allergies, and intolerances, specifically how to recognize it and heal it.
- **Enteric Nervous System (Chapter 10):** The gut has more nerve endings than the spine and more neurotransmitters than the brain. Here we look at the role of neurotransmitters, stress, and their role in digestive health.
- **Laboratory Testing (Chapter 11):** This chapter includes information on common Functional Laboratory testing, plus questionnaires and self-tests to help you determine where you are out of balance.

Finally in this section, functional laboratory testing and self-tests are also discussed. If you read only one section, read Part II.

In Part III, you will find the specifics about bringing your body back into balance: Wellness as a lifestyle, food as your best medicine, therapeutic diets for gut healing, use of restorative foods for malnourishment and malabsorption, and tools for managing stress and detoxification. Excellent health begins with the basics: food, sleep, movement, laughter, friendship. This section dives deeply into the many ways that we are empowered to change our lifestyle to optimize health. This section also looks deeply at healing foods and therapeutic gut healing diets.

Part IV offers specific healing methods for a wide number of digestive health conditions. We begin with the mouth and traverse the entire digestive tract, discussing each organ in turn. Here you'll get specific ideas about what to do about heartburn, irritable bowel syndrome, bad breath, and so much more.

And finally in Part V, we explore systemic illnesses that have digestive components. Specific research is discussed along with specific healing modalities and functional lab tests.

Throughout the book are exercises and questionnaires designed to increase your self-awareness of mind and body; this awareness will help you shop more wisely, breathe more deeply, relax more fully, and live more freely. Even though we may not be aware of it, we all practice medical self-care. When we get a headache, we take an aspirin, lie down, or go for a walk. If we have indigestion, we take an antacid, eat an umeboshi plum, or drink ginger tea. We know when we're too sick to go to work. Most of the time, we make our own assessment and treatment plan, expecting that the problem will pass with time. When these plans fail, we seek professional help. This book will expose you to more plans, new ideas, and the tools to be your own health expert. Just as one tool won't work for every job, not all of these tools will work for you. But some will, and even the failures may give you useful information.

Digestive Wellness is about taking control of your lifestyle to increase your chances of getting healthier and more vibrant each year. It's informative and practical, and it puts you in the driver's seat. Since the first edition, many thousands of people have been helped from its pages. I hope that you and your loved ones will be among them.

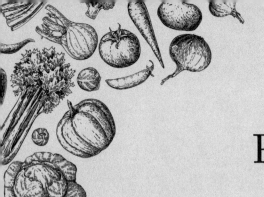

Fundamentals

In Part I, we begin to look at the digestive system in all its glory and wonder. In Chapter 1, you'll hear about the role it plays in our overall health, metabolism, and immunity, and what can push it out of balance. You'll also find questionnaires that help you examine your lifestyle and your digestive health. Take the time to fill these out to gain insights into which sections of the book may be most helpful to you personally. If you'd rather print these out, you can download these from the book's website: www.digestivewellnessbook.com

In Chapter 2, join me as we take a voyage through the how the digestive system works. You'll learn more about the structure and function of the digestive organs and how they work in concert to keep us well.

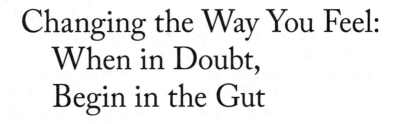

CHAPTER 1

Changing the Way You Feel: When in Doubt, Begin in the Gut

"All Disease begins in the gut."

—Hippocrates

When working with clients, I always begin by looking at simple solutions. Recently, a woman in her mid-50s came to see me. Her neck, back, and wrists hurt. She was losing strength in her right arm and hand and was experiencing numbness in her hand. Her memory was "going down the tubes." Her anxiety and stress levels were high, and she wasn't sleeping well. Her neurologist had diagnosed her with some sort of undifferentiated autoimmune disease. She was about 35 pounds overweight, which she wanted to lose to see if that made a difference in how she felt. Her lifestyle was terrific; she ate whole foods and a well-balanced diet. She taught Pilates and did gentle yoga practice daily. Over the past few months she'd been getting a massage weekly.

So, you're asking, what does this have to do with digestive wellness? Sometimes systemic pain and autoimmune disease can be modulated with changes in diet and lifestyle. The word *diet* comes from the Greek word *diata*, which literally means "our manner of living." Our diet consists of everything we take in. So, I recommended several things. First, I recommended that she see a chiropractor or osteopath to determine whether the weakness and numbness on the right side of her body could be helped with manipulative therapy. Second, I recommended that she go on an elimination diet for two weeks. Third, I recommended that she rest when tired. These are simple solutions.

After three weeks, her neck, arm, and hand pain were nearly gone, and her memory was improving. She lost four pounds, had better energy, and was sleeping better. It was hard to rest during the day, but she was doing it. We added some gut-supportive nutrients, and she continued with what she'd been doing.

When she walked into my office after three months, she had lost 22 pounds "without trying." Her energy level was high, and she was experiencing *no* pain at all anywhere in her body. She was sleeping well and felt entirely healthy. Even though she still had stress in her life, she felt terrific. When I asked about her autoimmune symptoms, she looked at me, threw her arms up, and said, "What autoimmune disease?"

Certainly not everyone gets such benefit from simple solutions, but people often do. This book gives you a step-by-step outline as to what you can do.

WHY DIGESTION?

There is currently an epidemic of digestive illness in our country, one that is directly related to the foods we eat and the way we live. According to the Digestive Disease Clearinghouse and Information Center, between 30 and 40 percent of us have diagnosed digestive issues. Also, 10 to 15 percent of us have irritable bowel syndrome (IBS). Other common digestive conditions include constipation, diarrhea, gastroesophageal reflux disease (GERD), inflammatory bowel diseases (IBDs) such as Crohn's and ulcerative colitis, liver conditions such as fatty liver and hepatitis, gallbladder problems, stomach and duodenal ulcers, esophagitis, pancreatitis, gastrointestinal (GI) infections, diverticular disease, and hemorrhoids.

This list doesn't even include the systemic health issues that have digestive components, such as autoimmune disease, migraines, skin problems, diabetes, and many others.

Healthy Digestion Is the Seat of Total Health

The digestive system is like a river that runs through us. Each day we put pounds of foreign substances (food, drinks, medications, and supplements) into our mouths hoping that our bodies will be able to sort out friend from foe. And generally our bodies do a terrific job, even though much of what we put in our mouths was foreign to the environment even 100 years ago. Because of this interface, the digestive system is the seat of our immune system, runs our metabolism, makes vitamins, and communicates with *every* other cell in our bodies. The purpose of the digestive system, also lovingly called "the gut," is to bring nutrients to each cell of your body. When this doesn't occur, we feel tired and sluggish, can't think clearly, and begin to develop symptoms of illness. If left untended, these symptoms can develop into full-blown health problems.

Surprising Information About Your Digestive System

Research into the functioning of the digestive system has yielded surprising results, turning the arena of digestive health on its head.

- If spread flat, your digestive system would cover a tennis court.
- Roughly 70 percent of your immune system is located in the digestive system.
- You have as many bacteria in your body as cells in your body, and billions of fungi and viruses. These microbes live in communities that live in symbiosis with you. The health of these communities determines your overall health. Collectively these communities are called the microbiome.
- You have 150 times more DNA in your microbiome than in the cells of your body. Put another way, less than 1 percent of the DNA in your body is human; the rest is microbial. The DNA in your cells and in your microbiome talk to each other.
- You have three and a half to four and a half pounds of bacteria in your digestive system that help to make vitamins, protect you against infection, and run your metabolism. Collectively this is called the GUT microbiome.
- The digestive system is often called the "second brain" because if the vagus nerve, which connects the brain and the digestive system, is cut, the digestive system functions fine on its own.
- Your gut manufactures significantly more neurotransmitters, such as serotonin, than the brain. In fact, 80 to 90 percent of your serotonin is made in the gut, and every class of brain neurotransmitter has been found in the gut. The many ways in which your gut and brain communicate is known as the Enteric Nervous System (ENS.)
- You eat food to ultimately nourish all of your cells. If you make poor food choices *or* if your body cannot digest, absorb, and utilize the food due to poor digestive function, you probably will eventually develop signs, symptoms, and finally a diagnosable illness. Digestive insufficiencies contribute to a wide range of health issues, including migraine headaches, depression, arthritis, foggy thinking, autoimmune illness, autism, fibromyalgia, chronic fatigue, multiple sclerosis, and more.
- And finally, foods that are terrific for others may or may not be healthful for you.

PERSONALIZED MEDICINE

A new era of individualized medicine is arriving under different names: Personalized Medicine, Network Medicine, Functional Medicine, Restorative Medicine, Integrative Medicine, Systems Biology. These medicines recognize that rather than focusing on a specific "disease" or "what's wrong," a systems theory model is utilized to explore YOU and your uniqueness to discover which modalities will move you into better health. The new medicine is patient-centered and uses a bio-social framework to balance body, mind and spirit. A diagnosis is a beginning point to explore what you need to optimize your health. The new medicine is based on a team approach, with you at the center. Seventy-five percent of why we seek medical care is due to stress in our lives. So looking at root causes and lifestyle imbalances at the core of this new medicine.

When I was in high school, I first learned about Gregor Mendel and the science of genetics. I was taught that our genes are our destiny, that they were set in stone. This was wrong. Based on research in identical twins, the expression of genes begins changing as our environment changes. One twin may be thin, another obese. One may have diabetes while the other doesn't. If genetics alone were responsible, identical twins would have identical health issues, and this is not so. The things that we do, say, are exposed to, feel, eat, and hang out with make up our environment. In Buddhist terms you might say that our "dharma," or the way we live our life, affects the way our genes react. (See Figure 1.1.) If you are an optimist, then your genes get happy messages. If you are depressed, your genes get unhappy messages. Dr. Candice Pert, in her groundbreaking book *Molecules of Emotion*, explained that when we are happy, dopamine sits on our receptor sites and blocks cold viruses from those sites. Therefore, happy people get fewer colds. In fact, subsequent research finds that

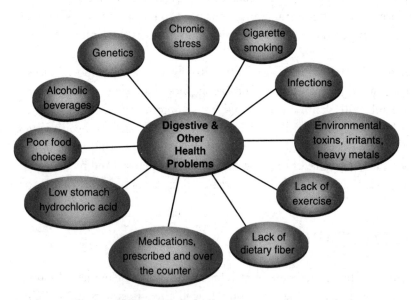

Figure 1.1 **Causes of digestive imbalance.**

happy people get 65 percent fewer colds than unhappy people do. This can be simpli-fied into the following equation:

$$Genes + Environment = Health\ Status$$

To illustrate this point, here are two studies on the effect of lifestyle and diet on how our genes behave. The Functional Genomics and Nutrition Study (FUNGENUT) looked to see whether different carbohydrate sources would change the way genes worked. Participants ate 25 percent of their calories either as rye bread and dark pasta or as oat-wheat bread and potatoes. Those who ate the rye and dark pasta diet had 62 genes that were up-regulated (turned on). The genes that were affected were related to better handling of stress and reductions in inflammatory markers. This study was done in Scandinavia; would the results be the same if this study was duplicated in an Irish population where oats and potatoes provide a large part of the starches in the diet is customary? We don't know because this study hasn't been done. Dean Ornish, MD, performed genetic testing on 30 men who had low-risk prostate cancer. Eighteen of these men's cancer-protective genes were down-regulated (turned off) and 388 of their cancer-promoting genes were up-regulated. For three months, they changed their lifestyles to include a low-fat, whole-foods, plant-based diet; daily stress-management techniques; moderate exercise; and participation in a support group. At the end of the study, the cancer-protective genes were significantly turned on and the cancer-promoting genes had been significantly turned off.

While so far no genetic studies of this type have been done on digestive issues, we can anticipate many of them in the future. The few studies that we do have illus-trate that small changes in lifestyle can have dramatic impacts on how genes express themselves and on how you feel.

Why is this important?

- Your genes are not your destiny. Even though certain "diseases" or "conditions" run in families, your own risk is largely in your own hands. This is known to be true for all of the major chronic health conditions, including heart disease, Type 2 diabetes, cancers, autoimmune conditions, and digestive illness.
- A diagnosis is also not your destiny. Most people can optimize health and feel better than they believed by changing their diet and lifestyle.
- A healthy gut reduces inflammation throughout your body and optimizes metabolism. This is true whether you have digestive issues, autoimmune condi-tions, mental health issues, kidney disease, and/or neurological issues.
- Finding what works for you is unique to you. This book helps you discover your own uniqueness.

EXERCISE 1: ASSESSING YOUR LIFE AND SYMPTOMS

This questionnaire provides the opportunity to consider areas in your life that provide the greatest leverage to move you toward optimal health. You'll also be able to better pinpoint which areas of your digestive system need support. Later sections of the book will provide more detail in how to best do this.

DIGESTIVE AND LIFESTYLE QUESTIONNAIRE

Date: _____

PART 1

This questionnaire will help you assess your lifestyle and digestive status. It is not meant as a replacement for a physician's care. The answers will help you focus your attention on specific areas of need.

MEDICATIONS CURRENTLY USED

Circle any of the following medications you are taking. Add to this list any other medications that you take.

Antacids	Aspirin	Prednisone
Antibiotics	Cortisone	Stool softeners
Antifungals	Laxatives	Tylenol
Anti-inflammatories	Oral contraceptives	Ulcer medications
Other _____		

FOOD, NUTRITION, AND LIFESTYLE

Circle if you eat, drink, or use:

Alcohol	Fast foods	Beans, lentils, and peas
Candy	Fried foods	Margarine
Chewing tobacco	Luncheon meats	Soft drinks
Cigarettes	Fresh fruits and vegetables	Sweets or pastries
Coffee	Nuts and seeds	

Circle if you:

Diet often

Do not exercise regularly

Are under excessive stress

Are exposed to chemicals at work

Are exposed to cigarette smoke

How often do you cook meals from scratch? _____

How often do you eat meals at home? _____

How often do you eat meals out? _____

INTERPRETATION OF QUESTIONNAIRE PART 1

■ Medications

- ■ Medications are good indicators that your body is in some sort of imbalance.
- ■ Medications have drug/nutrient interactions. Some nutrient needs may be increased, some decreased; some nutrients may block absorption or usefulness of the drug. You may want to read a book, ask your pharmacist, or look online for drug-nutrient interactions to see if there are specific nutrients or herbs that you *should* or *should not* be taking with your medications.

■ Foods, Drinks, Tobacco

- ■ Candy, alcohol, sweets, and soft drinks: These "empty-calorie foods" contain few nutrients; however, nutrients are needed to metabolize them, and they replace healthy foods in our diets. These foods have a detrimental effect on most digestive problems; for instance, simple sugars feed yeasts, bacteria, and parasites.
- ■ Cigarettes and chewing tobacco: Make sure to take a good antioxidant supplement and lots of vitamin C to compensate for the stress that tobacco causes. Tobacco has a negative effect on the digestive system, it ages you, and it increases your risk of lung cancer. Chewing tobacco increases the risk of oral cancers.
- ■ Luncheon meats, pastries, fast foods, and margarine: If you eat these foods you are probably getting too much of the wrong kinds of fat: restructured, nutrient-depleted fats. Margarine and most pastries also contain hydrogenated oils, which are absorbed into our cells but are detrimental to our health. They make the cell membranes stiff and stifle the intake of nutrients and outgo of wastes, promote free radical activity, and contribute to atherosclerosis and inflammatory diseases. New research even indicates that they may shorten your life.
- ■ The oils used in deep-frying are used over and over. This creates a breakdown of the oil and increases inflammation throughout your body. Eating fried foods on occasion won't hurt you, but as a part of your general diet, it's not recommended.
- ■ Coffee, tea, energy drinks, and soft drinks that contain caffeine are a mixed bag. On one hand, coffee and tea provide polyphenols and antioxidant nutrients. If you like drinking coffee or tea, that's fine. If you need to drink coffee or tea to maintain your energy throughout the day, that's an issue. Try snacking on healthful foods every few hours to see if that works as effectively. Take naps if you are tired, rather than pushing on.
- ■ As far as energy drinks and soft drinks, my opinion is that these are chemical soups, food-like substances that have no place in our diet. Live on the energy that you

have. Paying attention to what your body needs rather than what your mind wants is one of the keys to enduring health.

- Fruits and Vegetables: The more you eat, the better. Only 12 percent of us eat the minimum of five servings (about 2 1/2 cups) daily. Eating seven to twelve servings daily is optimal.
- Nuts and Seeds: Nuts and seeds are nutrient dense foods that contain healthful oils, fiber, protein, and micronutrients. A handful can be an excellent snack that will keep your blood sugar levels and energy steady.
- Beans, lentils and peas: These fiber-rich and microbiome-regulating foods can also regulate your blood sugar and cholesterol levels.

■ Lifestyle

- Diet often: Weight problems can be caused by a hypoactive thyroid, food sensitivities, poor food choices, sedentary lifestyle, imbalance in the gut microbiome, and emotional and social overeating. Chronic dieting leads to further metabolic slowdown. A wellness-centered approach works best for the overweight person.
- Lack of routine exercise: Exercise is the great stress reducer and enhances the health of our whole body, including our digestive system. Regular exercise at least three times a week for a total of 150 minutes can significantly reduce the risk of cardiovascular disease, help your bowels to move more regularly, and increase your total sense of well-being.
- High stress level: This indicates the need for a good exercise program, ways of nurturing oneself, and training to increase emotional heartiness. Food choices usually suffer during stressful periods, while nutrient needs are increased. Supplementation may be indicated. Read Chapter 13 for ideas on how to better handle and balance life's many stressors.
- Exposure to chemicals: Prolonged exposure to chemicals can cause environmental illness, which can manifest as obvious illness or as nondiagnosable complaints of confusion, chronic fatigue, headaches, or just not feeling right. Metabolic clearing and low-temperature saunas are important.
- Exposure to cigarette smoke: Research indicates that secondhand smoke is detrimental to a healthy respiratory system. If you cannot get away from smokers, buy them "smokeless" ashtrays, open windows whenever possible, and take antioxidant supplements.
- Cooking meals from scratch: Cooking is self-love. Home-cooked meals are generally less expensive, and depending on what you cook, they can be more nutrient dense. A simple meal can be made from scratch in 20 to 30 minutes.
- Eating meals out: If you eat out for most of your meals, make healthful selections. Choose restaurants that serve salads, vegetables, and high-quality food whenever possible.

PART 2

This part of the questionnaire will help you discover where your digestive system is having problems. It is a screening tool and does not constitute an exact diagnosis of your problem. However, it can point you in the right direction in determining where the highest priorities lie in your healing process.

Circle the number that best describes the intensity of your symptoms. If you do not know the answer to a question, leave it blank. Add the totals for each section to assess which areas need your attention.

0 = Symptom is not present/rarely present
1 = Mild/sometimes
2 = Moderate/often
3 = Severe/almost always

SECTION A: HYPOACIDITY OF THE STOMACH

1. Burping or feeling bloated right after eating	0	1	2	3
2. Feels like food sits in stomach	0	1	2	3
3. History of allergies or autoimmune disease	0	1	2	3
4. You easily get food poisoning	0	1	2	3
5. Stomach upsets easily	0	1	2	3
6. History of constipation	0	1	2	3
7. Known food allergies	0	1	2	3
8. Iron-deficiency anemia	0	1	2	3
9. Nausea after taking supplements	0	1	2	3
10. Undigested food in stool	0	1	2	3
11. History of small intestinal bacterial overgrowth (SIBO)	0	1	2	3
12. Age 75–80 = 2 points, over 85 = 3 points	0	1	2	3
13. Takes antacids or proton pump inhibitors (PPIs)	0	1	2	3
14. Pruritis ani (itchy anus)	0	1	2	3

Total: _____

Score 0–7: Low priority
Score 8–12: Moderate priority
Score 12+ High priority

SECTION B: HYPOFUNCTION OF SMALL INTESTINES AND/OR PANCREAS

1. Abdominal cramps	0	1	2	3
2. Indigestion one to three hours after eating	0	1	2	3
3. Fatigue after eating	0	1	2	3

		0	1	2	3
4.	Lower bowel gas	0	1	2	3
5.	Alternating constipation and diarrhea	0	1	2	3
6.	Diarrhea	0	1	2	3
7.	Roughage and fiber cause constipation	0	1	2	3
8.	Mucus in stools	0	1	2	3
9.	Stool poorly formed	0	1	2	3
10.	Shiny stool	0	1	2	3
11.	Three or more large bowel movements daily	0	1	2	3
12.	Dry, flaky skin and/or dry, brittle hair	0	1	2	3
13.	Pain in left side under rib cage or chronic stomach pain	0	1	2	3
14.	Acne	0	1	2	3
15.	Food allergies	0	1	2	3
16.	Difficulty gaining weight	0	1	2	3
17.	Foul-smelling stool	0	1	2	3
18.	Gallstones/history of gallbladder disease	0	1	2	3
19.	Undigested food in stool	0	1	2	3
20.	Nausea	0	1	2	3
21.	Acid reflux/heartburn	0	1	2	3
22.	Connective tissue disease: lupus, rheumatoid arthritis, Sjögren's	0	1	2	3
23.	Alcoholism, diabetes, osteoporosis	0	1	2	3

Total: _____

   Score 0–6: Low priority
   Score 6–10: Moderate priority
   Score 10 or above: High priority

SECTION C: GASTRIC REFLUX

		0	1	2	3
1.	Sour taste in mouth	0	1	2	3
2.	Regurgitate undigested food into mouth	0	1	2	3
3.	Frequent chronic coughing	0	1	2	3
4.	Burning sensation from citrus on way to stomach	0	1	2	3
5.	Heartburn	0	1	2	3
6.	Burping	0	1	2	3
7.	Difficulty swallowing solids or liquids	0	1	2	3

Total: _____

   Score 0–3: Low priority
   Score 4–6: Moderate priority
   Score 7 or above: High priority

SECTION D: ULCERS OR TOO MUCH STOMACH ACID IN THE WRONG PLACE

1. Stomach pains	0	1	2	3
2. Stomach pains before or after meals	0	1	2	3
3. Dependency on antacids for heartburn/acid reflux	0	1	2	3
4. Chronic abdominal pain	0	1	2	3
5. Butterfly sensations in stomach	0	1	2	3
6. Burping or bloating	0	1	2	3
7. Stomach pain when emotionally upset	0	1	2	3
8. Sudden, acute indigestion	0	1	2	3
9. Relief of symptoms by carbonated drinks	0	1	2	3
10. Relief of stomach pain by drinking cream or milk	0	1	2	3
11. History or family history of ulcer or gastritis	0	1	2	3
12. Current ulcer	0	1	2	3
13. Black stool when not taking iron supplements	0	1	2	3
14. Use or previous use of pain medications: aspirin, ibuprofen, etc.	0	1	2	3

Total: _____

Score 0–4: Low priority

Score 5–8: Moderate Priority

Score 9 or above: High priority

SECTION E: LIVER/GALLBLADDER

1. Trouble digesting food with fats and oils	0	1	2	3
2. Jaundice or yellow-colored whites of eyes	0	1	2	3
3. Nausea and vomiting	0	1	2	3
4. Feeling queasy after a fatty meal	0	1	2	3
5. Feeling of fullness with deferred pain to head, belly, shoulder blades	0	1	2	3
6. Have had your gallbladder removed or have gallstones	0	1	2	3
7. Light- or tan-colored, frothy stools, smell bad	0	1	2	3
8. Diarrhea	0	1	2	3
9. Gas and bloating	0	1	2	3
10. Low serum albumin levels	0	1	2	3
11. Bleeding tendency (Vitamin K deficiency)	0	1	2	3
12. Less than one bowel movement daily	0	1	2	3
13. Itchy skin	0	1	2	3
14. Lack of appetite	0	1	2	3
15. Dark-colored urine	0	1	2	3

16. Having a bitter or sour taste in your mouth after eating 0   1   2   3
17. Water retention in legs and ankles 0   1   2   3
18. Big toe painful 0   1   2   3
19. Pain radiates along outside of leg............................... 0   1   2   3
20. Dry skin/hair 0   1   2   3
21. Red blood in stool 0   1   2   3
22. Have had jaundice or hepatitis.................................. 0   1   2   3
23. High blood cholesterol and/or triglycerides 0   1   2   3

Total: _____

    Score 0–5: Low priority
    Score 6–11: Moderate priority
    Score 12+: High priority

SECTION F: ENZYME INSUFFICIENCIES

1. Lactose intolerance, fructose intolerance, or sucrose intolerance.. 0   1   2   3
2. Undigested food in your stools 0   1   2   3
3. Abdominal discomfort, bloating, gas 0   1   2   3
4. Bleeding tendency (Vitamin K deficiency) 0   1   2   3
5. Can't gain weight 0   1   2   3
6. Fatigue for no obvious reason 0   1   2   3
7. Food sensitivities.. 0   1   2   3
8. Transient low blood sugar 0   1   2   3
9. Malabsorption issues.. 0   1   2   3
10. Pale or tan-colored stools, may be frothy and smell bad 0   1   2   3
11. Stools that float 0   1   2   3

Total: _____

    Score 0–4: Low priority
    Score 5–8: Moderate priority
    Score 9+: High priority

SECTION G: FOOD SENSITIVITIES

1. Nausea 0   1   2   3
2. Diarrhea 0   1   2   3
3. Abdominal pain or discomfort.................................. 0   1   2   3
4. Neurological issues, including brain fog, depression, difficulty
   focusing or remembering 0   1   2   3

5. Rashes or hives	0	1	2	3
6. Unexplained fatigue, joint pain, or muscle pain	0	1	2	3
7. Diagnosed with autoimmune disorder	0	1	2	3
8. Digestive issues	0	1	2	3

Total: _____

    Score 0–4: Low priority

    Score 5–8: Moderate priority

    Score 9+: High priority

SECTION H: FOOD ALLERGIES

1. Itching, rash, hives, or flushing	0	1	2	3
2. Itching or tingling in the mouth or on tongue	0	1	2	3
3. Swollen lips, face, tongue, throat, etc.	0	1	2	3
4. Symptoms come on rapidly after eating	0	1	2	3
5. Chronic sinusitis	0	1	2	3
6. Nausea and/or abdominal cramping	0	1	2	3
7. Diagnosed with allergies (i.e., hay fever, asthma, eczema)	0	1	2	3
8. Diarrhea	0	1	2	3
9. Dizziness, fainting, lightheaded	0	1	2	3

Total: _____

    Score 0–4: Low priority

    Score 5–8: Moderate priority

    Score 9+: High priority

SECTION I: INTESTINAL PERMEABILITY/LEAKY GUT SYNDROME DYSBIOSIS

1. Constipation and/or diarrhea	0	1	2	3
2. Abdominal pain or bloating	0	1	2	3
3. Mucus or blood in stool	0	1	2	3
4. Joint pain or swelling, or arthritis	0	1	2	3
5. Chronic or frequent fatigue or tiredness	0	1	2	3
6. Food allergy or food sensitivities or intolerances	0	1	2	3
7. Sinus or nasal congestion	0	1	2	3
8. Chronic or frequent inflammations	0	1	2	3
9. Eczema, skin rashes, or hives (urticaria)	0	1	2	3
10. Asthma, hay fever, or airborne allergies	0	1	2	3

11. Confusion, poor memory, or mood swings 0   1   2   3
12. Use of nonsteroidal anti-inflammatory drugs (NSAIDs), such as
    aspirin, ibuprofen 0   1   2   3
13. History of antibiotic use 0   1   2   3
14. Alcohol consumption, or alcohol makes you feel sick 0   1   2   3
15. An autoimmune disorder including, but not limited to: . . . .
    Ulcerative colitis, Crohn's disease, celiac disease, Hashimoto's . . . . .
    thyroiditis, Graves' disease, multiple sclerosis, lupus, rheumatoid . .
    arthritis, etc. 0   1   2   3
16. Headaches or migraine headaches. 0   1   2   3
17. Chronic nasal congestion. 0   1   2   3

Total: _____

    Score 1–5: Low priority
    Score 6–10: Mild case
    Score 7–19: Moderate priority
    Score 20+: High priority

SECTION J: SMALL BOWEL BACTERIAL OVERGROWTH

1. Excessive gas/flatulence. 0   1   2   3
2. Abdominal bloating and distension, especially with sugar, fiber,
    or carbohydrates 0   1   2   3
3. Diarrhea 0   1   2   3
4. Abdominal pain, cramping, mucus or blood in stools. 0   1   2   3
5. Irritable bowel syndrome (IBS) 0   1   2   3
6. Fibromyalgia. 0   1   2   3
7. Restless leg syndrome. 0   1   2   3
8. Interstitial cystitis 0   1   2   3
9. Chronic constipation 0   1   2   3
10. Intolerance to probiotic supplements. 0   1   2   3
11. Scored 9 or more on section A 0   1   2   3
12. Currently taking antiacids or proton pump inhibitors (PPIs) 0   1   2   3
13. Fatigue/low energy 0   1   2   3
14. Depression or anxiety 0   1   2   3
15. Bad breath. 0   1   2   3

Total: _____

    Score 0–4: Low priority
    Score 5–9: Moderate priority
    Score 10+ High priority

SECTION K: DYSBIOSIS: FUNGAL OVERGROWTH

1. Recurring vaginal, nail, skin, or other fungal infections 0   1   2   3
2. Diarrhea, constipation, or both 0   1   2   3
3. Unexplained fatigue and/or brain fog........................... 0   1   2   3
4. Depression and/or anxiety....................................... 0   1   2   3
5. Chronic sinusitis.. 0   1   2   3
6. Itching in vagina, anus, ears, or other mucus membranes........ 0   1   2   3
7. Gas and/or bloating 0   1   2   3
8. Diagnosis of autoimmune disease 0   1   2   3
9. Skin issues: eczema, psoriasis, hives, rashes 0   1   2   3
10. Low blood sugar issues, mood swings 0   1   2   3

Total: _____

    Score 0–4: Low priority

    Score 5–8: Moderate priority

    Score 9+: High priority

SECTION L: CELIAC DISEASE, GLUTEN SENSITIVITY, WHEAT REACTIONS

Digestive

1. Bloating and/or gas 0   1   2   3
2. Constipation and/or diarrhea 0   1   2   3
3. Nausea 0   1   2   3
4. Weight trouble 0   1   2   3
5. Iron-deficiency anemia 0   1   2   3

Hormonal

6. Fatigue 0   1   2   3
7. Sleep problems 0   1   2   3
8. Depression, anxiety, and/or mood swings 0   1   2   3
9. Menstrual problems 0   1   2   3
10. Infertility 0   1   2   3
11. Thyroid problems 0   1   2   3
12. Osteoporosis or osteopenia 0   1   2   3

Neurological

13. Headaches and/or migraines 0   1   2   3
14. Memory problems 0   1   2   3
15. Joint pains or aches 0   1   2   3
16. Fibromyalgia 0   1   2   3
17. Brain fog 0   1   2   3

Immune System

18. Get infections easily 0   1   2   3
19. History or family history of arthritis, any type 0   1   2   3
20. History or family history of cancer 0   1   2   3
21. History or family history of autoimmune disease 0   1   2   3
22. History or family history of celiac disease 0   1   2   3

Total: _____

   Score 0–6: Low priority

   Score 6–10: Moderate priority

   Score 10 or above: High priority

The section on gluten intolerance was adapted with permission from: Drs. Vikki and Richard Petersen, DC, CCN, *The Gluten Effect,* True Health Publishing, 2009; http://www.healthnowmedical.com. Sunnyvale, CA.

SECTION M: COLON/LARGE INTESTINE

1. Seasonal or recurring diarrhea 0   1   2   3
2. Frequent and recurrent infections (colds) 0   1   2   3
3. Bladder and kidney infections 0   1   2   3
4. Vaginal yeast infection 0   1   2   3
5. Abdominal cramps 0   1   2   3
6. Toe and fingernail fungus 0   1   2   3
7. Alternating diarrhea and constipation 0   1   2   3
8. Constipation 0   1   2   3
9. History of antibiotic use 0   1   2   3
10. Meat eater

      Never = 0   Rarely = 1   Often = 2   Daily = 3

11. Rapidly failing vision 0   1   2   3
12. Recurrent stomach pain 0   1   2   3
13. Blood or pus in stool 0   1   2   3
14. Family history of inflammatory bowel disease 0   1   2   3

Total: _____

   Score 0–5: Low priority

   Score 6–9: Moderate priority

   Score 10 or above: High priority

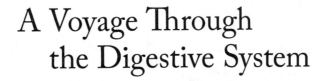

CHAPTER 2

A Voyage Through the Digestive System

"The surface area of the digestive mucosae, measuring up and down and around all the folds, rugae, villi, and microvilli, is about the size of a tennis court."

—Sidney Baker, MD

The digestive system is self-running and self-healing. Because this beautiful, intricate system works automatically, the average person knows very little about it. Let's take a trip through the digestive system to see what miraculous events occur inside us every moment of our lives.

The digestive system (also called the alimentary system, the gut, and the gastrointestinal system) comprises the mouth, pharynx, esophagus, stomach, small intestine, and large intestine (colon) (see Figure 2.1). There are also accessory digestive organs that are outside the digestive tract, including our teeth, tongue, salivary glands, gallbladder, pancreas, and liver. Think of the digestive tract as a 16- to 23-foot tubular set of muscles that runs from the mouth to the anus. At its most basic, its function is to turn food into molecules that our cells can use for energy, maintenance, growth and repair, and waste products. On a deeper level it helps run our metabolism and protects us from infections and foreign substances that may come in via our food.

The digestive system is like an irrigation system. A large source of water gets narrower and narrower, finally getting water to each tiny portion of a field. If the water becomes blocked upstream, the plants wither and die. In the body, the unblocked flow of nutrients is critical for optimal health and function. Along the way, the body breaks down food protein into amino acids, starches into glucose, and fats into fatty acids and glycerol. Enzymes, vitamins, and minerals are also absorbed. The cells use these raw materials for energy, growth, and repair. If digestive wellness is compromised, our cells lose their capacity to function fully. Unlike a field, the body is innovative and will try

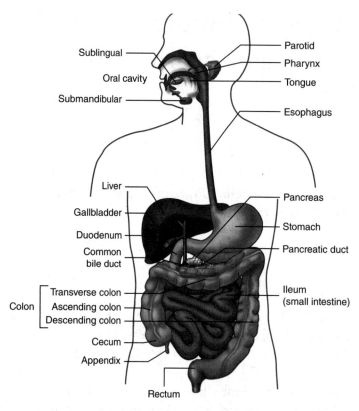

Figure 2.1   **The digestive system.**

THE DIGESTIVE SYSTEM IS WEBLIKE

The digestive system is complex. While we think of it as just something that digests food, here are some of its other less obvious functions:

- **Muscular:** The digestive structure is made of muscles.
- **Immune:** Most of the immune system lies in the digestive system.
- **Neurological:** The enteric nervous system has more nerve endings than our spines and more neurotransmitters than our brains. There is a direct gut–brain connection.
- **Endocrine:** There are more than 16 known digestive hormones, such as gastrin, ghrelin, and secretin.
- **Cardiovascular:** Probiotic bacteria help normalize cholesterol and triglyceride levels.
- **Metabolic:** The commensal bacteria in the digestive system drive the body's metabolism.

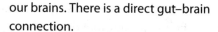

to find ways to make things work. Eventually, however, its ability to seek new pathways fails, and we feel unwell. This is especially apparent in the lining of the digestive tract, which repairs and replaces itself every three to five days.

YOU AREN'T ONLY WHAT YOU EAT

Eating healthful foods is the right place to start, and that's where we focus much of our attention, but many people eat all the "right" foods and still have digestive and other health problems. Typically we digest and absorb 90 to 97 percent of the food that we eat. The rest is typically plant fibers that serve to create bulk and synthesize short-chain fatty acids in our colon. Yet the best diet in the world won't help if you aren't digesting properly. You must be able to digest foods; break them down into tiny particles; absorb the food mash; take that through the intestinal lining and into the bloodstream; assimilate nutrients and calories into the cells where they can be used; and eliminate waste products through the kidneys, bowels, lymph system, and skin. Health can and does break down at any of these phases. For example, people with lots of intestinal gas are often fermenting their food rather than digesting it. Difficulty with absorption can cause people to have food sensitivities, fatigue, skin rashes, and migraine headaches. In people with celiac disease, the gut may be so inflamed that they have malabsorption issues. Diabetics have a problem with assimilation of glucose into the cells. Constipation and diarrhea are problems of elimination.

A GUIDED TOUR THROUGH THE DIGESTIVE SYSTEM

To gain a thorough understanding of how the digestive system works, let's take a guided tour, starting at the brain and ending at the colon.

Brain
Before you even put food into your mouth, any sound, sight, odor, taste, or texture associated with food can trigger the body to prepare for the food that will arrive. If you imagine eating a piece of pizza, you can taste the tangy sauce and creamy cheese and feel the texture of the crust. Digestive juices, saliva, enzymes, and digestive hormones begin to flow in anticipation of the food to come. As a result your body "revs up" to prepare for the work of digestion, and your heart rate and blood flow can change. (See Chapter 10, "The Enteric Nervous System," for more information.)

THE DIGESTIVE PROCESS

Eating (also called ingestion or the cephalic phase) is voluntary and begins when materials are put in the mouth. This is our portal for all nutrients to enter the body and involves the mouth, teeth, tongue, and parotid and salivary glands. Food choices are related to lifestyle, personal values, and cultural customs.

Digestion occurs in the mouth, stomach, and small intestine and requires cooperation from the liver and pancreas. Mechanically, foods are chewed in the mouth and churned in the small and large intestines to break the foods into small pieces so that they can be fully digested. Proper levels of stomach acid, bile, enzymes, and intestinal bacteria are critical for full digestive capacity.

Secretion is ongoing. Every day the walls of the digestive tract secrete about seven quarts of water, acid, buffers, and enzymes into the lumen (inside) of the digestive tract. Secretion occurs throughout the entire digestive tract. These secretions help maintain pH levels, send water into the gut to lubricate it and keep things moving, and trigger enzymes to digest foods and facilitate the digestive process. Hydration is essential for this phase of digestion to work properly.

Mixing and Motility are muscular functions. Whatever we eat is squeezed through the digestive system by a rhythmic muscular contraction called peristalsis. Sets of smooth muscles throughout the digestive tract contract and relax, alternately, pushing food through the esophagus to the stomach and through the intestines. (Think of a snake swallowing a mouse.) When the food has been swallowed, it is acidified, liquefied, neutralized, and homogenized until it's broken down into usable particles. From the time you swallow, this process is involuntary and can occur even if you stand on your head. (When my son, Arthur, was seven years old, he demonstrated this by eating upside-down. Yes, the food went down—or rather, up—as usual!)

Absorption occurs when digested food molecules are taken through the epithelial cell lining of the small intestine into the bloodstream and through the portal vein to the liver, where they are filtered. From the bloodstream they pass to the cells. Until food is absorbed, it is essentially outside the body—in a tube going through it. If the gut is inflamed, as with gluten intolerance or celiac disease, there can be malabsorption, which is typified by an inability to gain weight, lack of growth in children, anemia, and diarrhea.

Assimilation is the process by which fuel and nutrients enter the cells. Technically this isn't part of the digestive system, but it is the ultimate goal of the digestive process.

Elimination is the last step. In digestion we excrete wastes by having bowel movements (defecation). These wastes are comprised of indigestible food components, waste products, bacteria, cells from the mucosal lining that are being sloughed off, and food that has not been absorbed.

Mouth

The main function of the mouth is chewing and liquefying food. The salivary glands, located under the tongue, produce saliva, which softens food, begins dissolving soluble components, and helps keep the mouth and teeth clean. Saliva contains amylase, an enzyme for splitting carbohydrates, proteases for splitting proteins, and lipase, a fat-digesting enzyme. Only a small percentage of starches are digested by the amylase in your mouth, but they continue to work for about another hour until the stomach acid inactivates the enzymes. On the other hand, the lipases become activated once reaching the stomach, beginning the process of fat digestion. Saliva also has clotting factors, helps to buffer acids, allows us to swallow, and protects our teeth, oral mucosa, and esophagus. Saliva also reabsorbs nitrates from our foods, primarily green leafy vegetables and beets. These nitrates are converted into nitrites by bacteria on our tongues, concentrating this a thousand times greater than those found in plasma. When this nitrite-rich saliva gets swallowed into acidic gastric juics, it converts into nitric oxide (NO), reducing inflammation throughout the body and protecting the cardiovascular system.

Chewing also stimulates the parotid glands, behind the ears in the jaw, to release hormones that stimulate the thymus to produce T cells, which are the core of the protective immune system.

Healthy teeth and gums are critical for proper digestion. Many people eat so fast, they barely chew their food at all and then wash it down with liquids. That means the stomach receives chunks of food instead of mush. This undermines the function of the teeth, which is to increase the surface area of the food. These people often complain of indigestion or gas. In *May All Be Fed*, John Robbins describes three men who survived in a concentration camp during World War II by chewing their food very well, while their compatriots perished. Simply by chewing food thoroughly, we can enhance digestion and eliminate some problems of indigestion.

The most common problems that occur in the mouth are sores on the lips or tongue—usually canker sores or cold sores (herpes)—and tooth and gum problems.

Esophagus

The esophagus is the tube that passes from the mouth to the stomach. Here peristalsis begins to push the food along the digestive tract. Well-chewed food passes through the esophagus in about six seconds, but dry food can get stuck and take minutes to pass. At the bottom of the esophagus is a little door called the cardiac or esophageal sphincter. It separates the esophagus from the stomach, keeping stomach acid and food from coming back up. It remains closed most of the time, opening when a peristaltic wave, triggered by swallowing, relaxes the sphincter. The most common esophageal problems are heartburn (also called gastroesophageal reflux disease, or GERD), hiatal hernia, Barrett's esophagus, and eosinophilic esophagitis (EE).

Stomach: The Body's Blender

The stomach is the body's blender. It chops, dices, and liquefies as it changes food into a soupy liquid called chyme, which is the beginning of the process of protein digestion. The stomach is located under the rib cage, just under the heart.

After reaching your stomach, your food may stay in the top part for up to an hour. Here the salivary amylase continues to break down starches. Most food stays in the stomach two to four hours—less with a low-fat meal, more with a high-fat or high-fiber meal. Chronic stress lengthens the amount of time that food stays in the stomach, while short-term stress usually shortens the emptying time. Most of us have experienced a nervous stomach, or a feeling in the pit of the stomach, or a stomach that feels like it's filled with rocks. When the stomach has finished its job, chyme (the mixture of food mash and gastric juices) has the consistency of split-pea soup. Over several hours it passes in small amounts through the pyloric valve into the duodenum, the first 12 inches of the small intestine.

Once food enters your stomach, gentle mixing waves begin chopping up your food and increasing surface area. The hormone gastrin is also produced in the stomach and stimulates the production of gastric juices. Gastric juices are comprised of enzymes, hydrochloric acid, hormones, and intrinsic factor. Gastric acid, also called stomach acid, is comprised of hydrochloric acid, potassium chloride and sodium chloride. For example, protein molecules are composed of chains of amino acids—up to 200 amino acids strung together. The stomach produces a hormone called pepsinogen. When pepsinogen is exposed to hydrochloric acid, it turns into pepsin, which begins protein digestion, breaking the protein you eat into short chains called peptides.

Hydrochloric acid (HCl), produced by millions of parietal cells in the stomach lining, begins to break apart these protein chains. The parietal cells use huge amounts of ATP energy to concentrate acids to the low pH of about 1, which is required by the stomach. HCl also kills microbes that come in with food, protecting us against food poisoning, parasites, and bacterial infections. The HCl in your stomach is so strong that it would burn your skin and clothing if spilled on you. Yet, the stomach is protected by a thick coating of mucus (mucopolysaccharides), which keeps the acid from burning through the stomach lining. When the mucous layer of the stomach breaks down, HCl burns a hole in the stomach lining, causing a gastric ulcer. The bacteria, *Helicobacter pylori*, is the main cause of this disrupted mucosal layer and stomach ulcers. HCl production is stimulated by the presence of gastrin, acetylcholine (a neurotransmitter), or histamine. The stomach also produces small amounts of lipase, enzymes that digest fat. Most foods are digested and absorbed farther down the gastrointestinal tract, but alcohol, water, and certain salts are absorbed directly from the stomach into the bloodstream. That's why we feel the effects of alcohol so quickly.

Intrinsic factor is made in the stomach in the parietal cells, and it binds vitamin B_{12} so that it can be readily absorbed in the intestines. Without adequate amounts of intrinsic factor, we do not utilize vitamin B_{12} from our food, and pernicious anemia may occur. The main symptoms are dementia, depression, nervous system problems, muscle weakness, and fatigue. This is why many people benefit from vitamin B_{12} injections, under a physician's care, or use of sublingual B_{12} or even B_{12} in a nasal spray. I remember one elderly woman who had normal serum B_{12} levels, but she felt enormously different when B_{12} shots were added to her regimen. This simple, inexpensive therapy can dramatically affect quality of life for those who need it. By the time serum B_{12} levels are low, your tissues are depleted of vitamin B_{12}. A newer test to detect early B_{12} deficiencies is called the methylmalonic acid test (MMA, also called methylmalonate). Levels of MMA rise when our bodies cannot transform vitamin B_{12} to create energy. High levels of MMA indicate early B_{12} insufficiency. Recently, researchers have remarked that probably the best test for B_{12} is just taking sublingual B_{12} supplements or a trial of B_{12} shots to see if you feel better. I have seen this to be true; when people need B_{12} and take it, their energy and sense of well-being soar. People who try B_{12} and have sufficiency already don't notice a thing.

Hydrochloric acid is also produced by the parietal cells. As the parietal cells become less efficient, the production of both hydrochloric acid and intrinsic factor falls. As many as 90 percent of people diagnosed with pernicious anemia have anti-parietal cell antibodies. These antibodies are associated with higher incidence of other autoimmune conditions and occur years before pernicious anemia is evident.

The most common problems associated with the stomach are upset stomach, gastric ulcers, and underproduction of hydrochloric acid.

Small Intestine

The small intestine is hardly small. If this coiled-up garden hose were stretched out, it would average 15 to 20 feet long. If spread flat, it would cover a surface the size of a tennis court. Food is digested inside the lumen and moved through the epithelial cells, called enterocytes, into the bloodstream. Each enterocyte is covered with hundreds of small, finger-like folds, called villi, which are covered, in turn by millions of microvilli. (Think of them as small loops on a towel that then have smaller threads projecting from them.) The enterocyte layer is only one cell layer thick, but it performs multiple functions of producing digestive enzymes, absorbing nutrients, and blocking absorption of substances that aren't useful to the body.

The intestinal wall has a paradoxical function: It allows nutrients to pass into the bloodstream while blocking the absorption of foreign substances found in chemicals, bacterial products, and other large molecules found in food. Some foods we eat and medications we use irritate the intestinal wall, and it can lose the ability to discern between nutrients and foreign substances. When this occurs, there is a problem of increased intestinal permeability, commonly known as "leaky gut syndrome." This syndrome contributes to autoimmune and skin problems, food sensitivities, osteoarthritis, migraine headaches, and chronic fatigue syndrome. (See Chapter 4.)

The small intestine has three parts: the duodenum, the jejunum, and the ileum (see Figure 2.1). The duodenum is the first 12 inches of the small intestine, the jejunum composes about 40 percent of the digestive system (about 11 feet), and the ileum composes the last segment (about 8 feet). The jejunum and ileum are connected by the ileocecal valve. Each nutrient is absorbed at specific parts of the small intestine. The duodenum has an acidic environment that facilitates absorption of some minerals, including chlorine, sulfur, calcium, copper, iron, thiamin, manganese, and zinc. We also begin the process of absorbing fat-soluble vitamins (A, D, E), fats, and some water-soluble vitamins (B_1, B_2, B_6, C, and folic acid). People with low hydrochloric acid levels may become deficient in one or more of these nutrients because they need acid for absorption. In the jejunum, we continue absorption of nutrients plus sugars, proteins, and amino acids. The ileum and large intestine are connected by the ileocecal valve. In the ileum, we finish the job of digesting many nutrients and add absorption of cholesterol, B_{12}, and bile salts. And finally, in the colon, we absorb potassium, water, salt, vitamin K, and short-chain fatty acids. If you look at the nutrient absorption chart in Figure 2.4, you can see specifically where each nutrient is absorbed along the digestive tract.

The Gut Mucosa or GALT

The GI mucosa, depicted in Figure 2.2, is the inner lining of the digestive tract. It consists of the lumen, which is the space inside the digestive tube; the epithelial layer; the lamina propria; and the muscularis mucosae, or smooth muscles. The entire mucosa is a large mucous membrane, not unlike the tissues inside your nose. It is here that our food makes contact with us and is eventually absorbed in the intestines. It is home to trillions of bacteria and fungi and is the center of our body's immune system. It is your body's first line of defense against infections and other invaders.

The primary layers of the gut mucosa (also called gut-associated lymphoid tissue, or GALT) include the epithelium, the lamina propria, and the muscularis mucosae.

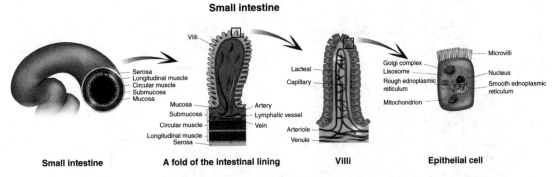

Figure 2.2 **Small intestine.** In this figure, the drawing on the left represents the lumen. Inside this lumen, like the inside of a hose, is where the small intestine selectively brings substances into the bloodstream. The second picture shows the structure of the small intestine, which looks a lot like the brain, with many folds. On it, a single villi is labeled, which is expanded in the third drawing. On the villi is a single layer made up of individual epithelial cells, called enterocytes. This layer renews itself every 5 to 7 days. On each enterocyte are thousands of smaller, fingerlike projections called the microvilli, depicted on the far right, where digested foods and other substances pass into the bloodstream through capillaries and fats to pass into the lymphatic system directly. (*Shutterstock*)

The epithelium is comprised of a single layer of cells, called enterocytes, that come into direct contact with your food. This layer of cells is held together in tight junctions that prevent molecules from moving between the cells. (See Chapter 4.) This epithelial layer replaces itself every five to seven days and uses glutamine as its primary energy source. There are exocrine cells among the epithelial cells that secrete mucus and fluid, as well as endocrine cells that release hormones.

The lamina propria connects the digestive system to the lymphatic system for digestion of fats and to the blood for absorption of nutrients (Figure 2.3). The lamina propria is where lymphatic nodules, lymphocytes, plasma cells, and macrophages form the first line of defense against infections. These are lymphatic nodes (like the ones that swell in your throat when you have a bad cold) that run throughout the digestive system but are most prominent in the tonsils, small intestine, appendix, and large intestine. The lymphatic system circulates fluids throughout your body; drains excess fluids from the fluid between cells (interstitial fluid); initiates immune response against infection and allergy; transports the fat-soluble vitamins A, D, E, and K; and brings digested fats into the bloodstream, among other things.

The lamina propria is also where cytokines, such as IL-6, IL-10, TNF-α, and others, are produced. Some cytokines are inflammatory, while others are healing.

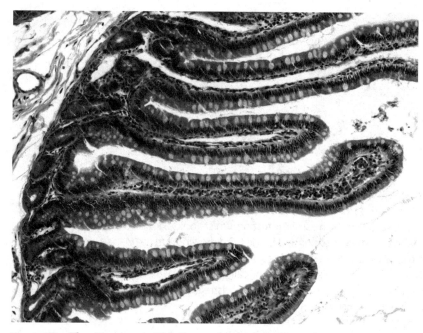

Figure 2.3   **The GI mucosa.** This figure shows the villi on the enterocytes (cells that line the small intestine). On each villi are tiny microvilli, which create the surface through which we absorb food into the bloodstream. *(McGraw-Hill/Al Telser photographer)*

The final layer of the GALT is the muscularis mucosae, which is a thin layer of smooth muscle that runs from the stomach through the small intestine. (See Chapter 9.)

Pancreas

The pancreas has two main roles: to aid in the digestion of food and to produce produce hormones such as insulin and glucagon, which regulate blood sugar levels, thereby maintaining both digestive and global function.

When food passes from the stomach to the duodenum, cholecystokinin, a gut hormone, is secreted and enhanced by secretin. This stimulates the pancreas to secrete bicarbonate-rich alkaline fluid, essentially baking soda, which neutralizes the acidity of the chyme. The hydrochloric acid has already finished its work, and a more neutral pH is where the rest of the digestive system functions best. The pancreas also manufactures and secretes specific digestive enzymes. Pancreatic amylase digests starches and sugars. The protein-splitting enzymes are called trypsin, chymotrypsin, carboxypeptidase, and elastase (also called pancreatic elastase). Pancreatic lipase and colipase break fats into fatty acids and glycerol. Ribonuclease and deoxyribonuclease

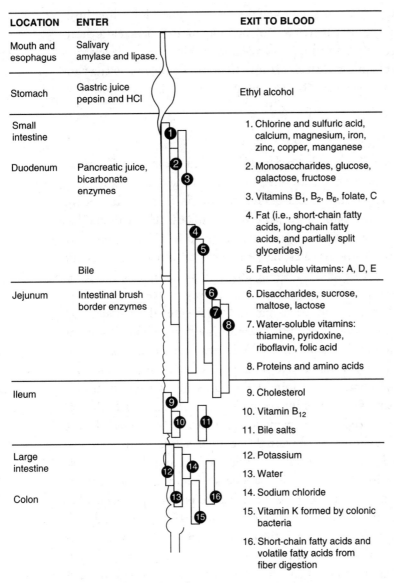

LOCATION	ENTER	EXIT TO BLOOD
Mouth and esophagus	Salivary amylase and lipase.	
Stomach	Gastric juice pepsin and HCl	Ethyl alcohol
Small intestine		1. Chlorine and sulfuric acid, calcium, magnesium, iron, zinc, copper, manganese
Duodenum	Pancreatic juice, bicarbonate enzymes	2. Monosaccharides, glucose, galactose, fructose
		3. Vitamins B_1, B_2, B_6, folate, C
		4. Fat (i.e., short-chain fatty acids, long-chain fatty acids, and partially split glycerides)
	Bile	5. Fat-soluble vitamins: A, D, E
Jejunum	Intestinal brush border enzymes	6. Disaccharides, sucrose, maltose, lactose
		7. Water-soluble vitamins: thiamine, pyridoxine, riboflavin, folic acid
		8. Proteins and amino acids
Ileum		9. Cholesterol
		10. Vitamin B_{12}
		11. Bile salts
Large intestine		12. Potassium
		13. Water
Colon		14. Sodium chloride
		15. Vitamin K formed by colonic bacteria
		16. Short-chain fatty acids and volatile fatty acids from fiber digestion

Figure 2.4 **Nutrient absorption chart.**

digest old RNA and DNA. Once our food has been fully digested, nutrients can be absorbed into the bloodstream and used by the cells. Low secretion of pancreatic enzymes can lead to nutritional deficiencies. For example, vitamin B_{12} requires protein-splitting enzymes to separate it from its carrier molecule, so poor pancreatic function can lead directly to vitamin B_{12} deficiencies.

The second role of the pancreas is the production of hormones, including insulin, glucagon, somatostatin, and pancreatic polypeptide in the pancreatic islets (also called islets of Langerhans). Insulin is secreted when blood sugar levels rise; glucagon is secreted when blood sugar levels are low. Common problems in the pancreas are diabetes, which is a systemic disease, and pancreatitis (i.e., inflammation of the pancreas).

Liver: The Body's Fuel Filter

The liver is the most complex of the body's organs. It performs more than 500 functions and is critical to most of our metabolism. I once heard the dean of a medical school say, "I'd rather run all of the operations of General Motors for a day than be my own liver." Your four-and-a-half-pound liver manufactures 13,000 chemicals and has 2,000 enzyme systems, plus thousands of synergists that help with body functions. It regulates the metabolism of carbohydrates, fats, and proteins; it manufactures bile to emulsify fats for digestion; it makes and breaks down many hormones, including cholesterol, testosterone, and estrogens; it regulates blood sugar levels; it processes all food, nutrients, alcohol, drugs, and other materials that enter the bloodstream and lets them pass, breaks them down, or stores them. It is a storage house for many nutrients: glycogen, fats, vitamin B_{12}, vitamins A, D, E, and K, and zinc, iron, copper, and magnesium. Your liver can store five to seven years of vitamin B_{12}, four years of vitamin A, and up to four months of vitamin D. Proteins synthesized in your liver transport vitamin A, iron, zinc, and copper into your bloodstream. Practically all vitamins and minerals we take in need to be enzymatically processed by the liver before we can use them. Several vitamins are converted into their active forms: carotene to vitamin A, folic acid to 5-methyltetrahydrofolic acid, and vitamin D to its active form 25-hydroxycholecalciferol. Your liver also produces proteins and lipoproteins that allow your blood to clot. The liver can lose as much as 70 percent of its capability and not show diagnosable liver disease. It can also regenerate itself after being injured.

The liver breaks down toxins ingested with our foods and those that are produced by bacterial metabolism. With these chemicals and enzymes, it "humanizes" nutrients so that the cells can use them. If the liver becomes too congested to enzymatically process these nutrients, we do not get the benefit from them.

Bile, manufactured by the liver and stored by the gallbladder, buffers the intestinal contents due to its high concentration of bicarbonates. It also emulsifies fats. Bile is a soaplike substance made of bile salts, cholesterol, and lecithin. It makes fats more water-soluble, increasing their surface area so that the enzymes can split them for the cells to use. It's essential for absorption of fats, the fat-soluble vitamins A, D, E, and K, and some minerals. Bile also secretes immunoglobulins that protect our intestinal mucosa. In addition, it is an important mechanism for detoxification. Drugs and other toxins are eliminated from the liver through bile. The brown color of stool comes from the yellow color of bilirubin in bile.

The liver is also part of our immune system. The Kupffer cells filter bacteria and debris from the blood. The liver also stores environmental toxins like radioactive substances, pesticides, herbicides, food preservatives, and dyes. The liver will detoxify what it can, but if it can't break down a particular substance, it stores it there and in tissues throughout the body. The most common liver problems include fatty liver, hepatitis, and cirrhosis.

Gallbladder: A Holding Tank for Bile

The gallbladder is a pear-shaped organ that lies just below the liver. The gallbladder's function is to store and concentrate bile, which is produced by the liver. When you eat a food that contains fat, cholecystokinin is released from the duodenum, which stimulates the gallbladder and liver to release bile into the common duct that connects the liver, gallbladder, and pancreas to the duodenum. Bile emulsifies the fats, cholesterol, and fat-soluble vitamins you've eaten by breaking them into tiny globules. These create a greater surface area for the fat-splitting enzymes (lipase) to act on during digestion.

The most common problem of the gallbladder is gallstones. When bile becomes too concentrated, stones may form, which can cause pain, nausea, and discomfort. Another common issue is bile reflux, where bile backs up into the stomach. Gallbladder disease is directly related to diet.

CLINICAL CLUES OF BILE INSUFFICIENCY

- Have had your gallbladder removed or have gallbladder issues
- Liver disease
- Thyroid issues (hypothyroid or hyperthyroid)
- Ileostomy (removal of part of your ileum)
- Incomplete digestion/absorption of fats
- Steatorrhea (stools that have a lot of fat in them; they typically are frothy, smell bad, and are tan or light in color)
- Diarrhea
- Abdominal discomfort
- Gas and bloating

- Decreased absorption of nutrients
- Water retention
- Low serum albumin levels
- Bleeding tendency (vitamin K deficiency)
- Weight loss
- Growth failure in children
- Having a bitter taste in your mouth after eating
- Nausea and vomiting
- Feeling queasy after a fatty meal
- A constant feeling of fullness, and deferred pain to head, belly, shoulder blades, etc.

Appendix

The appendix is a small, fingerlike sac that extends off the beginning of the colon. Until recently, the function of the appendix was a mystery. Now we know it contains a great deal of lymphatic tissue and is important for fetal and early childhood development. Hormones produced in the appendix beginning about the 11th week of pregnancy help regulate fetal metabolism. The appendix contains a lot of lymphatic tissue and is especially important in immune health in the first decades of life. In the developmental years, the appendix produces secretory Immunoglobulin A(IgA) and helps with the maturation of B-lymphocytes (a type of white blood cell). These functions help to support local immune function.

Large Intestine or Colon

When all nutrients have been absorbed, water, bacteria, and fiber pass through the ileocecal valve to the large intestine and colon. The ileocecal valve is located by your right hip bone and separates the contents of the small and large intestines. The ileocecal valve can work improperly by not opening or staying open. An ileocecal valve that doesn't close properly can allow wastes to back up into the small intestine. This has been associated with increases in small intestinal bacterial overgrowth (SIBO).

The colon is short, only three to five feet long. Its job is to absorb water and remaining nutrients from the chyme and form stool. Two and a half gallons of water pass through the colon each day, two-thirds of which come from body fluids. The efficient colon pulls 80 percent of the water out of the chyme, which is absorbed into the bloodstream.

The large intestine has three main parts: the ascending colon (up the right side of the body), the transverse colon (straight across the belly under the ribs), and the descending colon (down the left side of the body) to the rectum, where feces exit the body. Stool begins to form in the transverse colon. If the chyme passes through the colon too quickly, water is not absorbed, causing diarrhea. Stool that sits too long in the colon becomes dry and hard to pass, leading to constipation. About two-thirds of stool is composed of water and undigested fiber and food products. The other third is composed of living and dead bacteria.

The large intestine contains the majority of the microbiome by far. In the colon, bifidobacteria and other microbes ferment fibers that become short-chain fatty acids (SCFAs): butyric, pripionic, acetic, and valerate. These SCFAs provide many benefits for the colon and systemic health. For instance, butyric acid provides 70 percent of the energy, maintenance, and repair of the cells of the colon. Butyrate also promotes neurotrophic substances, such as brain-derived neurogenic growth factor (BDNF), which are needed to support neurological health. On the other hand, low butyric acid levels or an inability of the colon bacteria to properly metabolize butyric acid has been associated with ulcerative colitis, colon cancer, active colitis, and inflammatory bowel disease.

When the stool is finally well formed, it gets pushed down into the descending colon and then into the rectum. It is held there until there is sufficient volume to have a bowel movement. Two sphincters—rings of muscle—control bowel movements. When enough feces have collected, the internal sphincter relaxes and your mind gets the signal that it's time to relieve yourself. The external sphincter opens when you command it. Because this is voluntary, you can have the urge to defecate but not do it right away. If you ignore the urge, though, water keeps being absorbed back into the body and the stool gets dry and hard. Some people are chronically constipated because they don't want to take the time to have a bowel movement or don't like to have bowel movements at work. This book is about listening to your body signals. Take the time when your body calls you, not when it's convenient or ideal.

Many health problems arise in the colon: appendicitis, constipation, diarrhea, diverticular disease, Crohn's disease, ulcerative colitis, rectal polyps, colon cancer, irritable bowel syndrome (IBS), parasites, and hemorrhoids.

WHAT GOES IN, MUST COME OUT!

We can learn a lot about ourselves from stool. Dennis Burkitt, MD, father of the fiber theory, found that on average people on Western diets excreted only 5 ounces of stool daily, whereas Africans eating traditional diets passed 16 ounces. Well-formed stool tells us when it wants to come out; we don't need to coax it. It looks like a brown banana with a point at one end, is well hydrated, and just slips out easily. Stool that looks like little balls all wadded together has been in the colon too long. The longer waste materials sit in the colon, the more concentrated the bile acids become; concentrated bile acids irritate the lining of the colon. Hormones that have been broken down by the body are also excreted via our feces. If the stools sit in the colon for too long, these hormones are reabsorbed into the bloodstream, increasing the risk for estrogen-dependent cancers. Betaglucuronidase, an enzyme that may activate formation of cancer-causing substances in the colon, can be measured in stool as a marker of hormone reabsorption.

Frequency of bowel movements is a good health indicator. How often do you have a bowel movement? People on good diets generally have one to three bowel movements each day. If you are not having a daily bowel movement, there can be many causes.

TESTING BOWEL TRANSIT TIME

Transit time is how long it takes from the time you eat a food until it comes out the other end. Buy charcoal tablets at a drugstore or health-food store, and take about 1,000 mg. Depending on the particular product, this can be two to four capsules. Note exactly when you took the charcoal. When you see darkened stool (charcoal will turn the stool black), calculate how many hours since you took the charcoal tablets. That is your transit time. You can also do the test with beets. Eating three or four whole beets will turn stool a deep garnet red.

The Results

- Less than 12 hours: This usually indicates that you are not absorbing all the nutrients you should from your food. You may have malabsorption problems.

- A range of 12 to 24 hours is optimal.
- More than 24 hours: This indicates that wastes are sitting inside your colon too long. Poor transit time greatly increases the risk of colon disease. Substances that were supposed to be eliminated get absorbed back into the bloodstream, and they can interfere with and irritate your system. Take action now! Increase your fiber intake by eating more fruit, vegetables, whole grains, and legumes. Drink lots of water every day. Get 30 minutes of exercise at least three times a week.

First, take a close look at your diet. You probably aren't eating enough fiber. If that's the case, increase your intake of fruits, vegetables, whole grains, and legumes. These foods are generally high in magnesium, which helps normalize peristalsis. Make sure that you are drinking enough fluids. Coffee and soft drinks don't count! And get regular exercise!

Another good indicator of your colon's health is your bowel transit time. (See Testing Bowel Transit Time.)

EXERCISE: CLEAN UP YOUR DIET!

Let's take a look at what foods you are eating and begin the process of cleaning up your diet. Take last week's food diary. Get out some crayons or markers. You're going to color! (If you don't already keep a food diary, you will find instructions on how to do so in Chapter 12.)

- **Circle the following foods red:** Sugar, caffeine, alcohol, fried foods, high-fat foods, microwave popcorn, highly processed foods, soft drinks, diet soft drinks, diet foods
- **Circle the following foods blue:** Dairy products: milk, cheese, yogurt, ice cream, frozen yogurt, ice milk
- **Circle the following foods green:** Fruits and vegetables
- **Circle the following foods yellow:** Protein foods: fish, poultry, beef, pork, lamb, veal, legumes, soy products
- **Circle the following foods purple:** Nuts and seeds, oils, butter, margarine
- **Circle the following foods black:** Grains: wheat, bread, cereal, corn, rice, millet, buckwheat, bulgur, quinoa, amaranth, barley, oats, rye

Look at those circles. Is there one food group that dominates your diary? If you eliminated one of these categories from your diet, which would be the easiest to give up and which would be the most difficult? Sometimes the ones that are the hardest to give up are the ones that are causing us the most trouble. They temporarily make us feel better, even though they are really making us sicker. Why? Our bodies may react negatively to dairy products, caffeine, sugar, wheat, pork, beef, citrus fruits, or any other foods, yet we crave them.

This week, focus on the foods you circled in red and eliminate them. Sugars ferment and can contribute to your digestive problems. Get rid of soft drinks, cookies, pastries, doughnuts, and sugar added to coffee or tea. We're not talking about perfection here. Let's just make some progress. Why? These foods make it harder for your body to be healthy. High-sugar foods deplete our nutrient stores. We need most of the B-complex vitamins, chromium, manganese, and potassium to metabolize these foods properly, but sweets don't have any of these nutrients. So we take nutrients out of storage, and eventually our tissues become depleted. Begin replacing these nutrient-poor foods with fresh fruit, vegetables, nuts, and seeds. Snack on hummus and vegetables, or nuts mixed with raisins.

After a couple of weeks, fruit begins to taste really sweet, which is just how it ought to taste. Once, I realized that it had been months since I had had any chocolate. I began to feel deprived, so I bought a big chocolate bar for my family and friends. I ate a few squares and was totally satisfied. I hope that eventually you can be satisfied with just a little bit, too. But if you can't, you're really better off without any. Once I was sick and was craving sweets like crazy. My doctor told me it was the bacteria—both good and bad—that wanted the energy. So starve those bad guys out. The helpful bacteria can thrive with real food.

The DIGIN Model
and the 5 Rs

In conventional medicine, a clinician makes a diagnosis and there are standard therapies for each diagnosis. In functional medicine, there is no cookie-cutter approach. Finding the underlying mechanisms of disease rather than focusing on symptom relief is the goal. Two people with the same diagnosis may need completely different therapies. At the same time, two people with completely dissimilar diagnoses may benefit from the same therapy. For example, irritable bowel syndrome (IBS), migraine headaches, attention deficit disorder, and fibromyalgia may seem like different diagnoses, but they may all have the underlying cause of leaky gut syndrome or food intolerances. On the other hand, three people with IBS could have completely different underlying causes, including small intestinal bacterial infection, a deficiency of protective bacteria, too little fiber, food sensitivities, lactose intolerance, celiac disease, imbalances in neurotransmitters, or stress-induced IBS, to name a few.

So how do we begin looking for underlying mechanisms? It's called the DIGIN approach. In the following chapters we'll explore each aspect of this model (see Figure II.1). I consider this section to be the heart of the book. No matter what the diagnosis, by looking at your symptoms and diagnoses through the DIGIN model, you'll find ways to move toward health.

THE DIGIN MODEL FOR ASSESSMENT OF DIGESTIVE ISSUES

DIGIN is an acronym for the five primary categories of digestive imbalances:

- **D**igestion/absorption
- **I**ntestinal permeability
- **G**astrointestinal (GI) microbiota

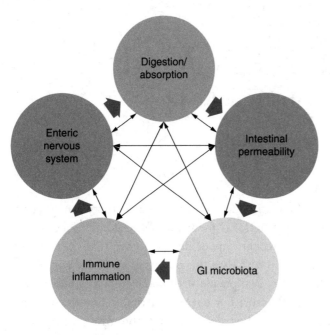

Figure II.1 **The DIGIN model.**

- **I**mmune function and inflammation
- Enteric **n**ervous system

By assessing each of these areas, you can discover how to best get your body back into balance.

THE 5 Rs

The principles of repair in functional medicine are fairly simple. As one of the pioneers in the field, Sidney Baker, MD, said: Get rid of what you don't need, and get what you do need. The 4 Rs were originally put together by Jeffrey Bland, PhD, and Metagenics. Recently at the Institute for Functional Medicine, we've updated this to the 5 R Program, which includes:

- **Remove:** Nutrient-depleted food, processed foods, poor-quality fats and oils, parasites, molds, metals, chemicals, infections, and foods that don't agree with us. Remove relationships and stressors that no longer serve us.

- **Replace:** Processed foods with whole foods, nutrients, digestive enzymes, hydrochloric acid (HCl), and bile salts. Also, replace poor lifestyle habits with better ones.
- **Reinoculate:** Beneficial probiotics and prebiotics from food and supplements.
- **Repair:** Using foods and supplements such as glutamine, gamma-oryzanol, duodenum glandular, N-acetyl glucosamine, fiber, boswellia, geranium, licorice, quercetin, goldenseal, wormwood, aloe, celandine, cranesbill, marshmallow root, bone stock, rice protein powders, essential fatty acids, okra, cabbage, fasting.
- **Rebalance:** Discover your "new normal," which may be the healthiest you've ever felt or not quite as great as you'd like. Investigate your lifestyle: stress management, sleeping seven to nine hours each night, regular exercise. What is your sense of purpose? How do you relax or have fun? Whom do you do these things with? Do you have a religious or spiritual connection, and if so, how do you renew it?

The 5 Rs are sprinkled throughout this section of the book and continue in Part III, "Coming Back into Balance."

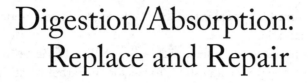

CHAPTER 3

Digestion/Absorption: Replace and Repair

"Things which matter most must never be at the mercy of things which matter least."
— Johann Wolfgang von Goethe

If you cannot digest and absorb your food, your cells won't get the nourishment that they need to function properly. Many health issues begin because people aren't fully digesting and/or absorbing their food. The primary areas to explore include:

- Poor chewing and rushed eating
- Gastric acid (HCl) insufficiency
- Bile salt insufficiency
- Enzyme insufficiency
- Lack of dietary fiber
- Hydration
- Motility

In today's rushed culture, we often don't chew our food well or even really pay much attention to what we are eating. I'm as guilty as anyone, reading while I eat or eating while driving in the car. Yet, the simple act of using our teeth for the purpose for which they were designed can dramatically improve our health.

Those pearly whites in your mouth, known as teeth, were designed for chewing. The act of chewing, or mastication, has many benefits. Most important, it mashes food into smaller pieces, which lessens the load on the rest of the digestive system and allows better absorption of nutrients. A study* published in the *American Journal of Clinical Nutrition* reports that young men who chewed each bite of food 40 times rather than 15 consumed fewer calories. Chewing also stimulated production of gut hormones that signal satiety.

Chewing also means more contact with saliva. Saliva lubricates our food and contains enzymes that begin the digestive process for fat, carbohydrate, and protein. Saliva also helps remineralize tooth enamel, has antimicrobial and antiviral properties, and enhances taste.

The Takeaway: Eating mindfully or consciously can help you digest food more efficiently and minimize digestive issues. It is an old custom to chew each bite 30 times. When drinking liquids, we also need to slow down and pay attention to pacing.

The human body is 70 percent water; being hydrated is important for proper cell function throughout the body. In the digestive system, adequate hydration helps to normalize gut motility and gastric emptying. It also acts as a lubricant and comprises the bulk of mucus, which is ever present throughout the digestive tract. Being well hydrated helps normalize stool transit time and emptying of the stomach (gastric emptying). Many people find that increasing fluid intake helps solve issues with constipation. We'll talk more about water and hydration in Chapter 13.

HYDROCHLORIC ACID

Hydrochloric acid (HCl), found in the stomach, is used to begin the process of protein digestion. The normal pH of our stomach is 0.8 to 1.5. If we poured this acid on our hands, we'd get burned. HCl is produced by the parietal cells in your stomach.

The parietal cells of your stomach use this pump to secrete gastric juice. Most of our body has a neutral pH of about 7.0, like water. In order to create HCl, our parietal cells concentrate our acid a millionfold. Small wonder that parietal cells are stuffed with mitochondria, our cellular energy factories, and use huge amounts of energy as they carry out this enormous concentration of protons.

The mucous layer in the stomach protects it from this acid. HCl utilizes the enzyme pepsinogen to synthesize pepsin. Pepsin cleaves large protein molecules so that they can be more easily broken down by digestive enzymes in the small intestine. In the duodenum, the high acid environment allows for absorption of minerals such as iron, calcium, magnesium, zinc, and copper. Stomach acid also provides our first defense against food poisoning, *Helicobacter pylori*, parasites, fungi, and other infections. Without adequate acid, we leave ourselves open to decreased immune resistance. A couple of tip-offs that people may have low stomach acid levels is that they often belch and burp, get food poisoning easily or repeatedly, or have been diagnosed with small intestinal bacterial overgrowth (SIBO).

In the current medical system, it is believed that excess stomach acid causes much disease. According to a Gallup poll, 44 percent of us experience heartburn at least once a month and 7 percent of us have it once a week or more. Many of us turn to antacids, like Tums or Rolaids, to buffer symptoms temporarily. Over-the-counter drugs, such as Tagamet, Zantac, Axid, and Pepsid, fall into the category of histamine 2 (H2) blockers. Their method of action is to lessen the production of HCl. Most physicians prescribe proton pump inhibitors (PPIs) which completely block the production of HCl. Common PPIs include Prevacid, Nexium, Prilosec, and Zegerid.

In 2017, the Food and Drug Administration (FDA) began to require new warning labels for PPIs due to the increased risk of osteoporosis and fracture with long-term use. This is true for all of us, and yet babies are increasingly being prescribed PPIs. Infants who take PPIs in the first 6 months of life have an increased risk of breaking a bone, and the longer they take them, the greater the risk. PPIs have also been associated with increased risk of death, pancreatic cancer, *Clostridium difficile*, kidney disease, inability to produce stomach acid, stomach infections, cardiovascular events, and more. If we recall that the acid is needed in the duodenum in order for us to absorb minerals, you can see that long-term use of PPIs could lead to mineral insufficiencies and many health conditions.

Chronic use of antacids and acid-blocking drugs contribute to long-term problems. They increase the incidence of SIBO; decrease mineral, folic acid, and B_{12} absorption; open us up to more food-borne infections; and cause dependence because when we stop using them we feel even worse than before we began. Jonathan Wright, in *Why Stomach Acid Is Good for You*, has found that many people with diseases such as type 1 diabetes, osteoporosis, childhood asthma, chronic fatigue, depression, and other illnesses have atypically low levels of HCl in their stomachs. When they are supported with HCl plus pepsin, digestive enzymes, nutrients, stress management, and other supportive treatment, their health issues improve or resolve.

Acid blockers and antacids *do* help us feel better. But is the cause too much acid or too much acid in the wrong place?

Between the esophagus and the stomach is a circular muscle called the lower esophageal sphincter (LES). It opens to allow food to pass from the esophagus into the stomach. In some people, the LES opens inappropriately for brief moments. This allows stomach acid to back up, or "reflux," into the esophagus. Even small amounts of this cause tissue damage and burning.

The problem, however, is typically due not to an overall excess of stomach acid, but to acid where it doesn't belong. As we age, stomach acid levels decline while heartburn increases. In addition, the LES works less effectively in many of us as we get older. Nicotine, caffeine, alcoholic drinks, high-fat meals, orange juice, tomatoes and tomato-based products like spaghetti sauce, and spicy foods, can weaken the LES. Carminitive herbs, such as peppermint and spearmint, also relax the LES and can increase acid reflux.

The symptoms of too little stomach acid and too much are similar. Typically I hear about belching, burping, and food that feels as if it sits in the stomach undigested for hours. Some clues that may indicate low stomach acid can be found in the following list.

CLINICAL CLUES OF LOW STOMACH ACID

- Bloating, belching, burning, and flatulence immediately after meals
- A sense of fullness after eating just a few bites of food
- Feeling as though food sits in stomach undigested for hours
- Indigestion, diarrhea, or constipation
- Multiple food allergies
- Nausea after taking supplements
- Itching around the rectum
- Weak, peeling, and cracked fingernails
- Dilated blood vessels in the cheeks and nose (in nonalcoholics)
- Acne
- Iron deficiency
- Chronic intestinal parasites or abnormal flora
- Undigested food in stool
- Chronic candida infections
- Upper-digestive-tract gassiness

The following are diseases associated with low gastric acidity:

- Addison's disease
- Asthma
- Celiac disease
- Chronic autoimmune disorders
- Chronic hives
- Dermatitis herpetiformis (herpes)
- Diabetes
- Eczema
- Gallbladder disease
- Graves disease
- Hepatitis
- Hyperthyroidism and hypothyroidism
- Lupus erythematosis
- Myasthenia gravis
- Osteoporosis
- Pernicious anemia
- Psoriasis
- Rheumatoid arthritis
- Rosacea
- Sjögren's syndrome
- Thyrotoxicosis
- Vitiligo

Used with permission from Michael Murray, ND, "Indigestion, Antacids, Achlorhydria and H. pylori," *American Journal of Natural Medicine* (January–February 1997): 11–16.

What causes too little stomach acid? Food sensitivities and stress play a role. Additionally, chlorine and fluoride in drinking water can block its production, and a stressful lifestyle can deplete acid output.

Testing for Low Hydrochloric Acid Levels

You can do a home test to determine whether your HCl levels are optimal. For definitive results, find a physician who can measure your HCl levels with a Heidelberg capsule test or the SmartPill test. (For self-testing and medical testing, see Chapter 11, "Functional Medicine/Functional Testing.")

Options for Increasing HCl Naturally

If you have determined through testing that your HCl levels are low, you can try the following:

- Take betaine HCl with pepsin with meals that contain protein. Dosage: 300 to 750 mg per capsule. Be cautious with taking betaine HCl. It is acid and you can create a stomach ulcer by taking too much. (See Chapter 11 for more insight.)
- Consider stress management to naturally allow your stomach to come into balance again.
- Chiropractic adjustments can improve blood flow to the stomach and help normalize HCl production. These are expecially useful in babies and children who experience gastroesophageal reflux disease (GERD).
- You can also stimulate HCl production by using bitters. Bitters have long been used to promote better digestion. They typically have gentian plus other herbs. They probably work by increasing saliva, HCl, pepsin, bile, and digestive enzymes. Swedish bitters (also called sweetish bitters) bitters can be found in health-food stores and some drugstores. Compari bitters are also effective and are found where alcoholic beverages are sold.
- Some people find relief by using diluted vinegar. Apple cider vinegar seems to work best. Begin with 1 teaspoon in 8 teaspoons of water. Gradually increase the amount of vinegar until you get the desired effect.
- Umeboshi plums are found in the Asian section of grocery and health-food stores. Umeboshi plums are salted, pickled plums that can relieve most indigestion and alkalize the body. They can be eaten whole or used as the base for tea, to replace salt and vinegar in salad dressings, or as umeboshi vinegar.
- Use protein-splitting enzymes to aid digestion of protein foods. The most common ones include bromelain (from pineapple stems), papain (from papaya), and mixed protease enzymes (also called proteolytic enzymes). (See the section later in this chapter on enzymes for more information.)

BILE SALTS

Bile is a soaplike substance secreted by the liver. Bile salts emulsify the fats from our food. By increasing the surface area of the molecules, our lipase (fat-splitting) enzymes can digest fats and absorb fat-soluble vitamins (A, D, E, and K) more efficiently. Bile is made from cholesterol; it sequesters cholesterol and is a main way in which we eliminate cholesterol from our bodies. Bile is also a main method used to remove metabolic wastes, excess hormones, and drugs, metals, and other artificial substances from our bodies. When our bile acid levels are high, our body stops making more cholesterol; conversely, when our bile acid levels are low, our bodies can make up to 15 times more cholesterol. Bile also helps make calcium and iron more absorbable. (See Figure 3.1.)

People who have had their gallbladders removed don't concentrate bile acids. They still produce bile, but it dribbles out in a constant, low stream rather than a burst of release when we eat fat. People with liver and gallbladder issues and people who have had their ileum removed often benefit from taking extra bile salts. While I haven't seen any studies on the supplemental use of bile to lower high serum cholesterol levels, it's something to consider.

Typical tests for bile acid insufficiency include endoscopy, or testing for fats in the stool at any lab or through a comprehensive stool test that looks more extensively at the composition of fatty acids.

If you have had your gallbladder removed, have liver disease, or experience a failure to absorb fats, consider using bile salts. A typical dosage would be between 200 to 1,000 mg with food. Taurine at dosages of 500 to 2,000 mg daily also enhances your body's ability to make bile salts.

Foods and herbs that help stimulate bile are called cholagogues. Cholagogic foods include radishes, dandelion, chicory, mustard greens, turnip greens, and

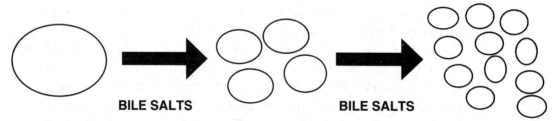

Figure 3.1   **Bile emulsifies fat molecules from food, making the surface area larger so that we can digest fats more easily.**

artichokes. You can often find cholagogue herbs in combination that will typically have dandelion and one or more of the following herbs: wormwood, greater celandine, boldo, blue flag, and fringe tree.

ENZYMES

An enzyme is a protein that catalyzes (triggers a change without being changed itself) a reaction to speed up, slow down, or change a small number of chemical reactions. Since each enzyme can make only a "small" change, we need many of them. Some enzymes also have a nonprotein part—a metal molecule, a vitamin, or another molecule attached to them. These are called coenzymes. Most of the B-complex vitamins are coenzymes.

Metabolic Enzymes

We have 75,000 known metabolic and digestive enzymes in our bodies. Enzymes are specific, each binding to a specific substance to perform a specific task. They are needed for *every* chemical reaction that occurs in the human body. We use them to make energy, think, and control blood sugar levels. We cannot utilize a vitamin, a mineral, or a fat; make or break down cells; or remove wastes without enzymes. Our immune system and nervous system cannot work without enzymes. We use them to build cartilage and bone, give our skin elasticity, keep our blood from clotting, build and break down hormones, and everything else. And if we don't have enough enzymes, we don't feel as well as we could. We make enzymes from the proteins we eat and by recycling them. In order for enzymes to work properly, they need to be synthesized correctly and be in a correct pH and temperature.

Digestive Enzymes

Our digestive system uses enzymes to break down the food we eat. (HCl and bile also help in the process of digestion.) We make most of our digestive enzymes in the pancreas, but enzymes are produced throughout the digestive system, beginning with amylase in our saliva. We have separate enzymes for digesting fats, carbohydrates, proteins, pectins, and phytic acid. The fat-splitting enzymes are called lipases, the carbohydrate-splitting enzymes are called amylases, and the protein-splitting enzymes are called proteases. Pectins are found in fruits, such as apples and pears. Pectinase enzymes help break them down. Phytic acid is found primarily in grains and beans. Phytic acid binds minerals, and we cannot use them if they are bound. Phytase enzymes help break them down, releasing minerals as a result.

Digestive Enzyme Insufficiencies. Many people have enzyme deficiencies, making them unable to adequately digest specific foods or food groups. Lactose intolerance, fructose intolerance, and lack of gluten-splitting enzymes are the most common of these.

- **Lactose intolerance:** It's estimated that about 25 percent of Americans and 75 percent of the world's population are lactose intolerant. It's most prevalent in people of Asian, African, or Mediterranean descent. In the United States, virtually all people of Asian ancestry and 80 percent of African Americans are lactose intolerant. Interestingly enough, most people can tolerate small amounts of dairy products. Even more can tolerate lactose-free milk or eat dairy products when they take lactase enzyme supplements. For many people, lactose-intolerance is due to increased intestinal permeability and/or dysbiosis. When the gut heals, people often become more lactose tolerant.

- **Gluten intolerance/celiac disease:** Celiac disease affects 1 in 133 people, 3 million Americans. About 40 percent of us have the correct genes to develop celiac disease, and it is estimated that up to 15 percent of us are gluten intolerant. People with celiac disease cannot fully digest gliadin, a protein found in wheat, barley, rye, spelt, and kamut. (See the section on celiac disease and gluten intolerance in Chapter 23.)

- **Fructose intolerance:** There are two types of fructose intolerance: inherited and acquired. Inherited fructose intolerance affects 1 in 20,000 people who have fructose 1-phosphate aldolase deficiency. This is typically found in infancy or early childhood with children who refuse to eat sweet foods or who get ill from them. Typical symptoms include vomiting, failure to thrive, liver changes, jaundice, acidosis, blood clotting disorders, hypoglycemia, and possibly seizures. Acquired fructose intolerance is much more common, affecting about 1 in every 3 people. Often people avoid fruit and juice because they notice that it makes them feel worse. Fructose intolerance is more common in women than men, and it looks a lot like the symptoms of IBS: constipation, diarrhea, abdominal spasms, gas, and nausea.

- **Disaccharide intolerance:** Some people lack the ability to break apart two-molecule sugars, such as lactose, maltose, and sucrose. These deficiencies are quite rare, yet many people with dysbiosis find that they benefit from the Specific Carbohydrate Diet until their gut has healed. The Specific Carbohydrate Diet (SCD) is a therapeutic diet that restricts disaccharides. It has been found to be especially useful in children and adults with Crohn's disease. It is discussed more fully in Chapter 14.

Enzymes in Our Foods

Foods can be a good source of enzymes if we are eating fresh, locally grown foods or if we are eating fermented or cultured foods. Enzymes are what ripen tomatoes or bananas sitting on our counter. Enzymes are also what continue to "compost" those tomatoes and bananas if we don't eat them fast enough.

Foods have the highest enzyme activity level when they are fresh or when they are fermenting. So, growing your own or buying local gives you the most enzyme activity. Raw fish, such as sushi or sashimi, is rich in active enzymes. Raw milk is high in enzymes. Fresh pineapple has bromelain enzymes, but canning or cooking deactivates the bromelain. Soy sauce is rich in enzymes to help digest the protein in the meal. Drinking kombucha and kefir, and eating kimchee, yogurt, sauerkraut, and other fermented foods can enhance enzyme intake.

Cooked, packaged, and processed foods are enzyme depleted. Cooking at temperatures as low as 118 degrees Fahrenheit destroys enzymes. If you regularly eat cooked, packaged and/or processed foods, you may benefit from enzyme supplementation and by including more raw foods into your daily diet.

Supplemental Enzymes and Their Clinical Use

Studies reveal that about 10 percent of 10-year-olds have enzyme deficiencies, 20 percent of 20-year-olds have enzyme deficiencies, 50 percent of 50-year-olds have enzyme deficiencies, and so on. This can occur from stress or low-grade inflammation in the stomach, called gastritis, and infections, such as H. pylori.

Enzyme deficiencies are obvious in children with cystic fibrosis but less obvious as a pivotal factor in type 2 diabetes and obesity in our children. Enzyme supplementation has been helpful in the treatment of these health problems.

Supplemental enzymes have also been used successfully to treat several types of arthritis in adults, working more effectively than drug treatment. Moreover, they have been used successfully to treat children and adults with food allergies, eosinophilic gastroenteritis, asthma, and other illnesses. Along with probiotics, they are the first thing I think of when working with children and adults who are failing to thrive.

Protein-splitting enzymes help the immune system to become hardier to IgG food sensitivities. The mechanism works by breaking down immune complexes. Other diseases for which enzymes have been used clinically include Crohn's disease, ulcerative colitis, hay fever, pulmonary fibrosis, sinusitis, multiple sclerosis, and bladder infections, Enzymes, specifically nattokinase and seratopeptidase, have been widely utilized to prevent and break up blood clots.

Protein-splitting enzymes also are used to reduce swelling and pain throughout the body and can be used to treat injuries. In one study, soccer players were given enzymes or placebos after they were injured. Injuries healed more quickly when enzymes were given, sometimes up to twice as fast. They can be used to reduce the time that bruises take to heal by about 50 percent.

Enzymes have also been used for decades in cancer treatment, especially in Europe. I recently heard oncologist Dr. Mahesh Kanojia speak at a medical conference. He said that use of Aspergillus-derived protein splitting, also called proteolytic enzymes, enzyme supplements lessens the side effects of chemotherapy, including hair loss, and enhances the results of the treatments. Nicholas Gonzales, MD, in New York, utilized pancreatic enzyme supplements as a critical part of his individualized programs for people with all types of cancers. The National Institutes of Health (NIH) was so impressed, they funded a study to reproduce his work. However, this study did not show the same effectiveness of Dr. Gonzales's treatments; According to Dr. Gonzales, patients put into the treatment and control groups were not evenly matched. Many more people who only a few weeks from dying were included in the enzyme treatment group. He discussed this in his 2012 book, *What Went Wrong*.

Categories of Enzyme Supplements

There are three major types of supplemental enzyme products: pancreatic enzymes, enzymes grown on a fungal base, and plant-based enzymes.

Pancreatic enzymes have been used and are part of common medical practice for illnesses such as cystic fibrosis. They are actually derived from animal pancreatic tissue. They work well to assist with digestion and to help stabilize blood glucose levels in people with diabetes and hypoglycemia. When I was in my 20s, I suffered from hypoglycemia; I took pancreatic enzymes several times a day for about a year and found my hypoglycemia to be nearly 100 percent gone. The difficulty with pancreatic enzymes is that they work in a limited pH range, at 8 or above. This pH is too alkaline to function in the stomach, where a large part of digestion takes place. In cystic fibrosis a small percentage of children become allergic to pancreatic enzymes.

More recently, enzymes have been grown on a fungal base of *Aspergillus niger* and *Aspergillus oryzae*. These enzymes have been used in food production for centuries and clinically for more than 50 years in Japan. There are hundreds of species of Aspergillus, but these two have been found to be completely free of mycotoxins (substances produced from fungi that are toxic). These enzymes are blended like wine to ensure that they work in the high-acid environment of the stomach and through the small and large intestines, which have a more neutral pH. They also are not derived from an animal protein and have been found to cause fewer allergic issues in people.

Plant-based enzymes, such as bromelain and papain, are protein-splitting enzymes. Bromelain is derived from the green stems of pineapple plants, and papain comes from green papayas. They are useful for reducing inflammation and pain and for digestion of protein.

Enzymes are rated by their activity level rather than by counting milligrams or micrograms of them. When you purchase enzyme supplement products, you will see units such as DU, HUT, FCCLU, CU, IAU, and many others to express the level of enzyme activity. If you look at an enzyme label and it measures the enzymes only in milligrams or micrograms, you cannot know if there are any active enzymes in the product at all. Enzyme supplements are very stable and will last for at least three years, so many labels do not have expiration dates.

MOTILITY

Motility refers to the way that food moves through the digestive tract. If motility isn't working effectively, we won't get the most benefit from our food. Common motility issues include GERD, gastroparesis, IBS, fecal incontinence, and chronic constipation.

We have several autonomic mechanisms that regulate motility: Drinking of fluids, chewing, swallowing, and peristalsis all move the food through the digestive system in a rhythmic way. In between meals, the migrating motor complex (MMC) sweeps food residues, debris, and microbes into the colon. The MMC is regulated by a hormone called motilin. Secretions from the pancreas and gallbladder stimulate the MMC. It's also stimulated when we fast and is one of the components of intermittent fasting. Many people find that eating two meals daily and fasting for 14 to 16 hours in between helps to stimulate the MMC.

Physicians often prescribe pro-kinetics drugs to stimulate motility. These include drugs such as Prucalopride, low-dose naltrexone, low-dose erythromycin, and metoclopramide. Natural prokinetics include magnesium supplementation, ginger, tryptophan, high doses of vitamin Cö, vitamin D, Swedish bitters, acupuncture and acupressure, breathing exercises, and exercise.

DIETARY FIBER

Insufficient dietary fiber intake is yet another reason people may not be absorbing or digesting their foods appropriately. In fact, most of us eat half as much fiber as our ancestors did. Soluble fiber, one category of prebiotic, (found in fruit, beans, barley, rice, flaxseed, and psyllium) helps bind bile acids, regulates cholesterol and blood sugar levels, and keeps our intestinal pH in balance. Insoluble fiber (found in bran, vegetables, whole grains, and carrots) helps keep us regular and normalizes peristalsis. Soluble fiber is fermented in our large intestines by beneficial bifidobacteria to produce butyrate and other short-chain fats that provide fuel and cell maintenance in our large intestines. By definition, soluble fibers are prebiotics, food for the microbiota. This is discussed more fully in Chapter 6. Soluble fiber helps to regulate both constipation-type and diarrhea-type IBS. Diets high in soluble fiber are helpful to people with IBS, Crohn's disease, hiatal hernia, and peptic ulcer. Dietary fiber also helps prevent obesity by slowing down digestion and the release of glucose and insulin. Fiber has been shown to normalize serum cholesterol levels. High-fiber diets reduce the risk of heart disease, high blood pressure, and certain types of cancer. (See Chapter 13 for more information on increasing high-fiber foods in your diet.)

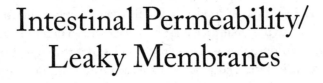

CHAPTER 4

Intestinal Permeability/ Leaky Membranes

The foot bone connected to the leg bone,
The leg bone connected to the knee bone,
The knee bone connected to the thigh bone,
The thigh bone connected to the back bone,
The back bone connected to the neck bone,
The neck bone connected to the head bone

—African American spiritual/children's song

*L*eaky gut syndrome is really a nickname for term *increased intestinal permeability*, which underlies an enormous variety of illnesses and symptoms. It's not a disease or an illness itself. It's a symptom of inflammation and imbalance that has many causes. The list of health conditions associated with increased intestinal permeability grows each year as we increase our knowledge of the synergy between digestion and the immune system. Currently there are more than 13,800 research articles on intestinal permeability.

The small intestines have a paradoxical function, allowing only properly digested fats, proteins, and starches to pass into the bloodstream, while providing a protective barrier to keep microbes, undigested food particles, metals, and chemicals from entering the bloodstream. It is tightly regulated by molecules such as zonulin, occludin, claudin 1, E-cadherin, JAM-1, catenins, cingulin, and actin. Most of the time, these tight junctions are closed to keep substances from passing through into the bloodstream. This is called the barrier function of the gastrointestinal mucosal lining. This surface is often called the brush border because under a microscope, its villi and microvilli look like bristles on a brush.

The cells of the small intestine are called enterocytes, lining the inside of the lumen. This cell lining is one cell thick and is the interface between our food and the bloodstream. The enterocytes are together by tight junctions, which prevent large molecules from passing into the bloodstream. The tight junctions selectively open to allow some molecules to pass, but they mainly stay closed. When the tight junctions become inflamed, they loosen up, and larger molecules pass through. The substances that pass through the intracellular junctions are seen by our immune system as foreign, stimulating an antibody reaction. Zonulin is a newly discovered (in 2000 by Dr. Allesio Fasano and his research team) molecule that signals opening of the tight junctions. (See Figure 4.1.)

When there is increased intestinal permeability, substances larger than particle size—bacteria, fungi, potentially toxic molecules, and undigested food particles—are allowed to pass directly through the weakened cell membranes into the bloodstream, activating antibodies and alarm substances called cytokines. The cytokines alert our lymphocytes (white blood cells) to battle the particles. Oxidants are produced in the battle, causing irritation and inflammation far from the digestive system.

Inflammation on this brush border can also prevent small nutrients and food molecules from passing into the gut lumen, causing malabsorption.

Intestinal mucus normally blocks bacteria from moving to other parts of the body. Small amounts of bacteria do move through the enterocytes in healthy people and are recognized and killed by our immune system. But when there is increased intestinal permeability, excessive amounts of bacteria can pass into the bloodstream, lymph, spleen, and kidneys and travel throughout the body. When intestinal bacteria colonize in other parts of the body, we call it bacterial translocation. Small intestinal bacterial overgrowth (SIBO) promotes bacterial translocation. Many of the microbes that migrate are gram negative and secrete lipopolysaccharides (LPS), which further increase intestinal permeability. Bacterial translocation can lead to infection and more rarely sepsis. For example, *Blastocystis hominis*, a bacteria that causes gastrointestinal (GI) problems, has been found in the synovial fluid in the knee of an arthritis patient. Surgery or tube feeding in hospitals can also cause bacterial translocation.

Here's a metaphor of how leaky gut syndrome can lead to food reactions. Imagine that your cells need a kernel of corn. They are screaming out, "Hey, send me a kernel of corn." The bloodstream replies, "I have an ear of corn but no enzymes to cut off individual kernels." So the ear of corn goes around and around while the cells starve for corn. Finally, our immune system reacts by making antibodies against the ear of corn, treating the corn as if it were a foreign invader. Your immune system has mobilized to finish the job of incomplete digestion, but this puts unneeded stress on it. The next time you eat corn, your body already has antibodies to react against it, which triggers the immune system, and so on. As time goes on, people with leaky gut syndrome tend to become more and more sensitive to a wider variety of foods and environmental contaminants.

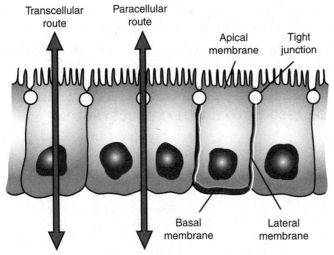

Figure 4.1   Healthy Gut Barrier.

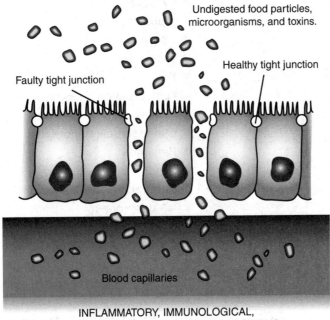

Figure 4.2

Depending on our own susceptibilities, we may develop a wide variety of signs, symptoms, and health problems. Leaky gut syndrome is associated with the following medical problems: allergies, celiac disease, Crohn's disease, HIV, and malabsorption syndromes. Leaky gut is a triggering factor in every autoimmune condition. These include multiple sclerosis, lupus, akylosing spondylitis, Sjögren's syndrome, rheumatoid arthritis, and psoriasis. It's also found in people with AIDS, liver diseases including hepatitis and cirrhosis, lung conditions including asthma and bronchitis, eczema, allergies, Reiter's syndrome, and other conditions.

SYMPTOMS AND DIAGNOSES ASSOCIATED WITH LEAKY GUT SYNDROME

- Abdominal pain
- Aggressive behavior
- Anxiety
- Asthma
- Bed wetting
- Bloating
- Chronic joint pain
- Chronic muscle pain
- Confusion
- Constipation
- Diarrhea
- Fatigue and malaise
- Fevers of unknown origin
- Fuzzy thinking
- Gas
- Indigestion
- Mood swings
- Nervousness
- Poor exercise tolerance
- Poor immunity
- Poor memory
- Recurrent bladder infections
- Recurrent vaginal infections
- Shortness of breath
- Toxic feelings

- Behcet's syndrome
- Burns (severe)
- Celiac disease
- Chemotherapy for cancer treatment
- Childhood hyperactivity
- Chronic fatigue syndrome
- Cirrhosis
- Crohn's disease
- Cystic fibrosis
- Diabetes type 1
- Eczema
- Endotoxemia
- Environmental illness
- Food allergy and food sensitivity
- Giardia
- Gluten sensitivity, nonceliac
- Hepatitis
- Hives
- HIV-positive status
- IgA nephropathy
- Intestinal infections
- Irritable bowel syndrome (IBS)
- Liver dysfunction
- Lupus (systemic lupus erythematosus, or SLE)
- Malnutrition
- Multiple chemical sensitivities
- Multiple sclerosis
- NSAID enteropathy
- Pancreatic insufficiency
- Psoriasis
- Schizophrenia
- Trauma
- Ulcerative colitis

The following are common clinical conditions associated with intestinal permeability:

- Acne
- Alcoholism
- Ankylosing spondylitis
- Arthritis
- Autism

The listed conditions can arise from a variety of causes, but leaky gut syndrome may underlie more classic diagnoses. If you have any of the common symptoms or disorders associated with leaky gut syndrome, ask your physician to order an intestinal permeability test to see if it is causing your problem.

TESTING FOR LEAKY GUT (INTESTINAL PERMEABILITY)

Many experienced clinicians do not routinely test for intestinal permeability. They utilize their clinical observations to determine the likelihood. Leaky gut is a symptom, not a cause. Does the client have food allergies or intolerances? Does he or she have parasites, yeast infections, or bacterial infections? Could high stress levels or medications be the cause of the leaky gut?

If so, do testing that explores the possible underlying causes and perpetuators. But for those of you who want something on paper proving that you have leaky gut, the lactulose-mannitol test has been the gold standard. Here are newer clinical tests that assess for intestinal permeability. (See Chapter 11 for details.)

- Lactulose-mannitol testing
- Zonulin-1 or zonulin antibody testing
- Serum diamine oxidase (DAO)
- Bacterial lipopolysaccharides (LPS)
- Indirect testing: food sensitivity testing—if a large number of foods are reactive, increased intestinal permeability can be assumed.

WHAT CAUSES LEAKY GUT SYNDROME?

Leaky gut syndrome has no single cause, but some of the most common are chronic stress, dysbiosis, environmental contaminants, gastrointestinal disease, immune overload, overuse of alcoholic beverages, poor food choices, presence of pathogenic bacteria, parasites and yeasts, and prolonged use of nonsteroidal anti-inflammatory drugs (NSAIDs). Let's discuss some of these one at a time.

Chronic Stress
Acute and chronic stresses change hormonal response and affect the immune system's ability to respond quickly and our ability to heal. It's like the story

of the boy who cried wolf. If we keep hollering that there's a wolf every time we're late for an appointment or we need to finish a project by a deadline, our bodies can't tell the difference between this type of stress and real stress—like meeting a vicious dog in the woods or a death in the family. Our body reacts to these stressors by producing less secretory IgA (sIgA) (one of the first lines of immune defense) and less dehydroepiandrosterone (DHEA, a antiaging, anti-stress adrenal hormone) and by slowing down digestion and peristalsis, reducing blood flow to digestive organs, and producing toxic metabolites. Meditation, guided imagery, relaxation, and a good sense of humor can help us deal with daily stresses. We can learn to let small problems and traumas wash over us, not taking them too seriously.

Dysbiosis

The presence of dysbiosis contributes to leaky gut syndrome. Lipopolysaccharides (LPSs) from mostly gram-negative bacteria increase permeability. Fungi, such as Candida, can also increase permeability by breaking down the brush borders. Blastocystis hominis, giardia, helicobacter, salmonella, shigella, *Yersinia enteroco-litica*, amoebas, and other parasites also irritate the intestinal lining and cause gastrointestinal symptoms.

Environmental Contaminants

Daily exposure to hundreds of household and environmental chemicals puts stress on our immune defenses and the body's ability to repair itself. This leads to chronic delay of necessary routine repairs. Our immune systems can pay attention to only so many places at one time, and parts of the body far away from the digestive system are affected. Connective tissue begins to break down, and we lose trace minerals like calcium, potassium, and magnesium. Environmental chemicals deplete our reserves of buffering minerals, causing acidosis in the cells and tissue and cell swelling. This is known as leaky cells—like having major internal plumbing problems!

Overconsumption of Alcoholic Beverages

People with alcohol dependence typically have increased permeability. Drinking alcoholic beverages can increase the number of gram-negative bacteria in the gut, increasing LPS, also known as endotoxin. LPSs increase production of zonulin, which opens the tight junctions. Alcohol is also metabolized by gram-negative bacteria in the gut lumen and can result in higher levels of acetaldehyde, which increases permeability. This becomes a vicious cycle because as people drink more, the liver becomes damaged, increasing leaky gut.

Poor Food Choices

Low-fiber diets cause an increase in transit time, allowing toxic by-products of digestion to concentrate and irritate the gut mucosa. In addition, diets of highly processed foods injure our intestinal lining. Processed foods invariably are low in nutrients and fiber, with high levels of food additives, restructured fats, and sugar. These foods promote inflammation of the GI tract.

It's also important to note that even foods we normally think of as healthful can be inflaming to the gut.

Use of Medication

Nonsteroidal drugs such as Advil, aspirin, and Motrin, damage brush borders, allowing microbes, partially digested food particles, and toxins to enter the bloodstream. Birth control pills and steroid drugs also create conditions that help feed fungi, which damage the lining. Chemotherapy drugs and radiation therapy can also significantly disrupt GI balance.

Food and Environmental Sensitivities

Food and environmental sensitivities are usually the result of leaky gut syndrome. The prevalence of these sensitivities is more widely recognized today than in the past; 24 percent of American adults claim they have food and environmental sensitivities. These sensitivities, also called delayed hypersensitivity reactions, differ from true food allergies, also called type I or immediate hypersensitivity reactions.

Lectins: Lectins are found primarily in legumes, grains, dairy products, and nightshade family foods: tomatoes, potatoes, eggplant, and peppers. Theoretically, lectins can increase inflammation, cause gas and bloating, cause joint pain, and increase leaky gut. We've all experienced the gas that can come from beans that haven't been well-cooked. Yet, the research to date has not looked at how people actually consume lectin-rich foods as part of a healthy diet. We have a large body of research demonstrating the health benefits of beans, peas, grains, dairy products, and nightshade family foods, so I'm not jumping on the bandwagon of the low-lectin diet, although there may be people who benefit.

We do have many anecdotal stories from people whose arthritis stopped when they gave up nightshade family foods. Other people find that eating a low-lectin diet helps with weight loss, energy, and mood. Currently, we don't have the research to understand why this might be so.

Endurance Exercise

Athletes who train and compete in endurance sports have been shown to have increased intestinal permeability. This resolves in a healthy athlete fairly quickly. We might think that aggressive training feels good—but your gut may feel differently.

RESTORING GUT INTEGRITY

If you believe you suffer from leaky gut, it's best to work with a health professional who can help you determine the underlying factors. Fortunately, you can find many ways to heal your gut. Some involve changing your habits, like chewing your food more completely; others involve taking specific supplements that will help your body repair itself. If you have food allergies or sensitivities, deal with them. Find out if you have an infection of some sort and get appropriate treatment. Replenish your bacterial flora with probiotics and prebiotics such as fructooligosaccharides (FOSs). You may need to support your digestive function with enzymes, bitters, or hydrochloric acid tablets.

The following are steps you can take to help repair your gut. Supportive foods and supplemental nutrients can help repair the mucosal lining directly. Cabbage juice, cabbage family foods, bone broths, vegetable broths, fresh vegetable juices, aloe vera juice, okra, and slippery elm tea and lozenges all have a healing effect on the small intestine.

Stop the Mediators that Perpetuate the Problem
- Stress
- Pain medications that injure the GI lining
- Environmental contaminants
- Overconsumption of alcohol
- Poor food choices
- Use of birth control pills or steroid medications

Dietary Recommendations

Diet will be discussed more fully later in the book (See Chapters 13 and 14). Key foods that can be helpful to heal increased intestinal permeability include:

- Bone broths
- Vegetables (steamed, raw, etc.) and vegetable juices
- Probiotic-rich foods
- Soothing foods such as okra, licorice tea, slippery elm tea, or marshmallow root tea

Avoid any foods you know you are sensitive to

Nutritional Supplements: *These can be taken individually or in products that combine several in one supplement.*

- **Glutamine** (also called: L-glutamine): Unlike the brain, which uses glucose for energy, the cells of the small intestine depend on glutamine as their main fuel and for maintenance and repair. Glutamine is the first nutrient I think of to repair a leaky gut. Glutamine is alkalizing to the body. It decreases the incidence of infection and stimulates the production of sIgA. Glutamine has also been shown to decrease the risk of bacterial translocation. Dosages can range from 1 to 30 grams daily, depending on your needs. Begin with 1 to 3 grams daily. Too much glutamine will probably constipate you, so that's a good gauge of how much you need. Many people find that they feel stronger and have more endurance when they take glutamine.
- **Zinc:** Zinc may be an essential nutrient for gut repair. The type that shows the most promise for digestive healing is zinc carnosine. A typical dose is 75 mg of zinc carnosine twice daily.
- *Lactobacillus plantarum:* L. plantarum is a probiotic that is specifically soothing to the small intestine. (See Chapter 6 for more on probiotics.)
- **Colostrum:** Colostrum is the first milk that a mammal produces after birth and provides immune support. In athletes, supplemental bovine colostrum has decreased the incidence of leaky gut, although not all studies show this. In people taking non-steroidal pain medications, like aspirin and Motrin, taking colostrum prevented leaky gut. Dosage: 1500-1700 mg daily of bovine or goat colostrum.
- **Quercetin:** Quercetin helps to heal leaky gut and also helps to modulate allergies by preventing histamine release. Be sure to get a high-quality quercetin

product. I use Perque Pain Guard and Repair Guard, which couples quercetin with grape-seed extract. The Repair Guard also contains pomegranate extract for antioxidant support. I wouldn't mention a brand, except in this case, it simply works better than other products. Take between 500 and 3,000 mg daily.

- **Aloe vera:** Although we have no specific research on aloe for leaky gut, it seems to work well for many people. Look for products that have the outer leaf removed. Use as directed.
- **Restore:** Restore is a soil-based extract lignite compound that is being promoted to heal leaky gut. No research has yet been done in people, though. One research group, including the founder of the company, has published two papers that report on Restore's protective effects on enterocytes when exposed to gliaden (a protein from wheat) and glyphosate. It would be good to see clinical and independent research on this product, but Restore seems to be protective of the gut membrane. The optimal adult dose is 1 teaspoon three times daily 30 minutes before a meal. If you are sensitive, begin with a smaller dose and work up.
- **Digestive enzymes:** Taking digestive enzymes with meals may ensure that all foods are completely digested. Take one to two digestive enzymes with meals.

Additional Supplements

- **Gamma oryzanol:** A compound found in rice bran oil, gamma oryzanol is a useful therapeutic tool in treating gastritis, IBS, and ulcers. It has a healing effect throughout the digestive tract and can help normalize cholesterol and serum triglycerides, menopausal symptoms, and depression. Take 100 mg three times daily for three weeks or longer.
- **Seacure:** Seacure is a supplement made from deep-ocean whitefish that has been broken down into peptides and amino acids. I don't know why, but the product is soothing and healing to the gut. This product is stinky; keeping it frozen can help with that. Take six capsules daily in divided doses.
- **Vitamin A:** Vitamin A is an essential nutrient for mucous membranes. Vitamin A is a two-edged sword, so monitor serum retinol levels and/or get your vitamin A from carotenoids, which can be converted into vitamin A in most, but not all, people. Plant foods that are rich sources of carotenoids are all green, yellow, and orange vegetables. Take 5,000 IU daily of preformed vitamin A and up to 25,000 IU carotenoids daily.
- **Vitamin C:** With its strong antioxidant properties, vitamin C binds viruses and toxins to chelate them out of the body. Take 500 to 10,000 mg or more daily.
- **Deglycyrrhized licorice:** Licorice root has many health-enhancing properties. It's soothing to the mucous membranes of the digestive tract, and chewable

licorice can help reduce inflammation and pain. It promotes healing of mucous membranes by stimulating production of prostaglandins that promote healing and cell proliferation. It also has antibiotic and antioxidant properties. Use only deglycerrhized licorice; whole licorice root can raise blood pressure levels and lower potassium levels. Take two tablets between meals as needed up to four times daily.

- **Antioxidant support:** Once the intestinal tract has been damaged, free radicals are often produced in quantities too large for the body to process. This causes inflammation and irritation, which exacerbate a leaky gut. So try eating antioxidant-rich foods like beans, fruits, vegetables, nuts, and seeds. Increasing use of antioxidant nutrients such as vitamin E, selenium, N-acetyl cysteine, superoxide dismutase (SOD), zinc (especially carnosine), manganese, copper, coenzyme Q10, lipoic acid, and vitamin C can help quench the free-radical fire.
- **Phosphatidylcholine:** Research indicates that phosphatidylcholine helps to reduce intestinal permeability. Phosphatidylcholine is found in the mucous gel of the intestinal lumen and protects the GI tract. Take 2,000 to 4,000 mg daily.

As you can see, increased intestinal permeability (leaky gut) can underlie many different health conditions and contribute to ill health. Taking the steps mentioned here can help renew your health, yet this is an often-overlooked factor in medicine today.

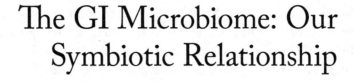

CHAPTER 5

The GI Microbiome: Our Symbiotic Relationship

"If you don't like bacteria, you're on the wrong planet."

—Stewart Brand (Editor of The Whole Earth Catalog, Founder of the WELL.)

After the Big Bang, the first life forms were microbes. They terraformed the planet and are the reason we breathe oxygen and plants utilize carbon dioxide. Microbes populate every niche that's been explored from Antarctica, to the oceans, and in the hot springs at Yellowstone National Park. Mitochondria, the energy factories in the nuclei of your cells, and most of the organelles in your cells were derived from bacteria long ago. Chloroplasts in plants were originally bacteria. These microbes consist of bacteria, fungi, viruses, protozoa, and helminths (parasites) weighing on average 3 to 7 pounds. Collectively, this "organ" is called the microbiome.

Although most of the press on microbes is about the ones that make us sick, most of these live in harmony with us and many provide us with benefits. There are three main types of microbes: pathogens that make us sick; commensals that enhance digestion of fats, protein, and carbohydrates and synthesize short-chain fatty acids (SCFAs) and vitamins; and symbiotic bacteria (also called probiotics), which provide a benefit to the host by making vitamins and regulating immune function.

In the last decade, research on the human microbiome has mushroomed. There are several emerging concepts and theories about the microbiome:

1. The emerging research suggests that the microbes that we evolved with play an enormous role in determining our overall health.
2. Having a wide diversity of microbes gives us great healthy resilience.
3. Modern people are missing chunks of microbes that used to give us greater diversity. Current research suggests that diversity is the key to optimal health.

The microbiome functions much like an organ, and it acts as a major part of the immune system. It protects us from microbial and parasitic diseases; influences the effects of drugs; affects whether we are fat or thin or happy or sad; determines our nutritional status and overall health; and contributes to our rate of aging.

You have the same number of bacteria in your gut that you have cells in your body. And the DNA in these microbes outnumbers your cellular DNA by 150 to 1. If only 1 percent of our DNA is human and 99 percent is microbial, you have to ask the question: Who's hosting whom? These bacteria are called your microbiota, and they live in your digestive tract, skin, eyes, airways, blood, mouth, and vagina. Each tissue in your body has its own microbiome; you have a microbiome of your tongue, lips, throat, lungs, several on your skin, and so forth. The microbes on your left and right hands are only 70 percent the same. This is true because we use each hand differently in our daily lives. The skin on the top of your arm has a different microbiome than the skin on the bottom side of your arm. Early research is beginning to demonstrate that there are distinct microbiomes in the brain, blood, and kidneys. As the research unfolds, I believe that we will discover microbiomes in every tissue and organ.

You have billions of microbes in your mouth, many billions in your small intestine, and hundreds of trillions in your large intestine (half of the colon's volume). It's estimated that we also have twice as many viruses as bacteria in our microbiome. Some of these helpful viruses are called phages, and they act as shepherds to keep the bacteria in balance and to cull the ones that can possibly make us sick. Each day, you produce several ounces of these microbes and eliminate several ounces in stool.

The microbiota function much like an organ, and they act as a major part of every system in your body. Ninety-nine percent of your metabolism is dependent on the microbes in your body, including how much energy (ATP) your mitochondria produce. They protect us from microbial and parasitic diseases and influence the effects of drugs.

Your microbiota is like a fingerprint; yours isn't exactly like anyone else's. Researchers are trying to determine whether there is a "core" balance that is common to all of us and what effects it might have on health.

WHERE DO THEY COME FROM?

Until birth, we receive predigested food from our mothers through the placenta. Until recently, it was believed that babies were born sterile, but newer research demonstrates that there are microbes transferred through the placenta into infants prior to birth. The colonization of these bacteria occurs after birth and matures over the first two years or so of life.

This process normally happens in a predictable way, and, once established, the colonies flourish. It is during this time when we set up our lifelong microbiota fingerprint which is the basis of our overall immunity and metabolism.

After birth babies are exposed to bacteria in breast milk and formula and when sucking on nipples, fingers, and toes. With every breath and touch, bacteria flock to an infant's skin and mucous membranes. In no time, every conceivable space in the colon is occupied by microbes. Within the first few days of life, colonization of *E. coli* and streptococcus occurs. Within a week of birth, *Bifidobacteria, Bacteroides*, and *Clostridium* are established in bottle-fed babies. Breast-fed infants have increased numbers of *lactobacillus* and *bifidobacteria* species. As babies begin eating solid foods, they begin developing a balance of microbes that are more like adults. Bacterial colonization patterns set up in infancy continue to prevail throughout our lifetime—and the foods and drugs to which we expose our children dramatically affect this delicate balance.

The balance of these microbes change dynamically depending on the mother's microbes, place of delivery, whether there was a vaginal or C-section birth, whether the baby came to full term or was premature, hygiene (which, when excessive, can disrupt normal balance), use of antibiotics, having siblings or not, whether a baby is breast-fed or bottle-fed, whether the infant is exposed to pets or farm animals, and the foods that are eaten.

Babies who are unable to properly colonize friendly flora, however, can become irritable and colicky and have gas pains, diaper rash, or eczema. Babies who don't develop the right balance of beneficial bacteria are also more susceptible as they age to diarrhea, constipation, irritable bowel syndrome, allergy, asthma, and eczema, and are more prone to acne and severe gingivitis.

In a study of growth rate and probiotic supplementation, babies given bifidobacteria showed better growth during their first six months of life; in another study, supplemental *Lactobacillus acidophilus and L. casei* decreased the severity and incidence of bronchitis and pneumonia in babies aged six months to two years. Adding probiotics to infant formula can reduce the need for antibiotics and can help prevent infections in preterm infants by giving their immune systems a boost. Probiotics can also calm babies with colic.

WHAT AFFECTS THEM?

The microbiota of modern humans has been influenced by what we eat, as well as our climate, and it differs from that of our ancestors, who traveled less and ate a more homogeneous diet. Medications, chemicals, C-section births, breast-feeding versus bottle-feeding, stress, diet, and lifestyle all affect the balance of these gut bacteria. Bacterial infections, antibiotics use, high stress levels, excessive alcohol intake, poor diet, and a number of other factors can disrupt the delicate balance of beneficial bacteria in our gut. Often, disease-producing bacteria and fungi will proliferate, causing symptoms such as diarrhea, bloating, and gas. If left unchecked, they can contribute to long-term conditions such as irritable bowel syndrome (IBS).

Bacteria "talk" to each other, and when there are enough of them, they begin to work as a group. This is called "quorum sensing." Quorum sensing is a process in both health and disease. It's like waiting until you amass enough troops to actually be effective before you try to scale the castle wall. It's believed that the cross talk between our genes and our bacteria runs our metabolism and modulates our immune system. Imbalances in the microbiome have been associated with the following conditions:

- Allergies
- Asthma
- Autism
- Autoimmune diseases
- Cancer
- Cardiovascular disease
- Celiac disease
- Diabetes
- Eczema
- Glaucoma
- Heart disease and lipids
- Heart failure
- HIV/AIDS
- IBS
- Kidney disease
- Liver diseases
- Mental health
- Mood disorders
- Neurological disease
- Obesity
- Oral health
- Rheumatic diseases
- Skin conditions
- Sleep disruption

THE GOOD, THE BAD, AND THE UGLY

You have somewhere between 500 and 1,000 types of bacteria in your digestive system, each type having hundreds of different strains. The average person has on average about 200 bacteria in his or her mouth and hundreds more in virtually every other tissue. I expect as our ability to sequence these microbes improves, these numbers will grow. These microbes have evolved with humans; they aren't different from us—they are us. They come in in cultured and fermented food, from putting our fingers in our mouths, through being born, and other events. Some are permanent residents; others are just passing through.

Although genetic research has discovered 40,000 different bacteria in the GI tracts of different people so far, 80 to 90 percent of these are from two bacterial families, or phyla. There are six predominant phyla of microbes in the human microbiome, although the great predominance is of Bacteroidetes and Firmicutes.

- Bacteroidetes include the families of Bacteroides, Prevotella, and Rilkenellaceae.
- Firmicute includes the families of Lactobacilli, Erysiopelotrichia, Lachnospiraceae, and Runinococcus.
- Actinobacteria, the third-most-abundant phylum, includes Bifidobacterium.
- Proteobacteria has the families of *Enterobacterium*, *Helicobacter pylori*, and *Escherichia coli*.
- Finally, there are the phyla of Verrucomicrobia and Euryarchaeota, which have not been well delineated yet.

The small intestine has relatively few microbes; the predominant species include *Lactobacilli*, *Erysiopelotrichia*, and *Enterobacteria*. The main families in the colon include *Bacteroides*, *Prevotella*, *Rilkenellaceae*, *Lachnospira*, and *Ruminococcus*. In the inner folds of the gut lumen, the main families include *Lachnospira* and *Ruminococcus*.

Collectively these bacteria are called commensals, which means they are the normal bacteria in your gut. There is much yet to be learned about the benefits of specific commensal microbes that live within us. In addition to commensal bacteria, you have probiotic bacteria, also called probionts, which are beneficial to you, as well as pathogenic or disease-causing bacteria. You also have fungi, viruses, and possibly some parasites in your microbiota.

Microbes that make us sick are called pathogens. When we think about bacteria, in our culture we mainly think about pathogens and use hand sanitizers, soaps, and household cleaners to protect ourselves from them. These microbes have names, like *Salmonella*, *Shigella*, *Pseudomonas*, *Vibrio*, and *Colostrum difficile*. They are single organisms that can overwhelm health. These can cause acute or chronic illness. Some bacteria are extremely virulent and cause sudden and violent illness. Our body reacts to virulent bacteria, such as Salmonella, with diarrhea, fever, loss of appetite, and vomiting. The body screams, "Get this stuff out of me!" and attempts to rapidly flush or starve it out. Most disease-causing microbes thrive at human body temperature, while fever kills them by overheating them. Some produce toxins that are more inflammatory than the bacteria. Many pathogens are less virulent, causing more subtle symptoms that we often learn to live with.

Bacteria that cause chronic illness are generally weak organisms of low virulence. They are often found in small quantities in all of us and have been assumed to be harmless. But when given the opportunity to thrive, they can and do cause illness.

BIOFILMS IN HEALTH AND DISEASE

Biofilms are starchy matrices that house microorganisms and exist pretty much everywhere on earth. Your microbiota live in biofilm communities. Biofilms are aggregates of bacteria, fungi, and other microorganisms that live in communities. They can be beneficial or harmful. They are integral in the human body and can be found in the mouth, lungs, digestive system, nostrils, genitourinary system, and more. Healthy people have healthy biofilms. Biofilms operate like corporations, banding together to do great work. They are well organized and help maintain our many microbiomes. For example the mucus in your nostrils is a biofilm. How would it feel to have completely dry nostrils? Can you imagine the lungs functioning without a mucous membrane? Or, in women, what would a completely dry vagina be like?

Studies initially focused on biofilms that showed up in water treatment facilities, hospital tubing, and industrial settings. Once this research blossomed, technologies to build healthy biofilms in these environments have been used successfully in water treatment plants and for cleaning up oil spills, groundwater contamination, and hazardous waste products; the "biomining" of minerals, such as zinc, copper, and gold, increases the yield in mining of minerals.

However, when biofilms become dysbiotic, they are difficult to eradicate. The starchy matrix protects the biofilm from its environment, making it less responsive to antibiotics and macrophages (white blood cells that are like Pac-Man, gobbling up everything in sight). Periodontal disease is a common example of what happens when a biofilm becomes dysbiotic. Biofilms have also been discovered on contact lenses, in wounds, in catheters, on knee and hip replacement pieces, on pacemakers, in machines, on ponds, and elsewhere.

It is believed that 70 percent of all bacterial infections in people are caused by biofilms. They've found a cushy place to thrive at our expense and are linked to lung infections in cystic fibrosis, periodontal disease, catheter infections, chronic wounds, chronic ear infections, implants, and Candida infections. Imagine, for example, that you've had a stent or pacemaker put into your heart and that it begins forming a biofilm that's loaded with Candida. These specific biofilms can cause endocarditis, an infection inside the heart chambers and valves. Infectious biofilms are resistant to antibiotics and can take 100 to 1,000 times the amount of antibiotics to eradicate compared to a regular infection. If your immune system isn't functioning well, these biofilms can cause infections that become life-threatening.

Little is known about the prevention and treatment of biofilms in people; research is just beginning to flourish in this field. Some of the ideas that are being studied include the following:

- Some researchers hypothesize that having an adequate amount of bile helps to keep biofilm formation from occurring.
- Dental research leads the way in the field of what works with people. Ozone therapy is being used in periodontal disease to eradicate biofilms and normalize oral microbiota. Probiotics, *Lactobacillus reuteri* and *Lactobacillus salivarius* (strain: W24) also produce healthful biofilms in the mouth and have demonstrated beneficial effects in people with gingivitis. Additional research shows promise with the use of polyethylene glycol, chlorexidine, and sodium hypochlorite in breaking up the biofilms that develop on our teeth, in root canals, and in other oral tissues.
- Others are looking at probiotic supplements to normalize biofilms. One group of researchers looked at the *E. coli* strain Nissle 1917 and found that it helped to form healthy biofilms that pushed out disease-causing *E. coli* bacteria. This could be especially useful in treating ulcerative colitis, which has been shown to respond well to *E. coli* Nissle.
- Other researchers report that use of prebiotics, such as inulin-type fructans such as fructooligosaccharides (FOS), support healthy biofilms and a healthy gut. One group of researchers has looked at components of oregano oil and thyme oil and found them to be effective at inhibiting biofilm formation.
- Chitosan, a product made from purified shrimp shells, has also been shown to break down biofilms in the heart composed primarily of a bacteria called Cryptococcus neoformans.
- Lactoferrin in our eyes helps prevent infection by binding to iron, which is needed for the growth and survival of disease-causing microbes. It also appears to inhibit the development of biofilms in the eyes. In addition, lactoferrin may help control oral biofilm development and is useful in people with gingivitis. Conversely, depleted levels of lactoferrin in the sinuses increase biofilm development and recurring sinus infections. You can increase lactoferrin levels by supplementing with whey, colostrum, or transfer factor.

■ Some integrative physicians are using chelation therapy with ethylenediamine-
tetraacetic acid (EDTA) to break up biofilms, although it hasn't been shown to
be terribly effective in dental biofilm research.

Integrative physicians have also been experimenting with a three-step approach
to eradicating disease-causing biofilms. In stage one, they combine the use of enzyme
products such as protein-splitting enzymes like serrapeptase, nattokinase, and proteases with oral EDTA and lactoferrin. They follow this with antibiotic treatment
with either herbs or medications and finally use insoluble fibers, charcoal, and pectin
to clean up the debris. I have heard good case reports but have not seen any large-
scale studies on this approach yet.

There is a lot of debate about whether it's best to "bust up" biofilms or to try to
optimize them with probiotics and prebiotics to support bile function. There probably isn't a one-size-fits-all approach, and yet I believe it's better to make love, not
war. When we break up biofilms, we also can disrupt healthy biofilms elsewhere in
the body. We don't yet understand all the ramifications of treating them.

BALANCING THE MICROBIOME

There are many things that affect the microbiome, and yet the quickest way to modulate it is with food. According to Benmark et al., 75 percent of food eaten in the Western diet gives little or no benefit to the microbiome. These foods have been stripped of
life and nutrients and have "new-to-nature" additives and pesticides. You can change
your microbiome in 24 hours by changing what you eat, but to change it permanently,
you need to change the foods you eat regularly. It's the life in food that gives us life.
We'll dive into this more deeply in Chapter 13.

Foods That Benefit the Microbiome
A diet that's loaded with vegetables, root vegetables, fruit, nuts, seeds, whole grains,
sea vegetables (like nori on sushi), lentils, and beans appears to be what the microbiome thrives on. These foods are loaded with prebiotics. Remember: It's the life in
food that gives you life.

■ **In healthy people, eating a Mediterranean-type diet is your best bet.** Mediterranean diets have been associated with reductions in cancers, cardiovascular
disease, diabetes, and virtually all chronic diseases. Part of this dietary approach
includes eating home-cooked meals most of the time and eating with friends
and family. Eating is historically a social event.

HUMAN–MICROBIOTA INTERACTIONS

What affects the balance of your microbiome?

WHAT AFFECTS THE MICROBIOME?

The microbiome is a dynamic group of organisms and is affected by everything we do.

For example, I moved into a brand new home a few years ago. When I had my microbiome tested, I discovered that I have microbes that are eating up formaldehyde I've been exposed to from cabinets in my kitchen and bathrooms. Much like using oil-eating microbes to clean up an oil spill, my body knew just what to do and increased bacteria to help break down chemicals found in my new home.

Your lifestyle affects your microbiome. Some of this is beyond your control, but you can control much of it. Here are things that we know contribute to changes in the microbiome:

- Mode of birth (vaginal delivery versus C-section)
- Breast-fed or bottle-fed as an infant
- Use of antibiotics and medications in the first three years of life
- Environment:
  - Temperature
  - What part of the world you live in
  - What culture you live in
  - How much time you spent outdoors in early childhood
  - How much time you spend outdoors now
  - Medication and recreational drugs
- Your genotype
- Diet/food:
  - o What type of soil your food was grown in
  - o How far it was shipped
  - o Whether it was organically or commercially grown
  - o How often you eat and your pattern of eating
- Prebiotics in food
- Probiotics in food
- Stress
- Dysbiosis/infection
- Exercise
- Smoking
- Alcohol consumption
- Sleep and circadian rhythm
- Hygiene: water supply, indoor toilets, handwashing, frequency of bathing
  - Herbicides, pesticides, fungicides
- Everyday chemicals in cosmetics, toiletries, cleaning supplies, furniture, plastics, and more items

THE MICROBIOME AFFECTS ALL ORGANS AND TISSUES AND METABOLISM

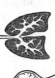
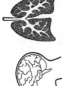

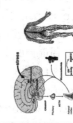
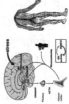

Regulates
Short-Chain Fatty Acids (SCFAs
Branched-chain amino acids
Hormone/gut hormones
Brain function
Inflammation/immune
neurological function
Dysbiosis and endotoxins
TMAO levels
Blood sugar and insulin regulation

- **Eat some prebiotic-rich foods at every meal.** Prebiotics are substrates in food that provide benefits to the microbiota. Until a consensus review paper was released in 2017, prebiotics were considered to be only soluble fibers, such as those found in oatmeal, beans, and root vegetables. Simply said: Prebiotics are food to your microbes, feeding lactobacilli, bifidobacteria, and other microbes. By eating prebiotics in food, you also get a blend of soluble and insoluble fiber, which gives the best outcome.

  Your microbiota and prebiotic-rich foods evolved together and need each other to perform. The prebiotic-rich foods feed the microbes creating SCFAs. These SCFAs are the main fuel sources for your colon, which is home to the bulk of the microbiome. They provide energy, maintenance, and repair for the colon, which is key to your overall well-being. (A full explanation of prebiotics and a list of prebiotic-rich foods is found in Chapter 6.)

- **Caveat about taking supplemental prebiotics:** Research published in October 2018 reports that when mice were given supplemental prebiotics without insoluble fiber, the risk of developing liver dysfunction and liver cancer increased. Supplemental prebiotic supplements and added to foods are rapidly becoming widely available, yet this paper gives us pause: Singh et al. state: "Its benefits notwithstanding, enrichment of foods with fermentable fiber should be approached with great caution as it may increase risk of hepatocellular carcinoma (liver cancer)." This brings us back to food: Eat real foods and do so in balance.

- **Cultured and fermented foods:** Cultured and fermented foods such as yogurt, kefir, kimchee, sauerkraut, and miso also feed the healthy microbiome. (We'll discuss this more in Chapter 6, where there will be a list of probiotic rich foods as well.)

Foods That Disrupt the Microbiome

- These include highly refined and processed foods, which comprise about 75 percent of the standard Western diet: refined carbohydrates like white flour and many other refined grains that lack fiber and nutrients, such as white breads, cookies, pastries, many breakfast cereals, sugar, and high-fructose corn syrup. Sugar and high-fructose corn syrup encourage the growth of dysbiotic microbes throughout the body and increase overall inflammation.

- Eating fast food and high amounts of saturated fat also disrupts the microbiome. Fast food has repeatedly been shown to increase dysbiosis (imbalance of the microbiome). The main culprits are saturated fat, artificial sweeteners, and sugar. It has been shown in mice that the emulsifiers carboxymethylcellulose, polysorbate-60, and polysorbate-80 at very low concentrations increase the risk of developing inflammatory bowel disease (IBD). It's hypothesized that in people at genetic risk for ulcerative colitis or Crohn's disease, these emulsifiers may also trigger the disease. Not all emulsifiers pose a risk (e.g., lecithin is protective of the gut lining).

- **Artificial sweeteners:** Use of artificial sweeteners, such as aspartame (NutriSweet), sucralose (Splenda), and acesulfame potassium (Ace K, or acesulfame K), also has a direct effect on the microbiome. In some people, such substances have a direct effect on increases in blood sugar levels and obesity. It's ironic because most people use artificial sweeteners to control weight, and yet they have never been shown to actually help. New research indicates that they actually make us less sensitive to insulin, which can increase weight and lead to type 2 diabetes.

CHAPTER 6

The GI Microbiome: Prebiotics and Probiotics from Food and Supplements

Élie Metchnikoff won the Nobel Prize in Physiology or Medicine in 1908 for demonstrating that the *Lactobacillus bulgaricus* in yogurt prevented and reversed bacterial infection. He called these health-promoting microbes "probiotics," meaning "protecting/enhancing life." His work with rural Balkan people showed that these probiotics were of benefit to everyone, but they had their greatest effect in babies, toddlers, and the elderly. Yet, when I was in my teens, yogurt was not a common American food. I used to drive 15 miles to the nearest health food store to buy it. Now, 100 years later, the focus is back on these miraculous microbes and what they eat: prebiotics. The marriage of prebiotics and probiotics is like any other marriage: Each partner has its own strengths, and they are better together than alone. This chapter explores these concepts.

MUTUALISM OF PROBIOTICS AND PREBIOTICS

Your microbiota- and prebiotic-rich foods evolved together and need each other to perform. The prebiotic-rich foods feed the microbes, creating short-chain fatty acids (SCFAs). These SCFAs are the main fuel sources for your colon, providing energy, maintenance, and repair. Simultaneously, the plant pigments in prebiotic-rich foods aren't utilized well directly. About 95 percent of these pigments need to be transformed in order to become bioactive. As they are gobbled up, they are activated and reduce inflammation throughout the body. They also "talk" to your genes, modulating inflammation from the deepest level.

PREBIOTICS

You've heard about probiotics but may not have heard about prebiotics yet. Simply stated, prebiotics are the food for the microbiome. Prebiotics "are substrates in food that provide benefits to the microbiota." They nourish and stimulate growth of lacto-bacilli and bifidobacteria in the microbiome, while reducing disease-causing bacteria such as *Clostridium difficile, Klebsiella,* and *Enterobacter.*

We, as humans, cannot digest and utilize prebiotics, but our microbes do. The average American consumes 2 to 8 grams (1/2 to 2 teaspoons) of prebiotics from daily. The International Scientific Association for Probiotics and Prebiotics recommends between 15 to 20 grams daily. We find these in foods such as vegetables, fruits, tubers, roots, nuts, seeds, lentils, and beans.

Until an expert consensus paper in 2017 sponsored by the International Scientific Association for Probiotics and Prebiotics was published, prebiotics were considered to be only soluble fibers, such as those found in oatmeal, beans, and root vegetables. The newer definition also includes plant polyphenols, which get activated as the microbes munch on them; fats, including conjugated linoleic acid (CLA) and polyunsaturated fats; and human milk oligosaccharides found in breast milk. I'm excited by this new definition because it expands the concept of what your microbiome thrives on.

Prebiotic Categories:

- Breast milk oligosaccharides and colostrum (current supplemental sources include cow or goat milk)
- Conjugated Linoleic Acid (CLA)
- Oligosaccharides
- Plant polyphenols and phytonutrients
- Polyunsaturated fats
- Soluble fiber

RESEARCH BENEFITS OF PREBIOTICS

Prebiotics benefit virtually all of your organs, tissues, and cells. They are the subtrate that the microbes use to synthesize SCFAs that keep your colon and microbiome healthy. SCFAs are critically important to overall health, having genomic functions, playing a role in drug metabolism, restoring energy production in oxidative phosphorylation and the citric acid cycle, modulating oxidative stress, and promoting neurotrophic growth factors.

SCFA Production in Colon

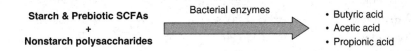

Starch & Prebiotic SCFAs
+
Nonstarch polysaccharides

Bacterial enzymes →

- Butyric acid
- Acetic acid
- Propionic acid

Prebiotics promote the growth of bifidobacteria and lactobacilli, while protecting us from pathogenic microbes and reducing disease-causing bacteria such as *C. difficile, Klebsiella, Salmonella, Listeria, Campylobacter, Shigella,* and *Vibrio.* They help build bone, keep blood sugar and insulin levels regulated, lower ammonia levels in people with liver disease, normalize serum triglyceride levels, prevent constipation and diarrhea, and protect against colon cancer. As little as 2.5 grams (a bit more than a half-teaspoon) of fructoligosaccharide (FOS) has demonstrated these benefits. Honey works, as well as FOS, galactooligosaccharides (GOS), and inulin in promoting the production of SCFAs.

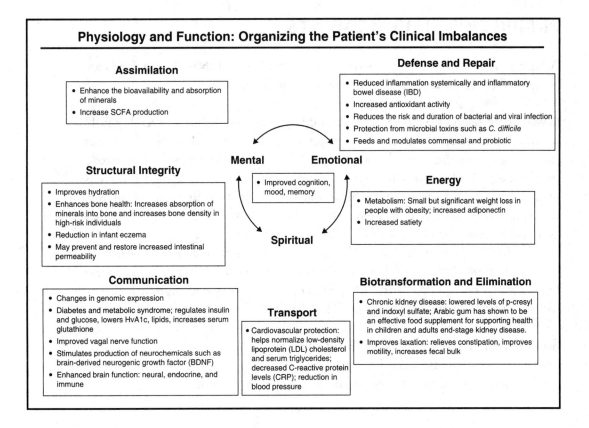

Physiology and Function: Organizing the Patient's Clinical Imbalances

Assimilation
- Enhance the bioavailability and absorption of minerals
- Increase SCFA production

Defense and Repair
- Reduced inflammation systemically and inflammatory bowel disease (IBD)
- Increased antioxidant activity
- Reduces the risk and duration of bacterial and viral infection
- Protection from microbial toxins such as *C. difficile*
- Feeds and modulates commensal and probiotic

Mental — Emotional
- Improved cognition, mood, memory

Structural Integrity
- Improves hydration
- Enhances bone health: Increases absorption of minerals into bone and increases bone density in high-risk individuals
- Reduction in infant eczema
- May prevent and restore increased intestinal permeability

Energy
- Metabolism: Small but significant weight loss in people with obesity; increased adiponectin
- Increased satiety

Spiritual

Communication
- Changes in genomic expression
- Diabetes and metabolic syndrome; regulates insulin and glucose, lowers HvA1c, lipids, increases serum glutathione
- Improved vagal nerve function
- Stimulates production of neurochemicals such as brain-derived neurogenic growth factor (BDNF)
- Enhanced brain function: neural, endocrine, and immune

Transport
- Cardiovascular protection: helps normalize low-density lipoprotein (LDL) cholesterol and serum triglycerides; decreased C-reactive protein levels (CRP); reduction in blood pressure

Biotransformation and Elimination
- Chronic kidney disease: lowered levels of p-cresyl and indoxyl sulfate; Arabic gum has shown to be an effective food supplement for supporting health in children and adults end-stage kidney disease.
- Improves laxation: relieves constipation, improves motility, increases fecal bulk

Prebiotic-Rich Foods: Eat Some At Every Meal

- Artichokes
- Asparagus
- Avocados
- Bananas (under ripe)
- Barley
- Beet root
- Bran
- Burdock root
- Chia seeds
- Chicory
- Chinese chives
- Cocoa
- Dandelion greens
- Dairy products (CLAs), yogurt, cottage cheese
- Eggplant
- Flax seeds
- Fruit
- Garlic
- Green tea
- Honey
- Jerusalem artichokes
- Jicama
- Kefir
- Leeks
- Legumes
- Lentils
- Onions
- Peas
- Plantains
- Potatoes
- Radishes
- Root vegetables
- Rye
- Sea vegetables
- Soybeans
- Spices and herbs
- Sugar maple
- Sweet potatoes
- Tomatoes
- Vegetables
- Yacon root
- Yams

PREBIOTICS IN SUPPLEMENTS

A slew of new prebiotic supplements and prebiotics added to packaged foods are being marketed for the many health benefits of prebiotics.

Caveat about taking supplemental prebiotics: Research published in October 2018 reports that in mice, giving supplemental prebiotics without insoluble fiber increases the risk of developing liver dysfunction and liver cancer. Supplemental prebiotic supplements added to foods are rapidly becoming widely available, and yet there is research that should give us pause. Singh et al. state: "Its benefits notwithstanding, enrichment of foods with fermentable fiber should be approached with great caution as it may increase risk of hepatocellular carcinoma (liver cancer)."

So, this brings us back to food. While this study was done in mice, research on supplemental prebiotics is so new that we don't yet have a full story. As an educator, I'd rather be safe than sorry. My preference is that people change their diet to include a variety of prebiotic and insoluble fibers.

Some Of The Ingredients You'll Find Include:

- Inulin from Jerusalem artichoke, or agave
- Beta glucan from oats, barley, mushrooms, and baker's yeast

- Alcohol sugars such as xylitol and mannitol
- Pectin
- Gums such as acacia and guar gum
- Chia seeds and flaxseeds
- Larch arabinogalactins
- A wide variety of purified oligosaccharides, including fructiloogosaccharides (FOS), galactooligosaccharides (GOS), lactulose-derived galactooligosaccharides (LDGOS), xylooligosaccharides (XOS), arbinooligosaccharides (AOS), algae-derived marine oligosaccharides (ADMOs), and pectin-derived oligosaccharides (pAOSs)

Prebiotics work synergistically with probiotics and can be taken together for best results (together, they are called synbiotics). You will often find them in your probiotic supplements. Like probiotics, they acidify the intestinal environment, enhancing the absorption of essential minerals.

Start slowly: Many people experience gas and bloating when they start or increase prebiotic-rich food or begin taking prebiotics supplements, but these symptoms usually dissipate after a week or so; if they do occur, you can either continue your current dosage or lower the dosage and then increase it gradually. Human studies of prebiotic use show the greatest growth of helpful bacteria in the people who need it most, with benefits most evident at doses up to 10 grams daily. After you stop taking prebiotics, your internal bacteria will return to their previous levels in about two to three weeks. So, changing your diet to include more prebiotic-rich foods on a permanent basis is ideal.

PROBIOTICS

The section on probiotics is after the section on prebiotics for a reason: If you don't have a rich environment for your gut microbes, taking probiotics won't be all that helpful. So begin with prebiotic-rich foods.

People have eaten cultured and fermented foods since the beginning of time. We evolved with these microbes; they are found in our own homes, farms, and environment, as well as in our bodies. These enhanced foods are the product of the marriage of probiotic microbes and prebiotics, which is what the microbes eat. Olives, wine, bread, and cheese are mentioned in ancient texts. Cultured and fermented foods are eaten all over the world and in every culture. They improve food security and reduce hunger because they extend the shelf-life of food. Even that term denotes such a huge change from the root cellars, drying, pickling, and culturing of foods to secure their life.

Common microbes that ferment and culture in food include *Acetobacter, Lactobacill, Lactococcus, Pediococcus, Propionibacteriace, Leuconosto, Streptococcus,* and *Saccharomyces cerevisiae.* During the fermentation process, carbohydrates are converted to lactic acid and organic acids that are used in our bodies for energy production. The lactic-acid–producing bacteria also inhibit the growth of disease-causing microbes. *Lactobacillus plantarum,* one of the most soothing of all probiotics, creates the acid that's present in sour vegetables, such as sauerkraut. *Leuconostoc mesenteroides* is the main bacteria associated with sauerkraut and pickles. The Propionibacteriaceae family of bacteria provide the flavor and holes in Swiss cheese. The acetic-acid–producing bacteria, *Acetobacter,* change foods such as apples and grapes into vinegar.

Culturing and fermenting of food breaks down the polyphenols and plant polyphenols; increases vitamin content, enzyme activity, and amino acid production; and breaks down antinutrients in foods such as phytates, tannins, and oxalates. This became seemingly less important with the invention of food processing and refrigeration, which more easily extended the life of food.

These bacteria synthesize nutrients for their own benefit, but we can reap the rewards. Pretty much any food that is cultured or fermented has increased amounts of nutrients. By ingesting cottage cheese and yogurt rather than milk (see Table 6.1), sauerkraut rather than cabbage, tofu and tempeh rather than soybeans, and wine rather than grapes, we obtain higher levels of B-complex vitamins and Vitamin K.

Table 6.1   **Nutritionally Enhanced Dairy Foods**

Original Food	*Fermented/Cultured Food*	*Increased Nutrition*
Milk	Cheddar cheese	Vitamin B_1, 3x
Milk	Cottage cheese	Vitamin B_{12}, 5x
Milk	Yogurt	Vitamin B_{12}, 5–30x
Milk	Yogurt	Vitamin B_3, 50x
Skim milk	Low-fat yogurt	Vitamin A, 7–14x

Probiotic-Rich Foods: Eat Some Each Day

- Amasake
- Beer (microbrew)
- Black tea, oolong tea
- Buttermilk
- Cheese
- Chocolate
- Coconut
- Coffee
- Cottage cheese
- Fermented sausages and meats
- Fermented vegetables
- Kefir
- Kimchee
- Kombucha
- Lassi
- Leban
- Miso
- Natto
- Olives
- Pickles (brine cured, not vinegar)
- Pulke
- Raw vinegar
- Raw whey
- Root and ginger beers
- Sauerkraut
- Sourdough breads (traditionally made)
- Tempeh
- Wheatgrass juice
- Wine
- Yogurt

A FEW SPECIFIC FOODS AND THEIR HEALTH BENEFITS

Kefir

Kefir is a traditionally a fermented milk product, much like a more fluid yogurt. It can also be made from any "milklike" substance, such as nuts, beans, and seeds. It has more probiotic microbes in it than yogurt. Different brands and homemade versions vary on the number and which substances they contain, but they typically have 6 to 14 varieties of bacteria and yeast; and nearly 100 specific bacteria and yeast have been described in research papers. Kefir has antimicrobial properties, is supportive to digestive and immune function, protects against carcinogens, enhances wound healing, helps with allergies, digests lactose, and helps normalize cholesterol levels. Historically, it has also been used to treat ulcers, to lower blood pressure, and as a heart tonic.

Kimchee

Kimchee is a traditional Korean condiment made from Napa and other types of cabbage and other vegetables. It has nutritional effects; promotes healthy weight; helps with constipation; improves colorectal health; helps normalize serum cholesterol; has anticlotting effects; promotes brain, immune system, and skin health; and is an antioxidant with antiaging properties.

Miso

Miso is a fermented soybean paste that's common in Japanese cuisine. It is often the base for soup and is used as a spread on rice and vegetables and as the umami flavor in sauces. You may have had miso soup at a Japanese restaurant. Miso is nutrient rich and has sodium (it's really salty!), choline, manganese, copper, zinc, and protein and smaller amounts of B-vitamins, calcium, iron, magnesium, selenium, and phosphorus. Research on miso reports that it has over 161 different bacteria and yeast. *L. plantarum* bacteria in miso degrade histamine, which is helpful for people with allergies. Aki-zuki reported that after the second atomic bomb was dropped in Japan during World War II, with his clinic only 1.4 kilometers from the center of the damage, patients and staff who drank miso soup with wakame seaweed every other day had no effects from radiation. Miso appears to be cancer protective, in spite of it having such a high sodium concentration, which has been associated with high rates of stomach cancer in the Japanese population. Animal studies report a lowered incidence of lung, colon, stomach, and breast cancers, when fed miso that had been fermented for six months or longer. Yamamoto reported that Japanese women who drank miso soup regularly as opposed to not at all had a 50 percent reduction in breast cancer risk, while there was a total halving of breast cancer in all women, post-menopausal women had the the greatest reduction. In rats, miso lowers blood pressure, has diuretic properties, lowers blood pressure and strokes, and protects against radiation injury.

THE MANY BENEFITS OF PROBIOTIC BACTERIA

Intestinal microbes play an important role in our ability to fight infectious disease, providing a front line in our immune defense. Friendly microbes also manufacture many nutrients, including Vitamin K and several of the B-complex vitamins, including biotin, B1, B2, B3, B5, B6, B12, and folic acid. Certain acid-secreting species increase our absorption of minerals, including calcium, copper, iron, magnesium, and manganese.

Probiotics improve peristalsis, help normalize bowel transit time, and are also important in preventing traveler's diarrhea. If you travel outside the United States, take a probiotic supplement daily, as studies show that it significantly increases your ability to withstand the new microbes to which you will be exposed. Native and supplemental probiotics help us in many other ways. Some have antitumor and anti-cancer effects, and others help to keep our normal internal fungus population from proliferating out of control. Probiotics help us metabolize foreign substances like mercury and pesticides, protect us from damaging radiation and harmful pollut-ants, and recycle and metabolize hormones like estrogen and thyroid hormones. Although the mechanism is not yet understood, bacterial balance is also essential for healthy metabolism; many super-thin people have been able to gain weight through the use of probiotic supplements. Probiotics lessen the risk of infections in preterm infants by giving their immune systems a boost. I've seen colicky babies become calm in less than 24 hours when given *Bifidobacteria infantis*—what a blessing!

Selected Benefits of Probiotics:

Nutrition

- Aid in protein digestion
- Convert flavonoids to usable forms
- Increase our absorption of minerals, including calcium, copper, iron, magnesium, and manganese
- Manufacture essential fatty acids and SCFAs
- Minimize or eliminate lactose intolerance
- Synthesize vitamins: biotin, B1, B2, B3, B5, B6, B12, folate, and Vitamin K

Immune system

- Activate mucosal-associated lymphoid tissue (MALT)
- Break down bacterial toxins
- Break down and prevent synthesis of bacterial toxins
- Decrease the severity and duration of respiratory and other infections
- Have antitumor and anticancer effects
- Prevent and alleviating eczema, asthma, and allergies
- Prevent and control thrush, vaginal yeast infection, and bladder infection
- Prevent and treat diarrhea from antibiotics
- Prevent food poisoning
- Prevent infection by producing antibiotic and antifungal substances
- Protect against toxic substances
- Protect and modulate autoimmune diseases

Digestive system

- Balance intestinal pH
- Digest lactose
- Digest proteins to free amino acids
- Help normalize bowel transit time
- Improve or prevent IBS
- Protect against travelers' diarrhea
- Protect gums and teeth
- Reduce intestinal inflammation
- Regulate peristalsis and improve diarrhea, constipation, and IBS
- Stop diarrhea

Heart
- Normalize serum cholesterol and triglycerides
- Support healthy blood pressure levels

Metabolic system
- Break down and rebuild hormones
- Break down bile acids
- Manufacture 5 to 10 percent of all SCFAs
- Promote healthy metabolism and weight
- Promote optimal growth
- Reduce blood ammonia levels in people with cirrhosis and liver disease

Probiotic Supplements may be Beneficial and have been Researched for the Following Health Conditions:

Cardio-metabolic disease
- Dyslipidemia: High cholesterol or triglycerides
- Gout
- Obesity, type-2 diabetes, fatty liver, nonalcoholic steatohepatitis, prevention of hepatic encephalopathy in people with liver cirrhosis
- Polycystic ovarian syndrome
- Stroke

Ear-nose and throat
- Asthma
- Chronic lung disease
- Colds/flu
- Ear infections
- Gingivitis/periondotitis
- Pneumonia
- Strep throat/pharyngitis

Immune conditions
- Allergy
- Autoimmune disease
- Autoimmune encephalomyletis
- General immune support: probiotics modulate the immune system

- Myasthenia gravis
- Rheumatoid arthritis
- Systemic lupus
- Type 1 diabetes

Gastrointestinal (GI) system

- Bariatric surgery
- Celiac disease
- Crohn's disease
- *Helicobacter pylori* infection
- IBS
- Parasites
- Small intestinal bacterial overgrowth (SIBO)
- Ulcerative colitis

Genitourinary system

- Bacterial vaginal infections
- Bladder infections
- Candida infections/yeast infections
- Chronic kidney disease and people on dialysis
- Kidney stones and high oxylate levels
- Prostate infections
- Toxic shock syndrome

Infections/Immune System

- Colds and flu
- Ear infections Myalgic Encephalomyelitis/Chronic Fatigue Syndrome
- Epstein-Barr virus
- Flu
- Foot and mouth disease
- Hepatitis
- HIV/AIDS
- Lyme disease
- Mastitis (breast infection during lactation)
- Pneumonia
- Strep throat/pharyngitis

Mental health/neurotransmitters/stress
- Anxiety
- Attention deficit hyperactive disorder
- Autism
- Depression

Neurological system
- Age-related cognitive decline
- Cerebral ischemia and reperfusion
- Hepatic encephalopathy
- Multiple sclerosis
- Traumatic brain injury

Skin health
- Acne
- Eczema
- Psoriasis
- Reactive skin

Cancer
- Bladder
- Breast
- Cervical
- Colorectal
- Leukemia
- Liver
- Lung
- Lymphoma
- Vaginal

PROBIOTIC SUPPLEMENTS

In addition to getting probiotics naturally from our food each day, they can be obtained by taking probiotic supplements. I am frequently asked about which probiotics to take, when to take them, and what type of dosage is required.

Buying Probiotic Supplements

The many probiotic supplements on the market look similar but can be extremely different in their effectiveness. Consumer Lab tested 25 probiotic products. Eight of them contained less than 1 percent of the number of probiotic bacteria listed on the label. It is important to use well-researched probiotics that have been found useful in clinical settings. So how can you know which products are best? Always look for a batch number and expiration date. Purchase your products from a health professional or store where someone has done the research for you.

Typically I look for mixed probiotic supplements that contain *Lactobacillus acidophilus* plus *Bifidobacteria* strains. However, there are times when you may choose to use a specific strain or specific probiotic. For example, for chronic diarrhea, you may choose to use *Saccharomyces boulardii* by itself. If you are lactose intolerant, you may choose to buy a dairy-free probiotic. However, some people find that by using dairy-based probiotics, they become more lactose tolerant. The best test is to try them out and see what your body likes best. Research on who needs which probiotics at which moment in their lives doesn't yet exist. When we take probiotic supplements, we are mostly guessing about their specific benefits. However, as discussed in the previous section, they do have many regulatory benefits.

What Types of Microbes Am I Looking For? Look for the normal gut flora such as lactobacilli and bifidobacteria. Supplements may also contain the species *Lactobacillus casei, L. reuteri, Bifidobacteria longum, Bifidobacterium breve, Lactobacillus lactis, Lactobacillus rhamnosus,* and others (see Table 6.2). *Bifidobacteria infantis* is the most appropriate choice for a newborn and is also useful for children and adults who have IBS.

More is being learned about specific strains of probiotics. Just as a poodle is not the same as an English setter, two strains of acidophilus or bifidobacteria can be very different.

Some supplements contain soil-based or spore-based probiotics such as *Bacillus laterosporus, Bacillus subtilis,* and *Lactobacillus sporonges* (also known as *Bacillus coagulous*), A couple of studies demonstrate that spore-based probiotic supplements have similar properties to other probiotics such as: reducing inflammation, modulating immunity, and decreasing gut permeability. It makes sense to add microbes from soil; yet some strains of these organisms can cause disease. Only purchase these from a reputable company.

Viability and Potency. Most probiotics supply between 1 billion and 25 billion organisms per dose, and a few supply substantially more (up to 450 billion). The number, however, isn't the important thing, as some studies have shown supplements

Table 6.2   **Common Species of Yeast and Bacteria Found in Supplements and Food**

Bifidobacteria	Lactobacilli	Streptococcus	Saccharomyces
B. adolescentis	L. acidophilus*	S. cerevisaie	S. bayanus
B. angulatum	L. brevis*	S. cremoris	S. boulardii*
B. animalis	L. bulgaricus*	S. diacetylactis	
B. bifidum*	L. casei*	S. intermedius	**Enterococcus**
B. breve*	L. cellebiosus	S. jacium	E. faecium
B. cantenulatum	L. curvatus	S. jaecali	E. durans
B. infantis*	L. debreukii	S. lactis	
B. longum*	L. fermentum	S. salavarius* K12 and M18	**Escherichia** coli Nissle 1971
B. pseurocate-nulatum	L. gasseri*	S. thermophilus*	
B. thermophilum	L. helveticus		**Bacilli**
	L. johnsonii	**Lactococcus**	B. subtilis*
	L. kefir	Lactoccus lactis	B. laterosporus*
	L. lactis*		B. coagulans*
	L. paracasei	**Leuconostoc**	B. indicus
	L. plantarum	L. mesenteroides	B. licheniformis
	L. reuteri		B. clausii
	L. rhamnosus* GG		
	L. salavarius*		Pediococcus acidilactici
	L. yoghuni		

* = Common in probiotic supplements

to be effective even when they contain only millions of organisms. What matters is whether the product contains viable organisms that adhere to the gut lining, are not destroyed by bile, and have benefits once in your body. Yet there is still much to be learned. Research indicates that even dead probiotics can have profound effects on the immune system.

Probiotics come in two main types: those that need refrigeration and those that don't. I generally prefer the refrigerated varieties, although lately we are seeing more shelf-stable products on the market. These delicate bacteria must be refrigerated in shipping, at the store, and in your home to ensure their life span and greatest potency. Probiotics will maintain potency at room temperature for short periods of time; for instance, if you are on vacation for a week or two, you'll probably lose a few percentages of potency. If you left them out for several months, they'd be dead. I personally keep mine in the refrigerator and put a week's worth of probiotics in my supplement container so that I don't forget to take them.

Bacteria multiply very quickly, but they need enough food and protection to survive the trip through the stomach and into the intestinal tract, so many probiotic supplements also contain prebiotics such as FOS and inulin, which provide nourishment for the bacteria (see the section "Prebiotics" earlier in this chapter).

What to Look for in a Probiotic Supplement

- Look for *L. acidophilus* and *B. bifidum*.
- Choose an age-appropriate product. For a baby or toddler, *B. infantis* is appropriate; for children and adults used a mixed product that contains *Lactobacillus* spp and *Bifidobacterium* spp. Some products may also contain *Streptoccus* spp. *Saccharomyces boulardii*, and/or *Bacillus* spp.
- The best-studied probiotics include *L. acidophilus* DDS-1 (Culturelle), VSL#3, and *Saccharomyces boulardii* (first researched by the makers of Florastor and now copied by many.)
- Choose a product that is condition appropriate when it's available. There are now supplements that are specific for lactose intolerance, sugar malabsorption, IBS, and diarrhea. There may soon be other specific products for psoriasis, vaginal infections, IBD, and other health conditions.
- Most of the best products come refrigerated. However, there are some viable products on the market that are stored at room temperature.
- Bacteria multiply very quickly, but they need enough food once they reach the intestines. Some products contain inulin, FOS, or other prebiotics that help the flora grow. This can vastly improve the viability of the product. Just note that some people bloat from FOS.
- Combination supplements with several types of flora are helpful. Bacteria compete for the same food supply, so look for freeze-dried products. Freeze-drying puts the flora into suspended animation, keeping them dormant until placed in water or in your body.

Finding the Appropriate Dosage

There is no consensus on whether we all benefit from taking daily probiotic supplements. Some research points to no, but others to yes. If you choose to take them, as I do, my advice is to rotate products. Each product has different probiotic strains, with slightly different benefits. Use a bottle or two of one brand or type, and then switch to another.

Therapeutic dosages vary depending on the severity of the condition. You may find 1 billion or 2 billion organisms daily keep you well and rebalance you. Other people may need 25 billion to 100 billion organisms, or more. After antibiotics, I typically recommend doses between 30 billion and 100 billion organisms daily for 2 to 4 weeks afterward. There is research indicating that taking probiotics at a different time of day while you are on antibiotics may be of benefit. Typically, I recommend *S. boulardii*, which is a yeast, so it can be taken simultaneously with antibiotic medications. Studies on people with ulcerative colitis have found benefit in dosages of more than 2 trillion microorganisms daily.

Begin taking the probiotics at a low level and increase the dose slowly. If you experience bloating, diarrhea, gas, or worsening of symptoms, stop taking it. As the disease-producing bacteria and fungus are killed, they release chemicals that aggravate symptoms. Begin again with tiny amounts and build up your dosage slowly to avoid the die-off reaction. Symptoms like this usually tip you off that what you are doing is correct; however, if that's true, they begin to subside after a few days. Of course, if the symptoms continue, you should see a doctor.

PROBIOTIC RESOURCES

Here are two resources that stay current on research about the benefits of various probiotic supplements:

1. AEProbio publishes two clinical guides, one for the United States and one for Canada (http://usprobioticguide.com/PBCIntroduction.html). They are updated each year and evaluate the research evidence on many common probiotic supplements, foods, and functional foods.
2. The Probiotic Advisor has more global products (https://www.probioticadvisor.com/).

The GI Microbiome: Dysbiosis, a Good Neighborhood Gone Bad

Dysbiosis is defined as imbalances or changes in the microbiome that cause symptoms of illness. If the microbiome loses homeostasis, then it becomes dysbiotic. Dysbiosis is a broad term and includes imbalances in bacteria, viruses, parasites, and fungi, as well as genetic mechanisms that make a person more reactive to so-called normal microbes in the microbiome, and more. It can occur in the digestive system, as well as on your skin, vagina, lungs, nose, sinuses, ears, nails, or eyes. Typically dysbiosis doesn't appear as a classic type of infection. These imbalances generally simmer along. After all, if the microbes were too virulent, you'd die. It's in their best interests to learn to coexist with you and not make you too uncomfortable so that you also just learn to live with it! Dysbiosis may express itself as irritable bowel syndrome (IBS) in one person, migraines in another, eczema, psoriasis, autoimmune illness, depression, and other illnesses. Dysbiosis is associated with inflammatory bowel disease (IBD), multiple sclerosis, types 1 and 2 diabetes, allergies, asthma, psoriasis, Alzheimer's disease, Parkinson's disease, chronic fatigue syndrome, celiac disease, metabolic syndrome, cardiovascular disease, obesity, fatty liver disease, Hepatitis C virus, and various cancers, including ovarian, breast, and lung. Dysbiosis in the mouth has been found in people who have oral, head, and neck squamous cell cancers, pancreatic cancer, and lung cancer.

The term *dysbiosis* was coined by Dr. Élie Metchnikoff early in the 20th century. It comes from *dys-*, which means "not," and *symbiosis*, which means "living together in mutual harmony." Dr. Metchnikoff was the first scientist to discover the useful properties of probiotics. He won the Nobel Prize in Physiology or Medicine in 1908 for his work on lactobacilli and their role in immunity and he was a colleague of Louis Pasteur, succeeding him as the director of the Pasteur Institute in Paris.

Dr. Metchnikoff found that the *Lactobacillus bulgaricus* bacteria in yogurt prevented and reversed bacterial infection. His research proved that lactobacilli could displace many disease-producing organisms and reduce the toxins they generated. He advocated the use of lactobacillus in the 1940s for ptomaine poisoning, a widely used therapy in Europe.

In more recent decades, Metchnikoff's work has taken a back seat to modern therapies, such as antibiotics and immunization programs, which scientists hoped would conquer infectious diseases. Microbes are extremely adaptable. In our efforts to eradicate them, we have pushed them to evolve. Long before chemists created antibiotics, yeasts, fungi, and rival bacteria were producing antibiotics to ward each other off and establish neighborhoods. They became adept at evading each other's strategies and adapting for survival. Because people have used antibiotics indiscriminately in humans and animals, the bacteria have had a chance to learn from it, undergoing rapid mutations. They talk to each other and borrow plasmids, small bacterial bits of DNA, which are incorporated into their genetic structure. Think about the way that we forward texts, emails, and videos to friends because they teach us cool things. Bacteria do the same thing, shuffling their components and learning new evolutionary dance steps. Superstrains of bacteria have been created that no longer respond to any antibiotic treatment.

Dysbiosis weakens our ability to protect ourselves from disease-causing microbes, which are generally composed of low-virulence organisms. Unlike salmonella, which causes immediate food-poisoning reactions, low-virulence microbes are insidious. They cause chronic problems that go undiagnosed in the great majority of cases. If left unrecognized and untreated, they become deep-seated and may cause chronic health problems, including joint pain, diarrhea, chronic fatigue syndrome, or colon disease. Dysbiosis presents itself in many ways. The most commonly known include the following:

Fungal infections: Also called yeast infections or small intestinal fungal overgrowth (SIFO), these are commonly caused by an overabundance of *Candidia* species, *Rhodotorula*, *Cyryptococcus*, and others. (See the section on *Candida* later in the book, for more details.)

Small intestinal bacterial overgrowth (SIBO): SIBO is dysbiosis in the small intestines. It often characterized by gas, bloating, and bowel issues. It underlies more than half of cases of IBS. It's also associated with fibromyalgia, restless leg syndrome, interstitial cystitis, and dozens of other conditions. (See the section on SIBO, later in the book, for more details.)

Parasites: Part of many of our so-called normal microbiomes contain parasites with whom we live in harmony. Some parasites can become abundant, causing diarrhea, bloody stools, rashes, abdominal cramping, tooth grinding, an so on. (See the section on parasites, later in the book, for more details.)

The most common issues associated with dysbiosis include:

- SIBO, which underlies between 50 and 75 percent of all cases of IBS.
- Fungal overgrowth anywhere in the body.
- *Helicobacter pylori* infection. It's not clear whether *H. pylori* itself would be considered dysbiosis because it is a true infection, yet *H. pylori* does contribute to dysbiosis of the digestive system.

Published research has listed dysbiosis as the cause of arthritis, diarrhea, autoimmune illness, B_{12} deficiency, chronic fatigue syndrome, cystic acne, cystitis, the early stages of colon and breast cancer, eczema, fibromyalgia, food allergy or sensitivity, IBD, IBS, psoriasis, restless leg syndrome, and steatorrhea. These problems were previously unrecognized as being microbial in origin. Common dysbiotic bacteria are aeromonas, citrobacter, helicobacter, klebsiella, salmonella, shigella, *Staphylococcus aureus*, vibrio, and yersinia. *H. pylori* for example, is commonly found in people with ulcers. Citrobacter is implicated in diarrheal diseases. A common dysbiosis culprit, the candida fungus causes a wide variety of symptoms that range from gas and bloating to depression, mood swings, and premenstrual syndrome (PMS).

Common Symptoms and Diseases Associated with Dysbiosis

- Allergy
- Alzheimer's disease
- Arthritis
- Asthma
- Autoimmune diseases
- Bad breath
- Belching
- Bloating
- Bowel urgency
- Celiac disease
- Chronic fatigue syndrome
- Constipation, chronic
- Cramping
- Cystic acne
- Depression or anxiety
- Diabetes: Types 1 and 2
- Diarrhea, chronic
- Fatigue
- Fatty liver disease
- Fibromyalgia
- Food allergies, intolerance & Sensitivities
- Foul-smelling stools
- Frequent indigestion
- Gas
- Gastritis
- Hypertension
- Inflammatory bowel disease
- Interstitial cystitis
- Irritable bowel syndrome
- Itching in the vagina, anus, or other mucous membranes
- Metabolic syndrome

- Mucus or blood in stool
- Multiple sclerosis
- Nausea after taking supplements
- Obesity
- Parkinson's disease
- Rectal itching
- Restless leg syndrome

- Rheumatoid arthritis
- Sinus congestion, chronic
- Skin conditions: psoriasis, eczema, vitiligo
- Small intestinal bacterial overgrowth
- Undigested food in stool

- Weight loss due to malabsorption
- Yeast infections of vagina, nails, hair, skin, scalp and other areas of the body

COMMON PATTERNS OF DYSBIOSIS

The lines between these types of dysbiosis often blur, and people often have more than one of these patterns.

- **Putrefaction dysbiosis:** This occurs when you don't have enough digestive enzymes, hydrochloric acid, and probiotic bacteria to enable you to fully digest your proteins. High-fat, high-animal-protein, low-fiber diets predispose people to putrefaction due to an increase of bacteroides bacteria, a decrease in beneficial bifidobacteria, and an increase in bile production. Bacteroides cause vitamin B_{12} deficiency by uncoupling the B_{12} from the intrinsic factor necessary for its use. Research has implicated putrefaction dysbiosis with hormone-related cancers such as breast, prostate, and colon cancer. Bacterial enzymes change bile acids into 33 substances formed in the colon that are tumor promoters. Bacterial enzymes, such as betaglucuronidase, re-create estrogens that were already broken down and put into the colon for excretion. These estrogens are reabsorbed into the bloodstream, increasing estrogen levels. Putrefaction dysbiosis can be corrected by eating more high-fiber foods, fruits, vegetables, and grains, and fewer meats and fats.

- **Bacterial overgrowth:** Bacteria may move (translocate) from the colon into the small intestine, or they may grow in the small intestine due to low levels of hydrochloric acid. Slow motility, impaired migrating motor complex, low secretory IgA, an ileocecal valve that's stuck closed, bacterial translocation, pancreatic insufficiency, bile acid deficiency, structural abnormalities in the small intestine, chronic kidney disease, and hypothyroidism can all contribute to bacterial overgrowth of the small or large intestines. In the small intestine it's known as small intestinal bacterial overgrowth (SIBO). There are also people whose underlying cause or causes are unknown.

■ This is most commonly known as small intestinal bacterial overgrowth (SIBO) and can also occur less commonly in the large intestine. Over half of people diagnosed with IBS have SIBO. People experience this often as gas and bloating, diarrhea, discomfort, and sometimes constipation. Low carbohydrate diets, such as the FODMAP diet, Paleo-Immune, and Atkin's diet are typically recommended along with Rifaxamin or herbal treatments.

■ **Fungal dysbiosis:** We normally have a fair number of *Candida* species, a diploid fungus in the yeast family, in our natural microbiome. Antibiotics, stress, sugar, steroids, and other medications can give them the opportunity to quickly grow, causing a myriad of ill effects. True to dysbiosis, these yeasts can colonize on skin (athlete's foot, eczema, psoriasis), in the vagina, in the small intestine, in the nose (some chronic sinusitis), on the scalp (seborrhea, cradle cap), and elsewhere in the body. They are always coupled with fermentation dysbiosis. In fact, in rare instances, *Candida* manufactures enough alcohol to make people drunk. Candida is typically treated with a low carbohydrate diet coupled with anti-fungal medications and/or herbal products.

■ **Parasitic dysbiosis:** Many people have amoebas, fluke, cysts, other protozoa, and other parasites. These are diagnosed through a variety of stool and are treated with medication.

WHAT CAUSES DYSBIOSIS?

While there are many causes of dysbiosis, we generally bring it on ourselves through chronic stress, poor food choices, and the use of antibiotics, proton-pump inhibitors, and other medications. Some people have a genetic predisposition that gives them an exaggerated immune response to otherwise normal microbes of the microbiome. Constant high levels of stress, the use of antacids and proton-pump inhibitors (PPIs), exposure to manufactured chemicals, poor food choices, gluten sensitivity, chronic constipation, oral contraceptives, gastric surgery (including gastric bypass surgery), and the use of antibiotics and painkillers all change the healthy balance of the digestive tract.

Antibiotics

The most common cause of dysbiosis is the use of antibiotics, which change the balance of intestinal microbes. Not terribly specific, antibiotics simultaneously kill

Causes of Dysbiosis

- Aging
- Antacids
- Antibiotics
- Cancer treatment: radiation and chemotherapy
- Chronic constipation
- Chronic illness
- Chronic stress
- Diet high in refined grains, sugars, refined carbohydrates
- Exposure to chemicals
- Gastric surgery, for weight loss and resectioning
- Genetics
- Ileocecal valve not working properly
- Imbalanced lifestyle
- Leaky gut
- Low gastric acid
- Motility dysfunction
- Oxidative stress
- Parenteral and enteral feeding
- Proton-Pump Inhibitors (PPIs)
- Smoking

both harmful and helpful bacteria throughout our digestive system, mouth, vagina, and skin, leaving the territory open to bacteria, parasites, viruses, and yeasts that are resistant to the antibiotic that was used.

Antacids and Proton-Pump Inhibitors

Antacids and PPIs are designed to block hydrochloric acid (HCl) production in the stomach. This acid acts as a first line of defense against microbes that come in as guests with our food. When blocked, our defense is gone.

Endotoxins

Endotoxins are substances that are produced by microbes as they rupture or disintegrate. Endotoxins are typically lipopolysaccharides (LPSs), which can be confusing because carbohydrates naturally occur as polysaccharides. Endotoxins are typically LPS from gram-negative bacteria, which in small amounts can cause problems such as increased intestinal permeability (leaky gut), fevers, and lowered immunity to infection.

Common microbes that produce endotoxins include *Escherichia coli*, *Salmonella*, *Shigella*, *Nesseria*, *Haemophilus*, *Pertussis*, and *Vibrio*.

Diet

Poor diet also contributes to dysbiosis. High-fat, high-protein, and low-fiber diets can contribute to dysbiosis because these diets slow down bowel motility. A diet high in fat, sugar, and processed foods may not have enough nutrients to optimally nourish the body or repair and maintain the digestive organs. The nutrients most likely to be lacking are the antioxidants (vitamins C and E, beta-carotene, coenzyme Q10, glutathione, selenium, the sulfur amino acids, and zinc), the B-complex vitamins, calcium, essential fatty acids, and magnesium.

Ileocecal Valve Gets Stuck

Poor ileocecal valve function can contribute to dysbiosis. The valve's job is to keep waste matter in the colon from mixing with the useful material that is still being digested and absorbed in the small intestine. When this valve is stuck, either open or closed, dysbiotic problems can occur. Chiropractors can adjust the ileocecal valve to alleviate this problem.

TESTING FOR DYSBIOSIS OF ALL TYPES

This list offers the most common tests that are used to assess whether you have dysbiosis. With the advent of inexpensive genomic testing of the microbiome, more companies are offering microbiome analysis.

If your symptoms are in your stomach:

- Antigen tests for *H. pylori*

If your symptoms are in your small intestine:

- Crook's yeast questionnaire to screen for fungal infections
- Stool testing with culture microbiology
- Stool testing with metagenomic probes (PCR)
- Stool testing to detect short-chain fatty acids (SCFA)
- Breath testing for small intestinal bacterial overgrowth.

If your symptoms are in your large intestine:

- Stool testing for ova and parasites
- Comprehensive stool testing
- Microbiome testing
- Antigen testing for *Clostridium difficile* and other infections

You can find more detailed information on functioning testing in Chapter 11.

THERAPEUTIC DIETS FOR DYSBIOSIS

Many, many therapeutic programs are available for people to follow to rid themselves of candida, SIBO, and other bacterial infections. Remember that yeasts and bacteria eat sugars and carbohydrates, so all of these diets limit sugars and carbohydrates. Changing your diet for a moderate amount of time is essential in treating dysbiosis. It's important to starve out the microbes while you treat them with medications, herbs, homeopathic medicines, etc.

Diets such as the FODMAP diet, specific carbohydrate diet, gut and psychology syndrome diet, anti-candida diets, paleo-immune type diets, and more are used therapeutically to starve out symptom-producing microbes and to give your digestive system foods that support healing. These diets are used in the short term and will be discussed more thoroughly in Chapter 14.

TREATING DYSBIOSIS

You probably will use only some of these treatments. Choose one type of prebiotic fiber. Choose one type of herbal therapy *or* use a product that contains a combination of herbs.

Base your treatment on the 5 Rs. These are Remove, Replace, Repair, Reinnoculate, and Rebalance/Reconnect. Work with a clinician to create a plan that's customized for you and your situation.

Remove Infection

First, you need to find out if you have an infection. Then a treatment plan using antibiotics and/or antimicrobial herbs should be developed. Antimicrobial herbs may include the following:

- Aromatic oils, such as oregano, peppermint oil, thyme, lavender, lemon and lime oils, bitter orange, sweet fennel, star anise, Ajowan, and others.
- Herbs and food: Garlic, wormwood, berberine (from Oregon grape, barberry, goldenseal, goldthread), pau d-arco, dill seed, sage leaf, and others.

Herbal therapy treatments include the following:

- Garlic: Either several cloves of garlic eaten daily or standardized to 5,000 mcg of allicin potential three times daily

- Goldenseal or berberine: Standardized to contain 200 to 400 mg of berberine;
- 200 to 400 mg three times daily
- Wormwood or Chinese wormwood: 1,000 to 3,000 mg three times daily
- Grapefruit seed extract: 250 to 500 mg three times daily
- Oregano (*Origanum vulgare*) oil: 200 mg three times daily
- Thyme (*Thymus vulgaris*): Standardized to contain thymol, 100 to 200 mg three times daily.

Pharmaceuticals used for treating the infection may include the following:

- Rifaxamin (brand name: Xifaxan): 1,200 mg daily seven days (for SIBO)
- Ciprofloxacin (brand names: Cipro, Proquin): 250 to 750 mg every 12 hours
- Norfloxacin (brand name: Noroxin): 250 to 750 mg every 12 hours
- Co-trimoxazole (brand names: Septra, Bacrim): 500 to 875 mg every 12 hours
- Antiparasitic medications such as metronidazole and Alinia
- Antifungal medications such as Nystatin, Diflucan, etc.

Replace

- Digestive enzymes, bile, or support gastric acid if needed.
- Poor-quality food with natural foods.
- Poor sleep with improved focus on sleep.
- Poor exercise habits with regular exercise.
- Stress with relaxation to balance it.

Repair Barrier Function

See Chapter 4 for other tips on repairing gut peremability.

Reinnoculate

Typically probiotics and prebiotic-rich foods and supplements are recommended. However, depending on the phase of treatment, these may be ramped up or restricted.

- Lactobacillus: 10 billion to 100 billion live organisms or higher daily.
- *Saccharomyces boulardii:* 250 to 3,000 mg daily; use specifically if you are taking antibiotics or experiencing diarrhea.
- Bifidobacterium (various species): 10 billion to 100 billion live organisms daily
- Combination products that contain Lactobacilli, Bifidobacterium, and other probiotic species work well.

Feed the microbiome with prebiotics. These may cause increased gas and bloating initially, so begin slowly.

- Begin with prebiotics. (See Chapters 6 and 13 for more details.)
- Take fructooligosaccharides (FOSs) or inulin or larch arabinogalactins: 500 to 5,000 mg daily.
- Take modified citrus pectin: 3,000 to 5,000.

Rebalance/Reconnect:

After you've recovered, you will have a new "normal," which may be your healthiest self or may restrict your life in some ways. If you've been ill for a long time, your lifestyle may revolve around being ill; once you are well, your relationships and daily activities will change.

As you feel better, it's time to look at your lifestyle and see what more you can do to improve your health. Incorporate relaxation and fun into your life. Readjust your relationships. Discover your sense of purpose. (See more in Chapter 16.)

As you can see from these recommendations, dosages can be complicated. When treating dysbiosis, I would advise you to work with someone experienced in this area. I've seen too many of my own clients who have been put on medication after medication. While sometimes medication is necessary, first try to heal the environment with diet and lifestyle change. Dietary change can have the most profound effect of all; yet alone, it is typically not enough to permanently correct the dysbiosis. Use a combination of lifestyle change, diet, prebiotics and probiotics, and either herbal or pharmaceutical substances to get the best effect.

Newer Therapies for Dysbiosis

There is ongoing research in two areas that look promising, although we don't have enough research to endorse them broadly. What the first two therapies have in common is (1) they can quickly modulate the immune system and microbiome, and (2) most people are too grossed out to even consider them as a therapeutic option. Hopefully that will change as the research demonstrates specific and sustained healing. I look forward to learning more about these unfolding stories.

Fecal Microbiota Transplant (FMT)

Simply said, fecal microbiota transplant (FMT), also known as fecal transplant or fecal bacteriotherapy, is the process of taking fecal bacteria (otherwise known as poop) from a healthy person and using it to normalize someone else's microbiome by using it as an enema or given orally in freeze-dried capsules. There is a growing body of work on this ancient treatment. Although it sounds repellant, it's probably the quickest and most permanent method that we currently have to normalize the human microbiome.

FMT is the standard treatment of choice for recurrent *C. difficile* infection, and there is ongoing research suggesting that it is promising for people with IBD, Crohn's disease, and ulcerative colitis. Some people heal completely; others don't. Yet it seems like curing IBD with one to three treatments would be something that many people with IBD would be willing to try, once it's easily available.

We have a few research studies in humans reporting improvements in IBS, hepatic encephalopathy, constipation, and metabolic syndrome. All of these conditions are associated with dysbiosis.

Helminth Therapy

Helminth is a general term for microscopic worms. In this case, nonhuman helminths are utilized to stimulate an immune response. Because they aren't from humans, they don't cause infections in people. Emerging research indicates that helminths can modulate the balance of commensal and disease-causing microbes to balance the microbiome. (See Chapter 8 for more details.)

Biofilm Therapies

Research is emerging in this area of biofilms (which were discussed in Chapter 5), including supporting bile, the use of probiotics and prebiotics, stevia, and chelation drugs. But our understanding is limited at this point in time.

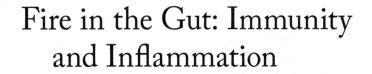

CHAPTER 8

Fire in the Gut: Immunity and Inflammation

"Our bodies respond to trauma or infection in a predictable manner, a phenomenon called inflammation. . . . Whether the stimulus is a laceration, a burn, or an inhaled speck of pollen by a person with atopic syndrome, a remarkably similar combination of signs is elicited."

—Robert Rountree, MD

"The gut immune system has the challenge of responding to the pathogens while remaining unresponsive to food antigens and the commensal flora. In the developed world this ability appears to be breaking down, with chronic inflammatory diseases of the gut commonplace in the apparent absence of overt infections."

—Thomas T. MacDonald and Giovanni Monteleone,
"Immunity, Inflammation, and Allergy in the Gut"

The function of the immune system is to determine what is us and what is not us: self from nonself. When exposed to a stimulus or event that our immune system interprets as nonself, it begins sending warriors to the rescue. Current research indicates that 70 percent of our immune system is located in or around the digestive system. This is because of the enormous amount of food and drink that we ingest, which is "foreign" material that needs to be sorted.

In fact, 99 percent of the time, it is the immune system's job *not* to respond. We develop what is called tolerance for our environment. Otherwise each time we ate an orange or inhaled some pollen, our immune system would be activated, much like the boy who cried wolf. Our bodies recognize what is similar to ourselves and what's not. When we eat foods high in antioxidants, nutrients, and polyphenols (colors), our immune system sighs, "All is well." But what if we eat foods that aren't really

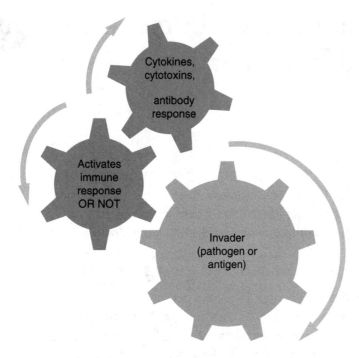

Figure 8.1   **Basic immune response.**

foods, for example, soft drinks, trans fats, artificial colors and flavors, and other food chemicals? Immune research indicates that our reaction to these "new-to-nature" foods is one of "nonself," which activates the immune system. Figure 8.1 illustrates the basic mechanism of an immune response.

The external manifestation of an immune system out of balance is inflammation, which we experience as swelling, heat, and/or pain. This reaction could be triggered by hay fever, a sprained ankle, acid reflux, or eating foods that disagree with us. In fact, inflammation is now believed to be the underlying cause of all disease.

Throughout our bodies, we have a continual communication that balances inflammation and healing. We are always walking a fine line between just the right amount of immune surveillance and inflammation, and not feeling well. When challenged, the immune system mounts a predictable response that is proportional to the threat. (See Table 8.1.) It produces inflammatory molecules such as cytokines; interleukins; chemokines; secretory IgA; IgG, IgE, and IgM antibodies; and others.

Table 8.1 **Causes and Degrees of Immune Vigilance**

	Stuff from Inside	**Stuff from Outside**
Vigilance	*(Cells, Molecules)*	*(Germs, Food, Pollen)*
Too little	Cancer	Infection
Just right	Self-knowledge	Environmental knowledge
Too much	Autoimmunity	Allergy

Used with permission from Sidney Baker, MD, Defeat Autism Now! conference, Dallas, October 2009.

IMMUNE IMBALANCES AND THE DIGESTIVE SYSTEM

When thinking about inflammation and immune imbalances in the digestive system, consider pain and discomfort: acid reflux; sores in our mouths; periodontal disease; inflammatory bowel diseases such as Crohn's and ulcerative colitis; irritable bowel syndrome (IBS); and dysbiosis. Also included are autoimmune diseases, such as type 1 diabetes, celiac disease, multiple sclerosis, lupus, Sjögren's disease, and rheumatoid arthritis. Inflammatory bowel diseases result from an exaggerated immune response to what would be normal bacteria in someone who has different genes. In the chapter on probiotics and prebiotics, we learned that their primary benefit is modulating the immune system. When we have a balance of probiotic, commensal, and few disease-causing bacteria, there is a balance between inflammation and healing. (See Figure 8.2.) When we have a lot of disease-causing microbes and few probiotic bacteria and commensal bacteria to balance that out, it leads to inflammation, pain, and disease.

THE IMMUNE SYSTEM 1.0

Our immune system has four basic parts. Our body's first response typically is to watch and be tolerant. When something unusual occurs, the immune system has an ordered way of responding that layers our defenses from simplest to most dire and then hopefully back to health again.

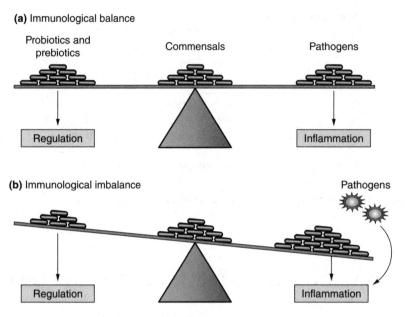

(a) Immunological balance

(b) Immunological imbalance

Figure 8.2 **How probiotics and prebiotics modulate the immune system.** (Adapted from Round, J.L., Mazmanian S.K. The gut microbiota shapes intestinal immune responses during health and disease. *Nat. Rev. Immunol.* 9, 313-323.)

- **Innate immune system:** This is our first line of defense against things that our bodies generally don't like, such as cancer cells, mold, mildew, yeast, and viruses. It responds quickly (within minutes or hours) to deal with bacteria, viruses, parasites, and other threats that can make us sick. Typically this is called a T-helper 1 cell response (Th-1 response). Some of the responses that are produced include interferon, defensins, lysozyme, complement (which activates the body to attack and kill cells), mast cells, polymorphonuclear lymphocytes, macrophages, dendritic cells, phagocytes, lactoferrin, reactive oxygen species (like hydrogen peroxide and superoxide radical), natural killer cells, and the interleukins IL-2, IL-12, and IL-18.

- **Adaptive immune system:** The second line of defense is our adaptive immune system. This is a slower response and is specific. Our bodies make a more careful examination to determine whether this is a friend or foe and then develop a specific response that is appropriate, most often an allergic response or antigenic. So, perhaps the first time we are stung by a bee, it's not so bad.

But then our body remembers that insult, and the next time we have a huge allergic reaction. If we are allergic to peanuts, our body produces an antigen that is specific to peanuts. Or if we have had the measles, our body will produce antibodies that are specific to measles. This is to help protect us from invaders with a long-term response. This level of immune response is also where food and environmental sensitivities reside. Typically this is a T-helper 2 (Th-2) response, where a specific response occurs to a specific challenge. Other cells involved are the antibodies IgA, IgM (memory antibodies), IgG (delayed sensitivities), IgE (allergy); T- and B-lymphocytes; and the interleukins IL-4, IL-5, IL-10, and IL-13.

- **Immune-inflammatory response:** In this response, our body overreacts and begins responding to our own tissues as if they were foreign. A combination of our genetics, our environmental exposures, and our overall immune balance will determine whether we trigger an autoimmune response. Increased intestinal permeability has been reported in all autoimmune conditions in which it has been studied, and it is believed to be a precondition for triggering autoimmunity. For example, virtually all people with celiac disease have HLA-DQ2 or HLA-DQ8 positive genes. When these people are exposed to gluten-containing grains along with a leaky gut, the grain triggers an immune and inflammatory response that is celiac disease. In other diseases, such as rheumatoid arthritis (RA) and ankylosing spondylitis (AS), genes (HLAB-27) meet bacteria (proteus in RA or klebsiella in AS), which sets off the immune response. The antibodies to these bacteria, which are typically non-disease-causing in most of us, set up an autoimmune response that causes inflammation, pain, and tissue destruction in people with the "right" genes and environment. In type 1 diabetes, either a virus or food sensitivities can trigger the disease. These are typically Th-17 responses and produce the interleukins IL-1, IL-17, and IL-22 and tumor necrosis factor alpha (TNF-alpha).
- **Regulatory system:** We also have a stop button, called the regulatory system, which suppresses our immune system and signals our body that all is well again. T cells are produced in the thymus and are called regulatory T cells (T-reg), also known as suppressor T cells, CD4, CD25, IL-10, and TGF-beta. T-reg cells are the brakes of the immune system. We want our bodies to react, but we also want them to stop reacting once the threat is gone. T-regs do this. Probiotics enhance T-reg production.

Of course, this all sounds nice and neat, but there is a lot of interplay and it's not all cut and dried.

THE GALT AND THE MALT

When microbes enter the digestive system, they are confronted with several non-specific and antigen-specific defense mechanisms (i.e., the innate immune system), including peristalsis, bile secretion, gastric acid, mucus, antibacterial peptides, and IgA. This stops most microbes and parasites from infecting the body.

Throughout our digestive systems, we have immune tissue called gut-associated lymphoid tissue (GALT). This underlies the single-cell epithelial lining and is comprised of 100–150 lymph nodes embedded in the gastrointestinal (GI) walls. Our tonsils, appendix, and Peyer's patches within the small intestine are examples of GALT. In the mucosal lining of the digestive lumen, we have mucosal-associated lymphoid tissue (MALT). MALT also encompasses our nose, our bronchia, and (in women) the vulvovaginal areas. All together, 70 percent of our immune system lies within the GALT and digestive MALT, and it protects us from antigens and other foreign invaders. The health of the GALT and MALT correlates with our own health. If these membranes are structurally strong, then we have greater resilience to disease. If these surfaces are compromised, then bacteria, antigenic food particles, and other inappropriate molecules get into our blood.

SECRETORY IgA (sIgA): Antibodies are produced as reactions to specific antigens as part of the adaptive immune system. Secretory IgA (sIgA) is the major way that MALT conveys the message of immune assault. This antibody comprises 80 percent of those in the digestive tract; like sentinels, it is on constant alert for foreign substances and blocks them from entering our bloodstream. When challenged by foreign molecules, sIgA forms immune complexes with allergens and microbes.

Deficiency of sIgA is the most common immunodeficiency. It's often found in infants, the elderly, malnourished people, and people with eating disorders. Low levels of sIgA make us more susceptible to infections in the lungs, gut, and genitourinary tracts. If low IgA levels persist, a chronic level of inflammation can occur, and it may be a fundamental cause of dysbiosis, asthma, autoimmune diseases, candidiasis, celiac disease, chronic infections, small intestinal bacterial overgrowth (SIBO), food allergies, Crohn's disease, rheumatoid arthritis, type 1 diabetes, viruses such as newborn rubella and Epstein-Barr virus, and more. Chronic stress, adrenal insufficiencies, oral bacteria, recurring infection, leaky gut, immune hypersensitivity, steroids, and anti-inflammatory drugs can lower sIgA. And if the sentry isn't standing at the gate, anyone can come in!

Some IgA-deficiency diseases include IgA nephropathy, vasculitis, lupus, rheumatoid arthritis, scleroderma, and Sjögren's syndrome. Immune complexes signal cytokines to begin an inflammatory process, which is designed to rid our bodies of antigenic materials, a response of the adaptive immune system. Without sufficient sIgA, MALT cannot work properly. A study examining people with Crohn's disease or ulcerative colitis found that all of them had low levels of sIgA. It concluded that raising sIgA levels might eliminate inflammatory bowel disease (IBD).

A high level of sIgA typically indicates a leaky gut, food sensitivities, or infection. High levels of sIgA are found in people who have chronic infections and whose immune systems are overloaded. It could also indicate malnutrition, malabsorption, lack of gastric acid production in the stomach, allergies, liver problems, parasites, or autoimmune conditions. It often accompanies chronic viral infections like cytomegalovirus (CMV), Epstein-Barr virus, and human immunodeficiency virus (HIV) and has been found in people with rare medical problems like Berger's nephropathy, dermatitis herpetiformis, gingivitis, hepatic glomerulonephritis, IgA neoplasms, parotitis, and antisperm antibodies. Factors that increase sIgA include acute stress, chronic infections, heavy smoking, alcoholism, periodontal disease, dental plaque accumulation, leaky gut, and throat cancer.

BALANCING sIgA: Lifestyle and nutritional factors can influence sIgA levels. For example, in people with IgA nephropathy, a kidney disease, 64 percent had decreases in sIgA-containing immune complexes on a gluten-free diet. Low sIgA levels can be normalized by a balanced lifestyle, which encompasses our ability to nurture ourselves; environmental considerations; exercise; good food choices; and moderate stress levels. Choline, essential fatty acids, glutathione, glycine, phosphatidylcholine, phosphatidylethanolamine, quercetin, vitamin C, and zinc are all required to maintain healthy sIgA levels. Detoxification programs and repair of intestinal mucosa help normalize sIgA. *Saccharomyces boulardii,* a nontoxic yeast probiotic supplement, has been shown to raise sIgA levels. A recent study showed that visualization and relaxation techniques significantly increase sIgA levels. Colostrum, transfer factor, fructooligosaccharides (FOSs), conjugated linolenic acid (CLA), medium-chain triglycerides, *Bifidobacteria longum, Lactobacillus casei,* EpiCor (beneficial yeast extract), astragalus, and Korean ginseng can all increase sIgA as well.

Additionally, the following can enhance sIgA production:

- **Rest and relaxation:** I often recommend that my clients rest for two hours during daylight every day. Typically, within a few weeks they are beginning to feel much better. (Radical, I know, but effective.) Rest also increases IgG and IgM antibodies.
- **Vitamin A:** A typical dosage is 5,000 IU daily. Taking high levels of retinol can be toxic, so if you increase the dosage, be sure to work with a health professional and have your serum retinol (vitamin A) levels monitored.
- **Bovine colostrum:** A typical dosage is 500 to 2,000 mg daily.

- **Transfer factor:** Dosage is 12.5 to 75 mg.
- **Medium-chain triglycerides (MCT) oil:** A typical dosage is up to 2 tablespoons daily. You can also eat coconut or drink coconut milk or fresh coconut juice.

PEYER'S PATCHES AND M-CELLS: Peyer's patches consist of lymphatic tissue that is mostly in the ileum. They have many B-cells, T-cells, and dendritic cells (cells that present antigens to the immune system and begin an immune reaction). Microfold cells (called M-cells) are found in Peyer's patches. M-cells help to control the flow of foreign substances, such as microbes and food particles, in the gut lumen. Antigenic substances are M-cells that carry antigens to the lining of the digestive tract. There, they are presented, or sampled, by Peyer's patches in the intestinal lining that alert B- and T-cells to begin processing the antigens.

TOLL-LIKE RECEPTORS (TLRs): We also have pattern-recognition substances, lectins, and toll-like receptors (TLRs), which help us recognize friend from foe. TLRs act as an antenna signaling the dendritic cells that start the immune cascade. Each type of TLR recognizes groups of pathogens that have structural shapes, called pathogen-associated molecular patterns (PAMPs), such as microbial lipopolysaccharides (LPSs). TLRs can also be stimulated from endogenous substances and trigger damage-associated molecular patterns (DAMPs) that alert the body to cellular and tissue injury. TLRs activate dendritic cells and turn on adaptive immune responses. When pathogenic microbes get through, TLRs stimulate production of pro-inflammatory cytokines by activation of NF-kappa B. One example of this occurs in Caucasian people with Crohn's disease. TLRs are altered due to changes in the NOD2 gene, which lead to an increase in inflammation from NF-kappa B and inflammatory interleukin molecules, while blocking anti-inflammatory IL-10 and defensins.

MICROBIOTA AND GUT IMMUNITY

As discussed in Chapter 5, the microbiome plays an enormous role in the gut-immune system. Commensal microbes provide nutrients, modulate inflammation, increased sIgA surveillance, activate T-regulatory cells, and mature dendritic cells.

PANETH CELLS

Paneth cells secrete antimicrobials that restrict their growth. They are found at the base of the enterocytes.

CAUSES OF DIGESTIVE INFLAMMATION AND IMMUNE IMBALANCE

Inflammation occurs when there is damage to cells or tissues. This is part of a normal response but can get out of control. Here are several factors that play a role.

- **The Hygiene Hypothesis:** It is believed that the constant exposure to microbes in infancy and early childhood contributes to the health and responsiveness of the adult immune system. This theory is called the Hygiene Hypothesis. In our culture, we don't challenge the immune system enough: We're too clean. We use antibacterial soaps and sponges in our obsession about microbes. As children, we don't play in the dirt; and we refrigerate, cook, and preserve our foods with chemicals, which lowers our exposure to microbes. We have good sanitation, we take antibiotics, and we don't eat fermented and cultured foods regularly. Children who have little opportunity to challenge microbes are at risk for allergy, eczema, and asthma, which may continue throughout their lifetime. Without these challenges, our immune system doesn't develop properly.
- **Genetics:** IBD, celiac disease, and arthritic diseases often have a genetic component.
- **Translocation of bacteria:** Even correct bacteria in the wrong place can cause problems.
- **Dysbiosis:** This occurs when the balance between probiotic and commensal organisms in the digestive system is overwhelmed by disease-producing microbes. Examples include bacterial, fungal, and parasitic infection.
- **Diet:** The standard Western diet, which is high in refined and poor-quality foods and low in fruits, meats, vegetables, nuts, whole grains, and seeds, increases inflammatory cytokines.
- **Leaky gut:** No matter what the cause, having a leaky gut leads to increased inflammation.
- **Stress:** This shunts blood away from GALT, impairs digestion and renewal of the gut epithelium, and alters the composition of the microbiome.

LABORATORY TESTING TO ASSESS GI INFLAMMATION

Calprotectin and lactoferrin are proteins found in stool. They are used to help discover whether there is inflammation in the large and are often elevated in IBD, postinfectious IBS, cancer in the digestive system, some GI infections, when people have caused damage from taking too many nonsteroidal anti-inflammatory medications, true food allergy, and chronic pancreatitis. When levels are high, it is a reliable marker to diagnose IBD. If you have IBD, these tests can be used to monitor the effectiveness of your chosen therapy. Stool testing is easy and certainly less invasive than scoping of the bowels.

Calprotectin binds both zinc and protein, so when levels are high, both can become depleted in our body. Since zinc is needed for healing of inflammation and calming the immune system, being deficient in zinc gives us a double whammy. Lactoferrin levels can be falsely elevated if we are using whey protein powders or taking lactoferrin, such as in colostrums or transfer factor.

Eosinophilic protein X is another marker of GI inflammation. It can be measured in urine or stool. It helps to determine whether there are either parasites or allergies associated with our health issues. It is commonly elevated when we have parasites, allergies, asthma, or eczema. It can also be used to monitor how effective treatment is. It is neurotoxic itself, so high levels increase inflammation.

Secretory IgA can be used to look at how well our immune system is responding. We can test for IgA in stool, saliva, and blood. (See Chapter 11 on Lab Testing for more information.)

REBALANCING THE GUT IMMUNE SYSTEM

In nearly all cases, probiotics and prebiotics help to dial down the inflammation and promote healing in IBD. They increase our T-regulatory response and IL-10, which also reduces inflammation. They also inhibit inflammatory cytokines, including TNF-alpha and NF-kappaB. Probiotics keep the membranes from becoming leaky, lessen muscle inflammation, and increase the production of mucin. (See Chapter 6 for more on prebiotics and probiotics.)

Try a Gut-Healing Therapeutic Diet
Elimination diets can be used temporarily to reduce inflammation and pain. (See Chapter 14.)

Eat a Rainbow: Polyphenols to Heal, Soothe, and Protect
Polyphenols are chemicals found in plant foods that have anti-inflammatory, prebiotic, and blood vessel protective properties. They are what give a rainbow of colors to our beans, spices, fruits, vegetables, nuts, seeds, and grains. They are among the reasons we

need to eat as many fruits and vegetables as possible, to focus on whole foods in general, and to season our food with herbs and spices. Eating just 10 cherries a day lowers inflammation. We should eat cherries, berries, and other high-polyphenol foods several times a day. Foods with the highest polyphenols include:

- Berries: strawberries, blackberries, raspberries, blueberries
- Fruits of all types: grapes (highest in red or purple), cherries, peaches, kiwis, apples, pears, plums
- Wine
- Tea: green (highest), black, rooibus, mint
- Chocolate
- Coffee (not a recommendation, but it is high in polyphenols)
- Onions, leeks
- Broccoli, cabbage
- Beans of all types, including soy
- Parsley, celery
- Millet, wheat
- Skin of citrus fruit
- Tomatoes
- Clover leaf tea

More Anti-Inflammatory High-Phenol Foods and Supplements

The use of nutritional supplements has been best studied in ulcerative colitis where inflammation can roar. Curcumin from turmeric, resveratrol from red wine and red grapes, Epigallocatechin gallate (EGCG) from green tea, and quercetin from maples, onions, leafy vegetables, and tea have all been shown to reduce inflammation in ulcerative colitis and throughout the body. Many high-polyphenol supplements, spices, and foods have been shown to decrease levels of NF-kappa B and to decrease inflammation. We can use many of these as foods, or they can be found singly or in combination in products that reduce inflammation.

- Curcumin: Curcumin is one of the main anti-inflammatory ingredients in turmeric root, and standardized curcuminoids can be purchased. Take 200 to 1,000 mg three times daily, or use 2 to 3 teaspoons of dried turmeric or 1 to 2 "fingers" of fresh turmeric juiced daily.
- Ginger: Drink as a tea or in fresh vegetable juice, eat crystallized ginger, use fresh or dried in cooking, or take 500 to 2,000 mg in capsule form daily.
- Boswellia (frankincense): Take 100 to 1,200 mg standardized extract daily.

- Green tea extract (EGCG) and green tea: Each cup of standardized green tea contains 100 to 300 mg of ECGC catechins. Drink green tea liberally throughout the day; decaffeinated is preferred. Or take EGCG in supplemental form at a dose of 100 to 400 mg once daily.
- Quercetin dihydrate: Take 500 to 1,000 mg three times daily.
- Wheatgrass: Drink up to 3.5 ounces daily. If you drink too much, it can cause intense nausea, so start slowly. Heidi Snyder, MS, a nutrition consultant on the faculty at Hawthorn University, suggests juicing gingerroot with wheatgrass to help the flavor.
- Bromelain: Best taken on an empty stomach to reduce inflammation; 200 to 500 mg one to three times daily.
- Carnosol: Found in rosemary leaf extract; take 200 mg one to three times daily.
- Grape seed extract: Take 50 to 200 mg daily.
- Probiotics: Take 1 billion to trillions of CFU. (See Chapter 6.)
- Alpha-lipoic acid: Take 100 to 1,200 mg daily.
- Resveratrol: Take 15 to 100 mg daily.
- Vitamin D: The Food and Drug Administration (FDA) states that 2,000 IU daily is a safe daily adult dose. If vitamin D levels are below 32, your clinician may recommend dosages of up to 10,000 IU vitamin D_3 daily for a short period of time. Prescription dosages of vitamin D_2 may range between 50,000 and 100,000 IU weekly or monthly. My preference is to use natural vitamin D_3.
- Omega 3 fatty acids: Fish oil capsules contain both eicosapentaenoic acid (EPA) and docosahexaenoic acid (DHA) fatty acids. Typical anti-inflammatory dosages are between 360 and 1,260 mg of EPA and 240 and 840 mg of DHA. Check the potency of your fish oil because it can vary widely. Most contain 180 mg of EPA and 120 mg of EPA. High-potency capsules can contain dosages as high as 650 mg EPA and 450 mg of EPA.
- Gamma-linolenic acid: GLA is found in evening primrose, borage, and sesame oil; take 360 to 720 mg daily.
- White willow bark: Take 60 to 120 mg as needed. White willow bark may cause stomach upset for some people, but it's less likely than with aspirin or other nonsteroidal anti-inflammatory drugs (NSAIDs).
- Devil's claw: Used as a digestive stimulant for digestive issues and for pain and arthritis; take 600 to 4,500 mg of powdered devil's claw daily or 200 mg of devil's claw standardized extracts up to three times daily.

Use of immune-supportive foods such as whey products, colostrum, or transfer factor may be helpful for healing. Whey can be consumed as a drink. Colostrum or transfer factor at levels of 1 to 2 teaspoons or more daily offers protective effects. Drinking raw cow's or goat's milk often can help healing for many people.

In herbal therapies, there is a group of herbs and foods called demulcents. Demulcents have a soothing effect on the GI system. Some of the most common demulcents include the following:

- Almonds
- Barley
- Borage: Available as a tea or a green
- Burdock root: A food also known as gobo root, which can be found in grocery and Asian stores
- Chickweed: A spring green easy to find in yards; terrific in a salad
- Coconut oil
- Coltsfoot: Typically is used as a tea or in cough syrups or lozenges
- Comfrey root: Used in teas
- Fenugreek: Best as a tea
- Figs
- Flaxseed
- Hops: Available as a tea or dried in capsules
- Licorice: Available as a tea, as "real" black licorice candy, in capsule or tincture, or as a chewable tablet; overuse of licorice, if it's not deglycyrrizinated licorice (DGL), can elevate blood pressure
- Mallow: Also called malva; available as a tea
- Marshmallow: Can be found as a tea or capsules
- Mullein: Found as a tea or compress
- Oats
- Okra
- Parsley
- Pomegranate seeds
- Prunes
- Psyllium: Plain or in products such as Metamucil
- Pumpkin
- Sage: Can be cooked or used as a tea
- Sarsaparilla and sassafras: Can be drunk as a tea after simmering roots for 20 minutes in water
- Slippery elm: Can be used in teas or soups or as lozenges
- Tapioca: Use as a flour or in pudding

HELMINTH THERAPY TO RESET THE IMMUNE SYSTEM: BIOME ENRICHMENT

Parasites evolved with humans over time. In hunter-gatherers, parasites live in symbiosis with us to a large extent. Much of our immune system's mechanisms were meant to deal with parasites. Today, in our so-called clean world (i.e., devoid of most parasites), the immune system often gets up to mischief, causing allergies and autoimmune conditions. I liken the immune system to a group of teenage boys on a summer day with nothing to do: They get into trouble! But one way to stop this trouble is by tricking these boys into doing something else...

This is where helminths come into the picture. Helminths trick the immune system by giving it a job. Basically, one takes serial doses of helminths that don't cause disease in humans. The immune system reacts to these for a couple of weeks, and allergies and other inflammation diminish. Most people react poorly to the idea of taking worms to feel better. So, the term "biome enrichment" is being used to soften the blow. Honestly, they are so small you can't see them, and they have no taste. The most common helminths used include *Trichurissuis ova* (TSO), which is a pig whipworm, and the cysticercoid developmental stage of *Hymenolepsis diminuta* (HDC), which are rat or beetle tapeworms.

Sidney Baker MD, a teacher of mine, first told me about the use of helminths. He began utilizing TSO whipworms and since has transitioned to the use of HDCs, which are rat tapeworms. He calls them "little dudes" and describes them as the most effective therapy in treating autistic children with GI issues. He has a lab where he grows and harvests these creatures. There is promise in this therapy. Of HDC, Woolsey et al. state:

> It is hoped that future clinical trials using this organism may shed light on the potential for helminthic therapy to alleviate inflammatory diseases. Further, it is hoped that studies with HDCs may provide a stepping stone toward population-wide restoration of the biota of the human body, potentially reversing the inflammatory consequences of biota depletion that currently affect Western society.

TSOs calm the immune system. These eggs of one of a dozen or so supposedly innocent worms that live in the digestive systems of pretty much all animals. The TSOs that are used therapeutically come from pigs. According to Dr. Sidney Baker, people occasionally can have some negative reactions to helminth therapy, including: digestive symptoms, a pungent smell to the urine, and rarely some aggravation of symptoms.

There is a good body of research indicating that TSO usage is safe. TSO treatment may help people who have conditions that involve chronic inflammation, oxidative stress, and problems with poor detoxification. Studies show benefits in people with ulcerative colitis, and while the results are mixed, some studies indicate benefits in people with allergies, multiple sclerosis, type 1 diabetes, and food sensitivities. People with Crohn's disease do not appear to benefit from this treatment.

Dr. Baker puts this into simple words: "The benefits are huge, the risk is nil, the odds are 50:50 that you'll improve (more in children than in elders), and the cost is tolerable." So why not consider it?

Further Resources
Moises Velasquez-Manoff's book, An epidemic of absence: *A New Way of Understanding Allergies and Autoimmune Diseases.* Scribner, NY, 2012.
"Exploring Helminth Therapy", *Natural Medicine Journal. Interview with Dr. Sidney Baker.* July 2018. https://www.naturalmedicinejournal.com/journal/2018-07/exploring-helminthic-therapy

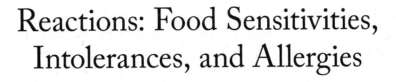

CHAPTER 9

Reactions: Food Sensitivities, Intolerances, and Allergies

"The gut is a major potential portal of entry into the body for foreign antigens. Only its intact mucosal barrier protects the body from foreign antigen entry and systemic exposure."

—Russell Jaffe, MD

Today one out of three people say that they have a food allergy or sensitivity and change their diet to reflect this. The average American eats about 2,000 pounds of food each which is why 2/3 of the immune system is located in the gut. Our body needs to determine whether what we ate is friend or foe.

Our immune system was designed to fend off infection, so if we have reactions to food or the environment, it's a signal that our body has become less tolerant. We must build tolerance so that we can live a normal and active life. Our tolerance of our foods and other environmental exposures is based on many factors, including genetics, age, gender, intestinal permeability (or increased permeability/leaky gut), infections, and balance of gut ecology as well as the type and dose of the particular substance or antigen. This can be provoked by foods, molds, pollen, chemicals, metals, and nearly any other substance. Fortunately, our body has mechanisms to bring us back into balance if we create the right conditions for it.

TRUE FOOD ALLERGIES

True food allergies—those that trigger IgE reactions—are rare, affecting only 0.3 to 7.5 percent of American children and 1 to 2 percent of adults. The foods that most often trigger true allergic reactions are eggs, cow's milk, nuts, shellfish, soy, wheat, and white fish.

Peanut Allergies

Allergy to peanuts has mushroomed since the late 1990s. In 2014, Bunyavanich and colleagues tested children for IgE reactions to peanuts and asked parents if their child had ever had any allergic reactions to peanuts. When asked, 4.6 percent of parents reported that their children had allergic reactions to peanuts; this was confirmed with tests reporting 5 percent of the same children had reactions to peanuts. In 1997, the rate of peanut allergy was 0.4 percent. In 2014 Bunyavanich studied 2128 American children from infancy for about 8 years for IgE reactions to peanuts. They also asked parents about peanut reactions. The results closely agreed, with 4.6 percent of parents reporting peanut allergy, and 5 percent of the children testing positive on testing. In 1997, the rate of peanut allergy was 0.4 percent.

In 2018 research by Tracy Pitt and associates analyzed peanut allergies in 342 Canadian families who had a family history of asthma or allergies. Women were enrolled during pregnancy. In this cohort 9.4 percent of the children had peanut reactions at age 7. Interestingly, in children whose babies ate peanuts in infancy and were exposed to peanuts via breastfeeding had only a 1.7 percent incidence of developing peanut allergy, compared with 5.6 percent in children who were not exposed to peanuts during infancy at all; 15.1 percent in babies who were exposed to peanuts through breastfeeding and 17.8 percent in infants who ate peanuts in infancy.

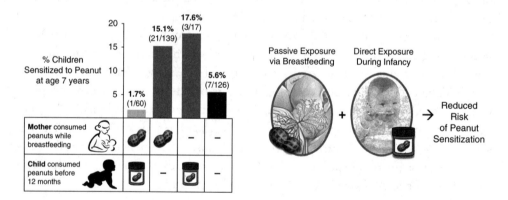

Probiotics also offer promise to children with peanut allergies. In a recent study, children received L. rhamnosus CGMCC at a dose of 20 bilion CFU daily or placebo. In children who received the probiotic, 89.7 percent were desensitized to peanuts, compared with 7.1 percent of children with placebo.

So what has changed between now and then? When my children went to school, everyone ate in the same lunch room. Today, children with food allergies must sit at a separate table from their peers, and very sensitive children may have to be in a different room altogether.

Peanut allergy can be so severe that a child may react if someone else recently ate peanuts or peanut butter in the room the child is in. Because of this, peanuts are no longer served on many airplanes and all nuts are banned in many schools.

Physicians diagnose food allergies using patch skin tests and radioallergosorbent test (RAST) blood testing, which are great for detecting food allergies. Yet research in eosinophilic esophagitis, which is equivalent to asthma of the esophagus, has demonstrated that an elimination diet can more accurately predict which foods a person is allergic to than IgE testing can. IgE antibodies attach to mast cells in mucous membranes and in connective tissues, stimulating the release of inflammatory cytokines and histamines. The resulting allergic response produces symptoms a few minutes to two hours after the food is eaten. Common symptoms include closing of the throat, fatigue, tearing, hives, itching, respiratory distress, watery or runny nose, skin rashes, itchy eyes or ears, and sometimes severe reactions of asthma and anaphylactic shock.

FOOD SENSITIVITIES

It is estimated that 10 to 20 percent of us have food sensitivities. Food sensitivity reactions, also called delayed hypersensitivity reactions and in the past called "serum sickness," occur when IgA, IgG, and IgM antibodies are triggered in response to foods, chemicals, and bacterial toxins. The most common antibody reactions are IgG to mold and foods; exposure to molds and foods is quite high compared to pollens. These IgA, IgM, and IgG responses are called delayed sensitivity reactions because the symptoms they cause can take from several hours to several days to appear, which makes it very difficult to track down the offending food or substance.

When antibodies bind to antigens, as in delayed food sensitivity reactions, they form immune complexes, which are clumps of molecules that the immune system disposes of. Large ones are eaten up by macrophages, the Pac-Man of the immune system. Smaller immune complexes, however, can bind to tissues, causing problems. Use of protein-digesting enzymes (also called protease enzymes or proteolytic enzymes) can help to clear the bloodstream of circulating immune complexes.

It is estimated that 95 percent of all food reactions are of this delayed type. IgM antibodies circulate temporarily, about three months, until IgG antibodies are mobilized to take over the fight. IgG antibodies are longer lasting, and we keep producing them as long as we eat the offending foods, have leaky gut, or are

SENSITIVITY SYMPTOMS

Professional evaluation is necessary to determine whether the following symptoms, which can be caused by many health conditions, are due to food and/or environmental sensitivities:

- **Head:** Chronic headaches, migraines, difficulty sleeping, dizziness
- **Mouth and throat:** Coughing; sore throat; hoarseness; swelling or pain; gagging; frequently clearing throat; sores on gums, lips, and tongue
- **Eyes, ears, nose:** Runny or stuffy nose; post-nasal drip; ringing in the ears; blurred vision; sinus problems; watery and itchy eyes; ear infections; hearing loss; sneezing attacks; hay fever; excessive mucus; dark circles under eyes; swollen, red, or sticky eyelids
- **Heart and lungs:** Irregular heartbeat (palpitations, arrhythmia), asthma, rapid heartbeat, chest pain and congestion, bronchitis, shortness of breath, difficulty breathing
- **Gastrointestinal tract:** Nausea and vomiting, constipation, diarrhea, irritable bowel syndrome (IBS), indigestion, bloating, passing gas, stomach pain, cramping, heartburn, gastroesophageal reflux disease (GERD), ulcers
- **Skin:** Hives, skin rashes, psoriasis, eczema, dry skin, excessive sweating, acne, hair loss, irritation around eyes

- **Muscles and joints:** General weakness, muscle and joint aches and pains, arthritis, swelling, stiffness
- **Energy and activity:** Fatigue, mental dullness and memory lapses, difficulty getting your work done, apathy, hyperactivity, restlessness
- **Emotions and mind:** Mood swings, anxiety and tension, fear, nervousness, anger, irritability, aggressive behavior, binge eating or drinking, food cravings, depression, confusion, poor comprehension, poor concentration, difficulty learning
- **Other:** Overweight, underweight, fluid retention, insomnia, genital itch, frequent urination, bed-wetting

In addition to the symptoms previously listed, children with food and/or environmental sensitivities may have:
- Attention deficit disorder
- Behavior problems
- Learning problems
- Recurring ear infections

Children with these problems will often benefit from a dietary evaluation and environmental sensitivity testing.

exposed to chemicals, bacterial toxins, or other foreign substances (antigens) that are challenging the immune system.

Although almost any food can cause a food sensitivity reaction, beef, citrus, dairy products, egg, corn, pork, and wheat provoke 80 percent of them.

Food sensitivities can underlie a huge variety of symptoms (see box). It's important to discover which foods we react to and to see what the underlying cause may be, such as parasites, candidiasis, bacterial or viral infection, pancreatic insufficiency, enzyme deficiency, medications, or poor lifestyle habits.

GLUTEN SENSITIVITY

Nonceliac gluten sensitivity (NCGS), also called gluten sensitivity and gluten intolerance, has overlapping symptoms with both celiac disease and irritable bowel syndrome (IBS). It appears that many people benefit from eliminating wheat and other gluten-containing grains from their diet, even though they do not have celiac disease. As the research unfolds, it has revealed that people can be reacting to gluten and gliadin proteins, wheat agglutinins (a lectin), amylase/trypsin inhibitors, glutenin, gluteomorphins, and prebiotic oligosaccharides in wheat. Based on the National Health and Nutrition Examination Survey, between 0.6 percent and 10.6 percent of us may be suffering from NCGS. The broad range is because when this data was collected, we didn't yet have reliable tests to diagnose NCGS easily. This is improving, with tests from Cyrex Labs, Cell Science/Alcat, Vibrant America, and other companies.

Still, the best test for NCGS is to scrupulously remove gluten-containing grains from your diet, such as in most of the plans listed in Chapter 13. This would be a relatively simple experiment and can provide a plethora of benefits. For many people who have NCGS, once they have gone gluten-free, subsequent eating of even small amounts of gluten can provoke dramatic distress. I had a client who had been gluten free for a couple of months celebrate with a piece of cake and be depressed and unable to get out of bed for several days. I had another client who got a smidgeon of soy sauce in a sushi roll, and it brought on a severe bout of cramping, bloating, and diarrhea.

We don't have research yet on whether NCGS can be reversed, allowing people to eat wheat again once the digestive system has been fixed, the gut barrier healed, dysbiosis treated, and microbiome rebalanced. I have a lot of faith in the ability of the body to heal, so I hope that NCGS can be reversed. The goal is always to broaden people's diets as much as possible in the long run. (See more on celiac disease and gluten sensitivity in Chapter 23 and on testing in Chapter 11.)

FOOD INTOLERANCES

Some people have intolerances to sugars or specific carbohydrates in certain foods. This means that they lack the enzymes that are needed to digest them. The most common ones include gluten intolerance, lactose intolerance, and fructose intolerance.

Lactose Intolerance

Lactose intolerance is common, affecting 25 percent of Americans and 75 percent of people globally and is highly prevalent in African Americans, Asian Americans, Caucasian Americans of Mediterranean and Jewish descent, Hispanics, and Native Americans. Lactose intolerance is not a milk allergy, which is the inability to digest milk proteins such as casein. Lactose intolerance is caused by a deficiency in lactase, an enzyme that digests lactose, which is a sugar naturally found in milk and milk products. After the age of two, our lactase production gradually tapers. Lowering of our ability to digest lactose can also occur from infections (bacterial, viral, parasitic, fungal), foods, and other substances that can injure the lining of the gut. Lactose intolerance causes a wide variety of symptoms, including abdominal cramping, acne, bloating, diarrhea, gas, eczema, headaches, and nausea. Often when dysbiosis is balanced, lactose intolerance becomes less of a problem.

Most people who are lactose intolerant can tolerate some dairy products, which makes figuring this out less obvious than one would think. Often, it's a matter of amount; sometimes it's a matter of which type of dairy product. I, personally, can eat kefir and some sheep's milk cheeses but cannot drink milk. Other people have told me that they can eat low-fat yogurt but not full-fat yogurt; and others just the opposite. Eliminating dairy completely from your diet for two to four weeks or doing a hydrogen breath test will give you a good idea whether dairy is for you.

A hereditary form of fructose intolerance occurs in 1 in 10,000 people and generally shows up when children are small. They naturally dislike sweets, juices, and foods that have fructose because it makes them sick.

Fructose Intolerance

But we can acquire fructose intolerance because of the high amount of fruit and sweeteners we eat. The average person eats 100 pounds of processed sugars in 2017 (down from 140 pounds in 2000) according to the U.S. Department of Agriculture. Each of us eats 39.8 pounds of fructose and 60.2 pounds of table sugar and sucrose, pushing many of us above the threshold that we can tolerate. Fructose is found in highest concentrations in table sugar, apples, pears, fruit juices, dried fruit, watermelon, honey, high fructose corn syrup, corn syrup solids, agave nectar, sorbitol, xylitol, and sweet wines. So, drinking sweetened teas and soft drinks is a big no-no!

The symptoms of fructose intolerance look like those of IBS. A third of people with IBS and 61 percent of people with Crohn's disease also test positive for fructose malabsorption. Common symptoms include loose stools or diarrhea, constipation, alternating diarrhea and constipation, gas, bloating, cramping, indigestion, depression, sometimes belching, nausea, and occasional vomiting. Testing for fructose intolerance is also done with breath testing.

If you have fructose intolerance, you'll want to avoid all foods that contain high amounts of fructose. You may also want to avoid foods with high fructan content including artichokes, asparagus, leeks, onions, and wheat products.

See Chapter 11 for more information on lactose, fructose, and gluten testing.

BIOAMINE AND HISTAMINE INTOLERANCE

More and more people are becoming intolerant to histamines and other bioactive amines: beta-phenylethylamine, tyramine, tryptamine, putrescine, cadaverine, spermine, and spermidine. Histamines and other bioactive amines are produced by a dysbiotic microbiota in the gut and can be too much for people to clear.

Although we associate histamines with allergy, histamine intolerance is not really an allergy because IgE antibodies are not involved in this process. This is a nonimmune problem. Rather, this is due to enzyme insufficiencies of diamine oxidase (DAO) and/or histamine N-methyltransferase (HMNT), dysbiosis in the gut, or a combination of the two.

These bioactive amines are naturally produced by microbes during fermentation, when foods have been stored too long, or when foods are decaying. Common food sources include fermented foods such as beer, wine, sauerkraut, yogurt, vinegar, cheese, salami, and sausages; leftover foods; fish that is not fresh; and milk. I first became aware of this years ago from my students, who discovered that their health issues resolved when high-histamine foods were eliminated from their diet.

Symptoms can be the same as allergy symptoms, or they may involve itching; hives; swelling of the face, throat, and mouth; drops in blood pressure; racing heartbeat (tachycardia); anxiety and/or panic attacks; chest pain; conjunctivitis; headaches; fatigue; confusion; irritability; digestive issues, especially heartburn, indigestion, and reflux; and rarely brief loss of consciousness for 1 to 2 seconds. In children, histamine intolerance often presents as diarrhea, abdominal pain, headache, and chronic intermittent vomiting.

Resources:

- Dr. Jonega, *A Beginners Guide to Histamine Intolerance and Histamine Intolerance: The Comprehensive Guide for Healthcare Professionals*
- Histamine Sensitivity.com website: https://histamine-sensitivity.com
- Jill Carnahan MD, Histamine Restricted Diet: https://www.jillcarnahan.com /downloads/Histamine RestrictedDiet.pdf

REACTIONS TO FOOD ADDITIVES

Many people also have reactions to common food additives such as sulfites, monosodium glutamate (MSG), food dyes, and benzoates.

Sulfites have been associated with the onset of asthma. Awareness of this grew in the 1980s as people ate at salad bars where lettuce and other vegetables were dipped in a sulfite wash to keep them from oxidizing/browning. Common food sources include wine, beer, cider, fruit juice, and dried fruit.

In some people, MSG has long been linked to asthma; headaches; hives; swelling, especially of the face, throat, and mouth; seizures; and rarely to rhinitis. MSG issues have been dubbed "Chinese restaurant syndrome" due to the widespread use of MSG as a flavor enhancer in Chinese food in the United States. It's also found in herb and spice blends, fish sauce, soy sauce, black bean sauce, tomato sauce, miso, marmite, and in dried soups.

In the United States, the use of food dyes has risen 500 percent, from 12 mg per person daily to 62 mg per person daily. Most of these substances are eaten by children. These dyes are used in foods, shampoos, cosmetics, drugs, and play dough, and are easily absorbed from foods and through the skin into the bloodstream. The relationship between food dyes and attention deficit hyperactivity disorder (ADHD) is strong. The Center for Science in the Public Interest has published several reports on this and petitioned the Food and Drug Administration (FDA) to change regulations for nearly a decade. Their effects are widespread. I remember a 12-year-old client who came into my office and notified me that if she ate a single yellow M&M, she would have a seizure within 20 minutes. According to Dr. Aristo Vodjani, food colorings are associated with liver toxicity and mitochondrial dysfunction, loss of oral tolerance, interference with digestive enzymes, increased intestinal permeability, hyperactivity, eczema, immune reactions to food, hypersensitivity, allergic rhinitis, asthma, and angioedema. In Europe, many of these dyes have been banned for a decade. Currently, Nestle's and Hershey have removed artificial dyes from their candy; and Mars is working on it.

Resource:

- Seeing Red: Time for Action on Food Dyes, *Center for Science in the Public Interest*, 2017. https://cspinet.org/resource/seeing-red-time-action -food-dyes

■ "Brand New Hue: The Quest to Make a True Blue M&M," *New York Times, Oct. 5, 2016.* https://www.nytimes.com/interactive/2016/10/09/magazine/blue-food-coloring-mars-company.html

Sodium benzoate and potassium benzoate are used commonly as food preservatives to inhibit mold. Virtually all pickles have sodium benzoate added to them. Both sodium and potassium benzoate can be found in salad dressings, sauces, jams, fruit juice, soft drinks, and spice mixes. Research loosely links benzoates to eczema, hives, asthma, rhinitis, and anaphylaxis.

LECTINS

Lectins, which are proteins in food that bind strongly to carbohydrates, are found everywhere in nature. Although much online material suggests that lectins are harmful, most research focuses on their benefits to immune recognition, reduction in inflammation, and cell defense. They are found in high amounts in all beans, peas, lentils, and peanuts, grains, and tubers. Plants produce lectins to protect themselves from being eaten, and lectins are involved in germination. In our own bodies lectins play a role in the immune system by recognizing carbohydrates that don't belong. On the other hand, they can wreak havoc if we don't have the enzymes to digest them: They bind to carbohydrate molecules in all tissues and cause them to clump together. They bind to the GI mucosa, which weakens it and allows it to become permeable (leaky). They degranulate mast cells, which causes them to produce IgE antibodies and set off allergic reactions.

Lectins, when not properly digested, can connect two IgE molecules, which triggers the release of histamines and begins an allergic reaction, mimicking food allergies. The digestive system and nervous system are especially sensitive to lectin reactions. This can appear as IBS, arthritis, or nearly any inflammatory condition. The people whose arthritis responds to elimination of the nightshade family of foods (potatoes, eggplant, tomatoes, peppers) probably have lectin sensitivities. Other people have symptoms that are identical to IBS, dysbiosis, and leaky gut syndrome. It's difficult to know whether this is specifically due to lectin reactions or not.

There is a lot of hype about lectins. Still, there is no risk limiting them in your diet for a few weeks and monitoring the results. Then, dive more deeply to see if you can restore the underlying imbalance. Using traditional cooking methods such as soaking, sprouting, cooking, and pressure cooking (hot pots such as Instant Pot) can break down lectins. Taking digestive enzymes can also help.

FOOD CRAVINGS AND EXORPHINS

Oddly enough, about half of people with food sensitivities and intolerances crave the foods that make them sick. This is because many foods, such as wheat and dairy products, produce protein molecules that are really similar to our natural endorphins, called exorphins. Endorphins and exorphins lessen pain and help generate a general sense of well-being in our world. So, even if we are intolerant of lactose, we crave it and even feel better when we drink milk . . . temporarily, that is. And then we crave some more.

ENVIRONMENTAL ILLNESS

Environmental sensitivities are another type of enzyme deficiency due to slow liver detoxification enzymes. (See Chapter 17 for more on detoxification.) Chronic exposure to food additives, household chemicals, building materials, contaminated recirculating air, and impure water can so depress and weaken a person's immune system that eventually exposure to even a small amount of a toxin can make one acutely or chronically ill. This condition, called environmental illness or multiple chemical sensitivities, is becoming more and more common. Two recent studies put its incidence at 12.9 percent and 15.9 percent in adults.

If blood testing shows that you have environmental allergies, or if you know that specific substances make you ill, it is essential that you avoid these substances. Regular use of low-temperature, infrared saunas can help to move these fat-soluble substances out of your tissues. You can read more about use of saunas in Chapter 17. Taking malic acid as a supplement can be helpful in neutralizing some of the reactions. Unfortunately, many people look fine and are treated as if they are depressed or psychotic. This is a serious illness and if you suspect environmental illness, it is also important to work with a health care provider who is educated in this area. Look for an MD who specializes in environmental medicine (http://www.aaemonline.org). Also, see information on testing for food reactions in Chapter 11.

HEALING OPTIONS FOR SENSITIVITIES AND ALLERGIES

With a holistic treatment program, you can become increasingly less sensitive to foods and environmental antigens over time. Begin by avoiding all substances you are sensitive or allergic to. Using the probiotics, anti-inflammatory nutrients, and herbs listed in this section will speed the process. Eating organically grown, nutrient-rich, natural foods promotes the body's self-repair. An exercise program and stress management also play a part in recovery. Also look at Chapter 13 to learn more about dietary approaches, which are your first line of therapy.

Do at least the first five of these recommendations for best results:

- **Avoidance:** For a period of 4 to 6 months, avoid all substances that cause you to have a sensitivity or allergic reaction, for a period of four to six months. To substitute for these, check out a health food store's plethora of options for people with food allergies. If chemical sensitivity is an issue, use natural household-cleaning products (it's good to use them anyway!). Some people also react to mattresses, gas stoves, paints, carpeting, and upholstery; avoiding these can be difficult. Consult a health care professional who can help with the details. See Chapter 17 for more on everyday chemicals.
- **Try an elimination diet:** See Chapter 13 for instructions.
- **Glutamine:** This is an amino acid that will help heal the intestinal tract. Take 500 mg once daily up to 15 grams daily, mixed in juice or water. Too much will be constipating. Many people discover that glutamine, also known as L-glutamine, gives them strength and endurance. If you have end-stage kidney disease, take only the lowest dosage of glutamine.
- **Probiotics:** Lactobacilli and bifidobacteria (see Chapter 6) protect the digestive tract's mucosal lining and limit damage caused by pathogenic bacteria. Take 10 billion to 50 billion colony-forming units (CFUs) daily with food.
- **Enzymes:** Digestive enzymes and proteolytic enzymes (protein-splitting enzymes) are very useful in helping normalize allergies. They are gentle and help in several ways. The digestive enzymes help the foods to be more fully digested. The proteolytic enzymes are taken between meals and break up immune complexes. Take one to two capsules of digestive enzymes with each meal and snack or one capsule of proteolytic enzymes at bedtime and upon rising.
- **Quercetin:** This bioflavonoid reduces pain and inflammatory responses and controls allergies. Take 250 to 1,000 mg one to four times daily.

- **Herbs:** Examples include milk thistle, dandelion root, and burdock, and they support the liver. These herbs can be used singly or in combination in tea or tinctures or capsules. Typical dosage for tea is 1 to 3 cups daily. For tinctures and capsules, use as directed on label.
- **Vitamin C:** This helps flush toxins. Take 500 to 3,000 mg or more of buffered ascorbate or Ester-C daily.
- **Mineral salts:** These contain bicarbonates of calcium, magnesium, and/or potassium (e.g., Alka-Seltzer Gold) to alkalize the stomach and to help minimize reactions. Use as directed on label.
- **Malic acid:** This acid naturally occurs in fruits and can be used to stop or slow reactions if you have eaten something questionable. Use as directed on label.
- **Four-day food-rotation diet:** If your test results indicate that you are sensitive to a wide variety of food, you still need to eat. A four-day rotation diet provides a temporary solution to this problem by allowing you to eat a broader variety of foods less often. This gives you a more balanced diet and a full complement of nutrients. This food plan is *only* for people who have a very limited diet because it is difficult to follow. It can be helpful to color code the foods you eat each of the four days. For example, put four different colors of stickers on the foods you will be eating on each of the four days—blue, purple, red, yellow or whatever colors you like. This will make it clear to you what is allowed each day as you rotate.

  In this protocol, you avoid eating any foods to which you had strong antibody reactions in the test and eat the remaining foods in a four-day pattern that helps prevent the development of sensitivity to those foods as well. This basically tricks the body into being more tolerant by rotating foods. When you eat a specific food that you are sensitive to, your body begins to produce antibodies against that food over the next 24 hours. If you eat the food again the next day, you will experience symptoms. If you don't eat it again for several days, those antibodies, which were ready for a fight, disappear as if it were a false alarm. When you restart the rotation and resume eating the food, the antibody-production process begins again, but you don't develop symptoms in response to the food because the antibodies are never present at the time you eat the food. Many labs supply customized rotation diets along with your results.

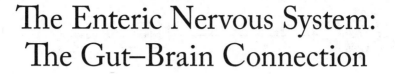

CHAPTER 10

The Enteric Nervous System: The Gut–Brain Connection

"If you have alterations in the brain, you will almost certainly have altered output to the gut because the two organs are that closely connected."

—Emeran Mayer, MD
David Geffen School of Medicine, UCLA.
Einstein, M. (2016) *Nature.* 533(7603) p. S104+. 19 May.

TWO BRAINS ARE BETTER THAN ONE

Do you have gut instincts? Do you get butterflies in your stomach when you're nervous? Have you experienced diarrhea from anxiety? Can a job interview cause you to have stomach cramps? These things happen because your nervous system and digestive system are intertwined. As mentioned in Chapter 1, the enteric nervous system (ENS) is often called "the second brain" because it has a mind of its own.

The ENS is the nervous system that runs through our digestive system. The ENS has about 100 million neurons (fewer than the brain and more than the spine). It is connected directly to the brain through the vagus nerve, although it can work entirely on its own. (In fact, before ulcer medications revolutionized the treatment of ulcer pain, surgeons cut the vagus nerve from the brain to the stomach, and the digestive system continued to operate completely!) It makes more neurotransmitters than the brain. This nervous system is found in sheaths of tissue lining the entire digestive system. Think about the taste, texture, smell, and feel of food on your tongue; in order to sense the qualities of food, we must have nerves. You've probably had a toothache, stomach cramp, or gas pains, so you know from direct experience that you have pain receptors and nerves in your digestive system.

Our brain talks to our gut; our gut talks to our brain. This is a two-way communication. When our behavior changes in a certain way, our brain sends a message

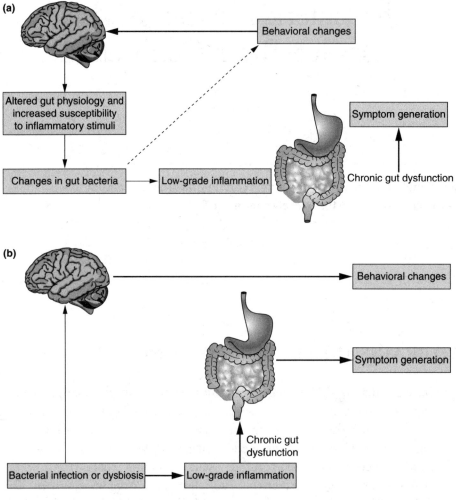

Figure 10.1   **The enteric nervous system.** (McLean, P., Calver, A., Alpers, D., Collins, S., Shanahan, F., & Lee, K. (2009). The emerging role of the microbial-gastrointestinal-neural axis. *Gastroenterology Insights*, 1(1), e3. https://doi.org/10.4081/gi.2009.e3)

that changes our gut bacteria, causing low-grade inflammation and possibly gastrointestinal (GI) distress. Similarly, if we have dysbiosis in our gut, it can lead to behavioral changes. (See Figure 10.1.)

We see that there is a high incidence of people who have mental health issues who also have digestive issues. For example, leaky gut increases the incidence of all sorts of mental dysfunction, including depression, fatigue, confusion, poor memory, and more. Seventy to ninety percent of people who have irritable bowel syndrome (IBS) also experience some sort of mood or anxiety disorder, including schizophrenia, major depression, and panic disorder. People with IBS are also more likely to experience migraines and fibromyalgia. It's estimated that about two-thirds of adults and children on the autistic spectrum have GI dysfunction. In the National Institutes of Health 2004 Consensus statement, ataxia, epilepsy, anxiety, depression, and migraine are all listed as associated diseases with celiac disease. In 2009, Burk and colleagues reported that in 72 people with celiac disease, 28 percent had migraines, 20 percent had carpel tunnel syndrome, 35 percent reported a history of psychiatric disease, and 35 percent had deep sensory loss.

The ENS consists of two layers in the intestinal wall: the myenteric plexus and the submucosal plexus. These two layers control muscles and secretion of neuro-peptides, neurotransmitters (serotonin, dopamine, acetylcholine), and nitric oxide. We synthesize the same neurotransmitters that work in our brain in our gut. Our neuro-transmitters can have local or systemic effects. For example, 90 percent of our serotonin is produced in our digestive system to help regulate peristalsis, smooth-muscle contraction, and mucosal secretions.

GUT HORMONES

For the ENS to control itself, it's necessary to monitor the intestinal lumen (the inside of the intestinal tube). There aren't nerves running through it; instead, it sends messages through intrinsic primary afferent neurons (IPANs). They do this by using a system of gut hormone–producing cells called enteroendocrine cells (ECs). These are distributed widely throughout the digestive system and secrete at least 16 hormones. These hormones are mainly found in the epithelium, but some are also found in the mucosal layer, neurons, central nervous system, and pancreatic islets. These are often called gut–brain peptides. These neurochemicals send messages to the gut, telling it to initiate peristalsis; relax; secrete enzymes, hormones, or hydrochloric acid; or respond in some other way.

Table 10.1 shows what's currently known about enteric hormones, where they are produced in your body, what stimulates their release, and what action they promote.

REST AND DIGEST: THE VAGUS NERVE AND THE SYMPATHETIC AND PARASYMPATHETIC NERVOUS SYSTEM

A large part of the communication between the digestive system and the brain runs through the vagus nerve at the brain stem (at the base of the brain).

Table 10.1 Enteric Hormones and Their Main Functions

Hormone	Where Produced	Stimuli for Release	Action
Somatostatin	D cells of pancreatic islet	Growth hormone and somatomedins, low pH	Inhibits insulin, thyroid-stimulating hormone, growth hormone, and glucagon secretion
Cholecystokinin (CCK)	Duodenum, intestinal mucosa	Partially digested fats and proteins in the duodenum	Inhibits gastrin production, slowing gastric emptying; stimulates gallbladder contraction; stimulates secretion of pancreatic enzymes; increases motility in the colon; increases satiety
Leptin	Adipose tissue, placenta, ovaries, muscle, stomach, breasts, bone marrow, long-term energy	Eating a meal, thyroid-stimulating hormone, insulin	Triggers sensation of satiety; suppresses appetite; mediates pituitary, liver balance; enhances weight loss; inhibits ghrelin
Ghrelin	Stomach, pancreas	Being hungry, not enough sleep, stress	Stimulates hunger and eating; promotes intestinal repair; promotes growth in fetuses
Gastrin	Stomach and duodenum	Peptides, amino acids, caffeine, some alcoholic beverages	Triggers secretion of HCl and pepsinogen in stomach; increases tone of esophageal sphincter
Secretin	Duodenum	Acid in small intestine	Stimulates enzyme and insulin release in pancreas; stimulates secretion bicarbonate, and enzyme secretion from pancreas; stimulates insulin release
Glucagon-like peptide (GLP-1)	Pancreas	Glucose, fat	Stimulates insulin release; inhibits glucagon
Glucose-dependent insulinotopic polypeptide (GIP)	Pancreas	Glucose, fat	Stimulates insulin release
Motilin	Stomach, small and large intestines	Gallbladder and pancreatic secretions, fasting	Promotes gastric emptying and GI motility

Ninety percent of the communication runs from the gut to the brain, and the remaining 10 percent from the brain to the gut. The vagus nerve gets its name from the Latin word for "wanderer." It wanders from the brain into all of the organs in the abdomen except the adrenals. The vagus nerve regulates homeostasis, heart rate, digestion, and breathing; reduces inflammation; and enhances mood. It also provides senses to the tongue for taste and senses in the throat, heart, lungs, and belly. It regulates muscles in the neck that are needed for swallowing and speech, as well as some reflexes.

Specifically in the digestive system, the vagus nerve stimulates the release of digestive enzymes, slows movement of the food out of the stomach, coordinates motility of the intestines, decreases inflammation and intestinal permeability, and enhances satiety. Figure 10.2 gives a pictoral version of this description.

The nervous system, like all systems in our body, needs balance. The sympathetic, "on-the-go" nervous system is where our activity originates. The parasympathetic, "chill-out" nervous system houses the vagus nerve, which is the largest in the body with this role.

When we are experiencing stress, such as eating on the run when driving through traffic, or are feeling fearful, anxious, or worried, our digestive capacity is

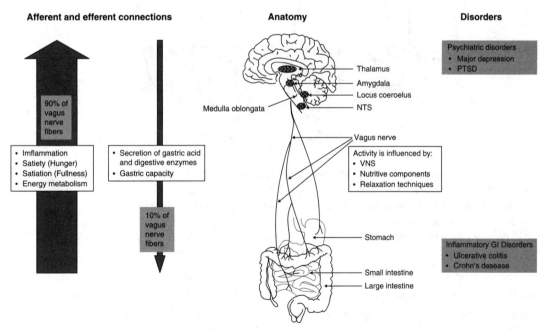

Figure 10.2 **Overview of the basic anatomy and functions of the vagus nerve.** (Breit S, Kupferberg A, Rogler G, Hasler G. Vagus Nerve as Modulator of the Brain-Gut Axis in Psychiatric and Inflammatory Disorders. Front Psychiatry. 2018;9:44. Published 2018 Mar 13. doi:10.3389/fpsyt.2018.00044)

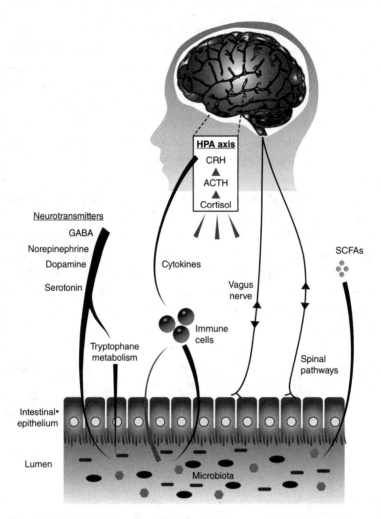

Figure 10.3 The Gut–Brain Bi-directional Routes of Communication. The multiple bidirectional routes of communication between the brain and the gut microbiota. These routes include the vagus nerve, the hypothalamic-pituitary-adrenal axis (HPA), cytokines produced by the immune system, tryptophan metabolism and production of short chain fatty acids. (Dinan, T.G., Stilling, R.M., Stanton, C. & Cryan, J.F., (2015) Collective unconscious: How gut microbes shape human behavior. *J of Psych.* Res. 63: 1-9.)

compromised. The sympathetic nerves slow GI secretions and motility. In extreme stress, they shut down digestion. Conversely, when we feel relaxed, our parasympathetic nervous system signals gut secretions and peristalsis, and digestion works easily. This is probably the origin of the after-lunch siesta.

Continued stress in our body and mind affects the body's ability to heal and perform. Because the digestive tract repairs and replaces itself every few days, it is one of the first places where our bodies alert us that all is not well. Stress and emotions play a major role in many digestive problems, such as ulcers, inflammatory bowel disease (IBD), irritable bowel syndrome (IBS), constipation, diarrhea, and gastroesophageal reflux disease (GERD), and these conditions often respond to stress-reduction techniques. Vagus nerve dysfunction has been associated with chronic fatigue syndrome, major depression, post-traumatic stress disorder, attention deficit hyperactivity disorder, cognitive disorders, weight management and leptin resistance, heart failure, high blood pressure, stroke, immune function, inflammatory bowel diseases, constipation, rheumatoid arthritis, and epilepsy. Rest and relaxation help to restore nervous-immune balance.

Deep breathing, meditation, prayer, spending time in nature, gardening, yoga, tai chi, painting, singing, playing music, acupuncture, *Bifidobacteria longum*, strength training, gargling vigorously several times a day, and other relaxing hobbies increases vagal tone, signaling to our body that all is well. We spend so much time in the outer world that taking time for our inner world brings us into better balance. My clients and I find that resting two hours each day during the daylight hours can do wonders for all sorts of health issues. Try it for three to four weeks and see what happens!

FOOD AND OUR BRAIN

Our relationship with food begins in the brain. Our body begins preparing for a meal when we begin thinking about that meal. Mostly, we eat when we are hungry. Yet many people eat when they are not hungry. We can eat mindlessly or because it's our typically response to our environment or to an emotional stressor. For example, you stop by a neighbor's house and they offer you something to eat and drink; you aren't hungry but eat because it's the neighborly custom. Or you are at work and people have brought food to share; as you walk by it, the cake or cookies scream out "eat some of me!"

We eat emotionally because we are upset, angry, lonely, depressed, happy, celebrating, procrastinating, rewarding ourselves, and a myriad of other reasons that have absolutely nothing to do with our body's need for nutrients.

Manufactured foods are designed to stimulate our tastes for fat, sugar, and salt. Layers upon layers of flavor "sing" to our brain a song that makes us feel rewarded and indulged. This stimulates the release of serotonin and dopamine, and then we want more of that food. So we continue to eat, even when we aren't hungry.

This emphasizes the importance of eating in a relaxed manner and appreciating the food you are about to ingest. Many people call this "mindful eating" or "gentle eating," which simply focuses our awareness on the flavors in each bite. Sounds pretty simple, yet most of the time we eat mindlessly instead. Some people find that taking time to say grace and to look at and smell the food, as well as making a special time and place for eating, can dramatically enhance their total digestive function more completely than can enzymes, bitters, or other digestive supplements.

PSYCHOBIOTICS

John Cryan, Ted Dinan, and their research group developed a new term in 2013: "psychobiotic." They define this "as a live organism that when ingested in adequate amounts, produces health benefits in patients suffering from a psychiatric illness. As a class of probiotic, these bacteria are capable of producing and delivering neuroactive substances such as gamma-aminobutyric acid and serotonin, which act on the brain-gut axis." Pulling this definition apart a bit, these are probiotic microbes that can modulate mood. The microbiota synthesize neurotransmitters, which modulate brain function. They also affect our reactions to stress via the vagus nerve and hypothalamus-pituitary-adrenal axis.

Early research on humans is demonstrating that probiotics can modulate anxiety and depression. In one study, women who received *Lactobacillus rhamnosus* HN001 during pregnancy had significantly lower amounts of postpartum depression and anxiety than controls. A group of people who experienced IBS, anxiety, and depression were given *Bifidobacterium longum* NCC3001 daily for 6 weeks. The probiotic group had reductions in depression and had improved quality of life compared to the control group, but there was no change in anxiety levels. One review paper reported that in healthy adults, taking probiotics had a significant improvement in psychological symptoms. Another paper associated probiotics with a significant reduction in depression. And yet another paper used the National Health and Nutrition Examination Survey (NHANES) data: Of over 18,000 people who were queried, 14.11 percent ate probiotic-rich foods such as yogurt, buttermilk, kefir, and kimchee on either of the two interview days where they were asked for dietary recall. Others had taken probiotic supplements at least once in the last 30 days. People who ate probiotic-rich foods or took probiotic supplements experienced significantly less depression. These people also ate more dietary fiber (think prebiotics) and fewer calories overall, and smoked less.

Although research on psychobiotics is still in its infancy, introducing prebiotics and probiotics into food and supplements and balancing the microbiome may be new ways to treat people with mood disorders and mental health issues. Two other probiotic microbes that are getting research attention are *Bifidobacterium longum* 1714 and *Lactobacillus reuteri.*

Neurotransmitters and Microbes

Neurotransmitters are chemicals that are released into the synapse (space) between nerve cells when a nerve fires. When the neurotransmitter diffuses across the synapse and touches the next nerve cell, it triggers that cell to fire. Balances and imbalances of neurotransmitters affect mood. Common neurotransmitters include acetylcholine; catecholamines such as epinephrine (adrenaline), norephinephrine (noradrenaline) and dopamine; GABA; serotonin; substance P, glutamate, and melatonin. Neurotransmitters affect gut motility; regulate blood flow; control absorption of nutrients; and modulate the innate immune system response in the digestive tract and the microbiome.

Table 10.2 Neurotransmitter Synthesis by Probiotic Microbes

Neurotransmitter	*Microbes That Synthesize This Neurotransmitter*
Acetylcholine	*Lactobacilli, Escherichia, Saccharomyces*
Catecholamines	*Escherichia, Saccharomyces, Bacillus*
Dopamine	*Bacillus* spp (including *Bacillus infantis*)
Gamma-aminobutyric acid (GABA)	*Lactobacilli,* including *Lactobacillus rhamnosis, Lactobacillus helviticus, Lactobacillus brevis, Lactobacillus plantarum, Lactobacillus delbrueckii* subsp. *Bulgaricus* *Bifidobacterium,* including *Bifidobacterium infantis, Bifidobacterium longum, Bifidobacterium dentium, Bifidobacterium infantis*
Melatonin	*Lactobacilli,* including *Lactobacillus bulgaricus, Lactobacillus delbrueckii* ssp., *Lactobacillus casei, Lactobacillus plantarum.* *Bifidobacterium,* including *Bifidobacterium longum, Bifidobacterium infantis, Bifidobacterium. breve Streptococcus salivarius* ssp.
Norphenephrine (= Noradrenalin)	*Escherichia, Sacchomyces, Bacillus* (specifically *Bacillus infantis* sp.)
Serotonin	*Candida, Saccharomyces, Enterococcus, Escherichia, Streptococcus*

Neurotransmitters are imbalanced in people with many conditions, including mental health and mood issues including depression and anxiety, pain response, strokes, Autism spectrum, brain injury, seizure disorders, Parkinson's disease, Alzheimer's disease, Huntington's disease, and inflammatory bowel disease. Microbes in your gut produce a significant percent of your neurotransmitters. Ninety percent of seratonin is produced in your gut. Here is just some of what's currently known.

Some of this research was done in mice. Many of the human studies were done by giving people fermented foods that contain these microbes and then measuring their levels of the neurotransmitters.

From this research, we know that:

- Be adequately nourished. Neurotransmitters are comprised of amino acids, primarily choline and tyrosine. Eating enough protein and virtually all other vitamins and minerals will ensure that you have the building materials to synthesize neurotransmitters.
- Drink black and/or green tea. Tea contains L-theanine which enhances synthesis of serotonin, dopamine and GABA.
- We should cultured and fermented foods to boost your neurotransmitter production.
- We should plant foods that are naturally rich in probiotic microorganisms.
- Probiotic microbes increase specific neurotransmitters and affect mood. There is ongoing research on these psychobiotics.

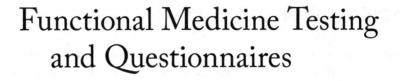

CHAPTER 11

Functional Medicine Testing and Questionnaires

> **"All truth passes through three stages: First, it is ridiculed; second, it is violently opposed; third, it is accepted as self-evident."**
>
> —Arthur Schopenhauer (1788–1860)

Modern medicine equates the absence of disease with health. Often people walk into a doctor's office feeling tired and run down, have an exam and a battery of tests that are normal, and are told that all is well. While it's good to know that there isn't anything serious wrong, they still don't feel well. This is where functional, complementary, and alternative medicines play a critical role. It's always important to treat the person and not the test. People often seek "alternative" treatment as a last resort, but the best medicine is medicine that combines what is the best of standard medicine care plus the best of functional and integrative care. It's in this way that the root causes of your issues can be resolved best.

Medical disciplines and medical testing are like the ancient East Indian folktale of the six blind men touching the elephant. We test for what we "see." But each of us is "blind" because no matter how much we know, there is still so much that is unknown to us. There are hundreds, if not thousands, of possible tests that clinicians can run to help diagnose what is going on with us. The art is in knowing which specific tests may be most useful in helping to optimize our health.

This chapter discusses testing that our own doctors may or may not be familiar with yet. Included are tests that are new and upcoming today but will become routine in the future. The results, taken in combination with how we feel, our family history, regular medical tests, and our symptoms can be a guide to putting the puzzle together to optimize our health.

TYPICAL MEDICAL TESTING

There are many medical tests that are done by most physicians. These include gastrointestinal scoping, ultrasound, and blood tests. Here are a few of the most commonly run tests.

Upper endoscopy (Upper GI): In this test a gastroenterologist will place a scope into the mouth; it runs through the throat, stomach, and into the duodenum, the upper part of the small intestine. This scope has a light and a camera so that the physician can literally see the inside of the GI tract. This test is used to determine the presence of stomach or duodenal ulcers, bleeding, esophageal issues such as eosinophilic esophagitis, gastrointestinal reflux and whether it's erosive or not, bile reflux, polyps, strictures, and tumors. It's typically done under anesthesia and biopsies may be performed. Some gastroenterologists may also perform additional tests to determine sufficiency of gastric acid (with a Smart Meter) and other tests.

Colonoscopy or sigmoidoscopy: These are also scoping tests utilized by gastroenterologists. A colonoscopy explores from the anus up to the ileocecal valve. A sigmoidoscopy checks only the rectum and the lower part of the colon. The most common reasons these tests are run are to rule out colon and rectal cancers, find and remove polyps, find and dilate strictures, discover the cause of rectal bleeding, find the cause of chronic abdominal pain, and treat bleeding diverticula (pockets in the colon).

Screening for Colorectal Cancers: The American Cancer Society recommends that people between the ages of 45 and 75 have periodic testing to detect colon cancer and rectal cancers. Until recently, a colonoscopy with bowel preparation and anesthesia was the only option.

Relatively inexpensive new tests can be used to screen for cancers instead. If these tests are abnormal, a follow-up colonoscopy or sigmoidoscopy is performed. Talk with your doctor about the pros and cons of each of these, and consult your insurance company to see if these newer tests are covered. Such tests include:

- Fecal immunochemical test (FIT): This test is covered by Medicare annually.
- Guaiac-based fecal occult blood test (gFOBT)
- Stool DNA test (Cologuard): This test is covered by Medicare every 3 years.
- CT colonographic (virtual colonoscopy): This test still requires a full bowel prep, exposes you to some radiation, and if positive still requires a traditional colonoscopy.

FUNCTIONAL MEDICINE TESTING

There are numerous tests used in the field of functional medicine which are not currently used in mainstream medicine. Functional medicine testing often leads the way, with conventional medicine adopting these tests over time. As such, you may need to teach your own doctor about these tests. If your own doctor is not willing or able to order these tests, look for a Functional Medicine clinician to work with you. You can find one by calling the lab to see who is in your area who orders these tests, or look online at: https://www.ifm.org/find-a-practitioner/. The following are the ones I've found to be most useful for digestive problems. Most of these are laboratory tests, but a few are home tests you can perform on your own!

The following tests are typically ordered by a physician. Many may be covered by insurance, with a moderate co-pay. Some are also covered by Medicare/Medicaid. Others may require an out-of-pocket payment. If you are willing to pay for these tests, you can order them yourself through companies such as DirectLabs, Any Lab Test Now, and Life Extension.

Table 11.1 lists lab testing companies and is divided into the DIGIN categories. It's not an all-inclusive list but rather a list of companies that I am currently familiar

Table 11.1 **DIGIN Model Icons for Testing**

DIGIN	*Tests*	*Labs Offering the Testing*
Digestion/ absorption	Breath testing for enzyme insufficiencies of lactose, fructose, sucrose, or d-xylose	■ Gastroenterology offices ■ Genova Diagnostics ■ QuinTron ■ Quest
	Stool testing often has digestion and absorption markers, such as pancreatic elastase, fecal fats, muscle (meat) fibers, vegetable fibers, and carbohydrates.	■ Doctor's Data Lab/Labrix ■ Genova Diagnostics
	Nutritional testing: vitamins, minerals	■ This can be ordered through local labs that your doctor uses. ■ Genova, Nutreval, ONE, or ION panels ■ Spectracell Labs ■ Quest Diagnostics/Cleveland HeartLab
Intestinal permeability	Lactulose/mannitol	■ Gastroenterology offices ■ BioHealth Lab ■ Genova Diagnostics
	Zonulin Zonulin/occludin/LPS	■ Doctors Data Lab/Labrix ■ Cyrex Labs ■ Dunwoody Labs

(continued)

Table 11.1 **DIGIN Model Icons for Testing** *(continued)*

Gut microbiome/ dysbiosis testing	Stool testing	■ BioHealth Lab ■ Diagnostic Solutions ■ Doctor's Data Lab/Labrix ■ Genova Diagnostics ■ Great Plains Lab
	Urinary organic acid testing	■ Genova Diagnostics ■ Great Plains Lab ■ US BioTek
	Breath testing (SIBO)	■ Gastroenterology offices ■ BioHealth ■ Genova Diagnostics ■ QuinTron
	Parasite testing: microscopic testing, genetic testing, and/or antigens in stool test	■ Diagnostic Solutions ■ Doctor's Data Lab/Labrix ■ Genova Diagnostics
	Fungal overgrowth: stool testing, antibody testing, urinary organic acid test	■ Traditional Labs ■ Genova Diagnostics ■ Great Plains Lab ■ US BioTek
	Screening for postinfectious IBS	■ Cyrex Labs
	Helicobacter pylori testing	■ This can be ordered through local labs that your doctor uses. The following companies include *H. pylori* tests as part of a broader panel of tests: ■ Diagnostic Solutions ■ Doctor's Data Lab/Labrix ■ Quest Diagnostics/Cleveland HeartLab
	Microbiome testing: general	■ uBiome ■ Viome
	Heavy metal testing	■ Doctors Data Lab/Labrix ■ Genova Diagnostics ■ Quicksilver Mercury Tri-Test

Inflammation/ immune function	Calprotectin, lactoferrin, or both	■ This can be ordered through local labs that your doctor uses. ■ Doctors Data Lab/Labrix ■ Genova Diagnostic
	Systemic infection	■ Cyrex Labs
	Predictive antibodies	■ Cyrex Labs
	Celiac disease testing	Celiac: ■ This can be ordered through local labs that your doctor uses. Celiac testing is also offered by ■ Doctor's Data ■ Genova Diagnostics ■ Cell Science ■ Quest Diagnostics/Cleveland HeartLab ■ US Biotek ■ Vibrant America ■ Cyrex Labs
	Gluten and wheat sensitivity testing	■ US BioTek ■ Vibrant America ■ Quest Diagnostics/Cleveland HeartLab
	Food allergies and sensitivities	■ Altesse ■ Cell Science Systems ■ Elisa Act ■ Genova Diagnostics ■ Great Plains Lab ■ Immuno Labs ■ KMBO Diagnostics ■ Meridian Valley Lab ■ MRT/LEAP ■ Vibrant America (IgE only) ■ US BioTek Lab
Enteric Nervous system/	Antigen testing	■ Cyrex

(continued)

Table 11.1   DIGIN Model Icons for Testing *(continued)*

	Neurotransmitter testing	■ Julia Ross/Mood Cure and Apex Energetics have excellent neurotransmitter questionnaires to reveal imbalances and needs.
		Urine testing: ■ Doctor's Data/Labrix ■ Dunwoody Labs ■ Life Extension ■ NeuroScience ■ Sanesco Labs ■ ZRT Labs
General genomic testing	Tests for SNPs/genomic strengths and weaknesses In order to complete these tests, all that is needed is a saliva sample or a cotton swab of your saliva. Some are direct to consumer and others require a physician to order testing.	■ 23andMe (does not provide clinical application) ■ Ancestry.com (does not provide clinical application) ■ Aperion ■ Cell Science ■ Diagnostic Solutions (with Opus23) ■ DNA Life ■ Genova Diagnostics ■ Great Plains Labs ■ IQYou ■ Livewello ■ Methyl Genetic Nutrition ■ Nordic Laboratories ■ NutraHacker ■ Nutrigenomix ■ Opus23 ■ Pathway Genomics ■ Prometheas (uses raw data from other testing) ■ PureGenomics

Starting from here, you'll see notations indicating which parts of the DIGIN model are most likely to be revealed from these tests. $\mathcal{Q}$ D I G I N with. If done correctly, breath testing offers uniform results. With all the other tests, each lab has slightly different markers and techniques. It's a bit like the Wild West, and no one test is foolproof. Still, you can gain information from these tests that can help you get well.

I remember working with a man who was an engineer. He drew a diagram that demonstrated an approximate 21-day cycle of his symptoms and subsequent resolution. This suggested a parasite infection to me. Yet the lab test didn't find any evidence of parasites. So, we sent it to a different lab. They reported finding an amoeba that typically wasn't found in humans. The point of this story is to keep looking if the results don't make sense.

COMPREHENSIVE STOOL TESTING: A PLACE TO BEGIN

Useful for anyone with digestive problems, comprehensive digestive stool analysis (called by various labs: CDSA, CSDA, CSA, stool profile, and GI-effects) is often where underlying issues can be found. If you choose to obtain only one test, make it a comprehensive stool test that includes parasitology screening (see later in the chapter). This is a home test kit; you will collect your own stool sample(s) and then ship it back to the lab. Shipping labels are included in the test kit, and the shipping cost is included in the price of the test.

A stool test is used to assess bacterial balance and health, digestive function, and dysbiosis. It identifies the types of bacteria and fungi present and measures the levels of beneficial, possibly harmful, and disease-producing microbes. Most labs do sensitivities on any bacteria or fungi (such as candida) that are found to determine what medications or herbs will be most effective against them. Some tests look at the diversity and balance of the microbiome. While this is very crude, it gives some indication of what is happening in your microbiome at that moment in time. Your microbiome is dynamic and changes somewhat throughout the day and week, depending on what you've eaten and your activities. These tests typically also measure calprotectin, lactoferrin, eosinophil protein X, and/or lysozyme levels to detect inflammation in the large intestine. Elevations could indicate ulcerative colitis, Crohn's disease, colon cancer, diverticulitis, or other inflammatory conditions. These markers can be used to find the inflammation without scoping, can help distinguish between irritable bowel syndrome (IBS) and more serious conditions, and can also be used to monitor whether the treatment or maintenance program you are using is effective for inflammatory conditions.

In addition, a stool test measures how well you are digesting fats, carbohydrates, and proteins; gives some indication of how well your pancreas is performing; and measures levels of butyric acid and short-chain fatty acids (SCFAs).

If candida is detected, it gives a good clinical picture. However, if it is not found in the stool, there still could be a candida issue. Organic acid testing (OAT) is the best measurement for candida and fungal infections.

These tests have morphed over the years, and many more companies offer them. Each company structures its tests differently; there currently is no standard test. Experienced clinicians may utilize three or four of these in their practice and choose the one that most likely will be of benefit to a specific patient.

When testing for dysbiosis or parasites, companies use microscopes, antigen testing, culturing microbes in petri dishes, genetic testing, and looking at metabolites. Each of these methods provides one piece of the puzzle.

H. PYLORI TESTING ⌕ DIGIN

H. pylori is the microbial culprit that drives stomach and duodenal ulcers. There are several ways to test for *H. pylori:* stool or blood antigens, urea breath testing, or genomic testing (polymerase chain reaction, or PCR). Blood testing is inexpensive and most commonly used. The American College of Gastroenterology recommends stool testing as the most specific and sensitive type, yet the cost is a lot higher. If people are taking proton-pump inhibitors (PPIs) or acid blockers, these tests may be falsely negative. These tests can be easily ordered through any physician or lab, and several of the functional labs also offer *H. pylori* testing.

CANDIDA ANTIBODY TESTS ⌕ DIGIN

Many labs, including regular medical labs, offer testing for candida antibodies. These tests can help to determine whether candida/yeast overgrowth is present. Another excellent way to determine whether there is fungal overgrowth is through organic acid testing. Dr. Crook's yeast questionnaire, presented here, is a good starting point. Many physicians will also use prescription medications to treat yeast overgrowth.

Candida Questionnaire
The following questionnaire can help determine whether candida is a factor in your own health. A candida questionnaire for use with children is presented next.

YEAST QUESTIONNAIRE—ADULT

Answering these questions and adding up the scores will help you decide if yeasts contribute to your health problems. However, you will not obtain an automatic "yes" or "no" answer.

For each "yes" answer in Section A, circle the points that correspond to that question. Total your score and record it at the end of the section. Then move on to Sections B and C and score as indicated.

Add your three scores to get your grand total.

SECTION A: HISTORY

Score

1. Have you taken tetracycline (Sumycin, Panmycin, Vibramycin, Minocin, and so forth) or other antibiotics for acne for one month (or longer)? 35

2. Have you, at any time in your life, taken other "broad-spectrum" antibiotics* for respiratory, urinary tract, or other infections (for two months or longer, or in shorter courses four or more times in a one-year period)? 35

3. Have you taken a broad-spectrum antibiotic drug,* even a single course? 6

4. Have you, at any time in your life, been bothered by persistent prostatitis, vaginitis, or other problems affecting your reproductive organs? 25

5. Have you been pregnant two or more times? 5

5a. One time? 3

6. Have you taken birth control pills for more than two years? 15

6a. For six months to two years? 8

7. Have you taken prednisone, Decadron, or other cortisone-type drugs for more than two weeks? 15

7a. For two weeks or less? 6

8. Does exposure to perfumes, insecticides, fabric shop odors, and other chemicals provoke:
   Moderate to severe symptoms? 20
   Mild symptoms? 5

9. Are your symptoms worse on damp, muggy days or in moldy places? 20

10. Have you had athlete's foot, ringworm, "jock itch," or other chronic fungus infections of the skin or nails? Have such infections been:
    Severe or persistent? 20
    Mild to moderate? 10

---

* Includes Keflex, ampicillin, amoxicillin, Ceclor, Bactrim, and Septra. Such antibiotics kill off "good germs" while they're killing off those that cause infection.

11. Do you crave sugar? 10
12. Do you crave breads? 10
13. Do you crave alcoholic beverages? 10
14. Does tobacco smoke really bother you? 10

Total Score, Section A _____

SECTION B: MAJOR SYMPTOMS

For each of your symptoms, enter the appropriate figure in the Score column:
   If a symptom is occasional or mild: 3 points
   If a symptom is frequent and/or moderately severe: 6 points
   If a symptom is severe and/or disabling: 9 points
   Total your score and record it at the end of this section.

                                                                                Score

1. Fatigue or lethargy .... _____
2. Feeling of being "drained" .... _____
3. Poor memory .... _____
4. Feeling "spacey" or "unreal" .... _____
5. Depression .... _____
6. Inability to make decisions .... _____
7. Numbness, burning, or tingling .... _____
8. Muscle aches or weakness .... _____
9. Pain and/or swelling in joints .... _____
10. Abdominal pain .... _____
11. Constipation .... _____
12. Diarrhea .... _____
13. Bloating, belching, or intestinal gas .... _____
14. Troublesome vaginal burning, itching, or discharge .... _____
15. Persistent vaginal burning or itching .... _____
16. Prostatitis .... _____
17. Impotence .... _____
18. Loss of sexual desire or feeling .... _____
19. Endometriosis or infertility .... _____
20. Cramps and/or other menstrual irregularities .... _____
21. Premenstrual tension .... _____
22. Attacks of anxiety or crying .... _____
23. Cold hands or feet and/or chilliness .... _____
24. Shaking or irritable when hungry .... _____

Total Score, Section B _____

SECTION C: OTHER SYMPTOMS*

For each of your symptoms, enter the appropriate figure in the Score column:

If a symptom is occasional or mild: 1 point

If a symptom is frequent and/or moderately severe: 2 points

If a symptom is severe and/or disabling: 3 points

Total your score and record it at the end of this section.

Score

1. Drowsiness . . . . _____
2. Irritability or jitteriness . . . . _____
3. Lack of coordination . . . . _____
4. Inability to concentrate. . . . . _____
5. Frequent mood swings. . . . . _____
6. Headaches. . . . . _____
7. Dizziness/loss of balance . . . . _____
8. Pressure above ears, feeling of head swelling . . . . _____
9. Tendency to bruise easily. . . . . _____
10. Chronic rashes or itching . . . . _____
11. Numbness, tingling . . . . _____
12. Indigestion or heartburn . . . . _____
13. Food sensitivity or intolerance. . . . . _____
14. Mucus in stools . . . . _____
15. Rectal itching . . . . _____
16. Dry mouth or throat. . . . . _____
17. Rash or blisters in mouth . . . . _____
18. Bad breath. . . . . _____
19. Foot, body, or hair odor not relieved by washing . . . . _____
20. Nasal congestion or postnasal drip . . . . _____
21. Nasal itching. . . . . _____
22. Sore throat. . . . . _____
23. Laryngitis, loss of voice . . . . _____
24. Cough or recurrent bronchitis . . . . _____
25. Pain or tightness in chest . . . . _____
26. Wheezing or shortness of breath . . . . _____
27. Urgency or urinary frequency . . . . _____
28. Burning on urination . . . . _____

* While the symptoms in this section commonly occur in people with yeast-connected illness, they are also found in other individuals.

29. Spots in front of eyes or erratic vision . . . . _____
30. Burning or tearing of eyes . . . . _____
31. Recurrent infections or fluid in ears . . . . _____
32. Ear pain or deafness. . . . . _____

Total Score, Section C _____

- Total Score, Section A
- Total Score, Section B _____
- Total Score, Section C _____
- Grand Total Score _____
- The Grand Total Score will help you and your physician decide whether your health problems are yeast connected. Scores for women will run higher than for men, as seven items in the questionnaire apply exclusively to women, while only two apply exclusively to men.
- Yeast-connected health problems are almost certainly present with scores higher than 180 for women and 140 for men.
- Yeast-connected health problems are probably present with scores higher than 120 for women and 90 for men.
- Yeast-connected health problems are possibly present with scores higher than 60 for women and 40 for men.
- With scores lower than 60 for women and 40 for men, yeasts are less apt to cause health problems.

YEAST QUESTIONNAIRE—CHILD

For each "yes" answer, circle the points that correspond to that question. Total your score and record it at the end of the questionnaire.

Score

1. During the two years before your child was born, were you bothered by recurrent vaginitis, menstrual irregularities, premenstrual tension, fatigue, headache, depression, digestive disorders, or "feeling bad all over"? 30
2. Was your child bothered by thrush?
   Mild? 10
   Severe or persistent? 20
3. Was your child bothered by frequent diaper rashes in infancy?
   Mild? 10
   Severe or persistent? 20
4. During infancy, was your child bothered by colic and irritability lasting longer than three months?
   Mild? 10
   Severe or persistent? 20

 5. Are your child's symptoms worse on damp days or in damp or moldy places? 20

 6. Has your child been bothered by recurrent or persistent "athlete's foot"
 or chronic fungus infections of his or her skin or nails? 30

 7. Has your child been bothered by recurrent hives, eczema, or other
 skin problems? 10

 8. Has your child received:
 Four or more courses of antibiotic drugs during the past year? Or has your
 child received continuous "prophylactic" courses of antibiotic drugs? 80
 Eight or more courses of "broad-spectrum" antibiotics (such as amoxicillin,
 Keflex, Septra, Bactrim, or Ceclor) during the past three years? 50

 9. Has your child experienced recurrent ear problems? 10

 10. Has your child had tubes inserted in his or her ears? 10

 11. Has your child been labeled "hyperactive"?
 Mild? 10
 Severe? 20

 12. Is your child bothered by learning problems (even though his or her
 early developmental history was normal)? 10

 13. Does your child have a short attention span? 10

 14. Is your child persistently irritable, unhappy, and hard to please? 10

 15. Has your child been bothered by persistent or recurrent digestive problems,
 including constipation, diarrhea, bloating, or excessive gas?
 Mild? 10
 Moderate? 20
 Severe? 30

 16. Has your child been bothered by persistent nasal congestion, cough,
 and/or wheezing? 10

 17. Is your child unusually tired, unhappy, or depressed?
 Mild? 10
 Severe? 20

 18. Has your child been bothered by recurrent headaches, abdominal pain,
 or muscle aches?
 Mild? 10
 Severe? 20

 19. Does your child crave sweets? 10

 20. Does exposure to perfume, insecticides, gas, or other chemicals provoke
 moderate to severe symptoms? 30

 21. Does tobacco smoke really bother your child? 20

 22. Do you feel that your child isn't well, yet diagnostic tests and studies
 haven't revealed the cause? 10

Total Score

- Yeasts possibly play a role in causing health problems in children with scores of 60 or higher.
- Yeasts probably play a role in causing health problems in children with scores of 100 or higher.
- Yeasts almost certainly play a role in causing health problems in children with scores of 140 or higher.

Source: Used with permission from William Crook, *The Yeast Connection and Women's Health.* Garden City Park, NY: Square One Publishers, 2003.

PARASITOLOGY TESTING $_Q$ DIGIN

Though we think of parasites as something we get from traveling in other countries, it's not true. According to the Centers for Disease Control and Prevention, parasites affect millions of Americans. Many of us live happily with parasites, but they can cause GI issues, seizures, blindness, complications during pregnancy, and even death. In 2014, the CDC targeted five parasitic infections that are either widespread or have severe consequences.

- *Trypanosoma cruzi.* This is the cause of Chagas disease, also known as American trypanosomiasis. In the United States 300,000 people are infected. About 300 babies each year are born with this infection. It's transmitted by insects called triatomine bugs who suck our blood and poop on us during sleep. They can also be passed through contaminated food, blood transfusions, organ transplants, and during pregnancy. The insects live in houses that are made from natural materials, such as mud, adobe, straw, and palm thatch. In the acute state, the infection can look like most others: fever, fatigue, body aches, headache, rash, loss of appetite, diarrhea, and/or vomiting. Children who rub bug feces in their eyes which causes their upper and lower eyelids to swell, which is called Romana's sign. Doctors may also pick up on this infection by noticing enlargement of the liver or spleen, swollen glands, or swelling at the site of the bites. Rarely, some children can die from this infection. When this infection becomes chronic, it can cause heart and GI issues. This is treated with anti-parasitic medications.
- *Taenia solium.* Over a thousand people are hospitalized each year for systematic cystericosis or the cysts that develop when we have tapeworms. It's passed through fecal-oral transmissions when people with an infection fail to wash their hands after going to the bathroom. Eggs subsequently get passed from their hands to

surfaces or can be passed through touch. One more reason to thoroughly wash our hands after using the bathroom. They form cysts (hence cysticercosis) in muscles, skin, rarely in the eyes, and in the brain and spinal cord. It can be treated with anti-parasitic medications. Sometimes the cysts are surgically removed.

- *Toxoplasma gondii.* This organism is responsible for toxoplasmosis, and typically we get it from cats' litter boxes, contaminated garden soil, undercooked meat that's been contaminated, lack of hand washing, contaminated cooking utensils, or contaminated drinking water. Infants whose moms are infected during pregnancy can be born with birth defects. People whose immune systems are weak, such as people with AIDS, those who have had organ transplants, or those currently being treated with chemotherapy, can have severe infections that can even cause death.

- *Trichomonas.* Trichomoniasis infections affect 3.7 million Americans. It is most commonly contracted sexually and can cause issues in pregnancy. It is easily treated and can be prevented with the use of condoms. Seventy percent of people who have Trichomoniasis have no symptoms. Others experience only mild irritation of the penis or vagina, or burning with urination; women may experience a change in vaginal discharge with increased volume or thinning of the discharge.

Genova Diagnostics Laboratory routinely surveys stool samples that come into the lab for parasites. Parasites were discovered in 23.5 percent of 14,000 stool samples that came from people who were experiencing symptoms of irritable bowel syndrome. The most common ones were *Blastocystis hominis* (12.5 percent), *Dientamoeba fragilis* (3.8 percent), *Entamoeba* species (3.4 percent), *Endolimax nana* (2.2 percent), and *Giardia lamblia* (0.7 percent). More than 130 types of parasites have been found in Americans. Parasites have become more prevalent for many reasons, including contaminated water supplies, day-care centers, ease of international travel, contaminated foods, increased immigration, pets, and the sexual revolution. Most people will meet a parasite at some point in their lives. Contrary to popular myths, having parasites isn't a reflection of your cleanliness.

If you have prolonged digestive symptoms, you should really consider having a comprehensive parasitology screening. Some symptoms of parasites can appear to be like other digestive problems: abdominal pain, allergy, anemia, bloating, bloody stools, chronic fatigue, constipation, coughing, diarrhea, gas, granulomas, irritable bowel syndrome, itching, joint and muscle aches, nervousness, pain, poor immune response, rashes, sleep disturbances, teeth grinding, unexplained fever, and unexplained weight loss. Most doctors use random ova and parasite (O & P) testing, which misses many parasites, so repeated testing is often necessary to get definitive results. For example, in order to definitively rule out giardia with O & P, eight tests would need to be performed.

Cryptosporidium, Giardia, and *Clostridium difficile* can easily be tested through stool antigen tests. The most accurate testing is done by laboratories that specialize in parasitology testing. Some labs recommend inducing diarrhea with an oral laxative in order to detect parasites that live further up the digestive tract. Other parasites may be found by using a rectal swab rather than a stool sample. Still others use PCR genetic testing.

PARASITE QUESTIONNAIRE
Check if yes.

1. Have you ever been to Africa, Asia, Central or South America, China, Europe, Israel, Mexico, or Russia?
2. Have you traveled to the Bahamas, the Caribbean, Hawaii, or other tropical islands?
3. Do you frequently swim in freshwater lakes, ponds, or streams while abroad?
4. Did you serve overseas while in the military?
5. Were you a prisoner of war in World War II, Korea, or Vietnam?
6. Have you had an elevated white blood count, intestinal problems, night sweats, or unexplained fever during or since traveling abroad?
7. Is your water supply from a mountainous area?
8. Do you drink untested water?
9. Have you ever drunk water from lakes, rivers, or streams on hiking or camping trips without first boiling or filtering it?
10. Do you use plain tap water to clean your contact lenses?
11. Do you use regular tap water that is unfiltered for colonics or enemas?
12. Can you trace the onset of symptoms (intermittent constipation and diarrhea, muscle aches and pains, night sweats, unexplained eye ulcers) to any of the above?
13. Do you regularly eat unpeeled raw fruits and raw vegetables in salads?
14. Do you frequently eat in Armenian, Chinese, Ethiopian, Filipino, fish, Greek, Indian, Japanese, Korean, Mexican, Pakistani, Thai, or vegetarian restaurants; in delicatessens, fast-food restaurants, steak houses, or sushi or salad bars?
15. Do you use a microwave oven for cooking (as opposed to reheating) beef, fish, or pork?
16. Do you prefer fish or meat that is undercooked, (i.e., rare or medium rare)?
17. Do you frequently eat hot dogs made from pork?
18. Do you enjoy raw fish dishes like Dutch green herring, Latin American ceviche, or sushi and sashimi?
19. Do you enjoy raw meat dishes like Italian carpaccio, Middle Eastern kibbe, or steak tartare?

20. At home, do you use the same cutting board for chicken, fish, and meat as you do for vegetables?
21. Do you prepare gefilte fish at home?
22. Can you trace the onset of symptoms (anemia, bloating, distended belly, weight loss) to any of the above?
23. Have you gotten a puppy recently?
24. Have you lived with, or do you currently live with or frequently handle pets?
25. Do you forget to wash your hands after petting or cleaning up after your animals and before eating?
26. Does your pet sleep with you in bed?
27. Does your pet eat off your plates?
28. Do you clean your cat's litter box?
29. Do you keep your pets in the yard where children play?
30. Can you trace the onset of your symptoms (abdominal pain, distended belly in children, high white blood count, unexplained fever) to any of the above?
31. Do you work in a hospital?
32. Do you work in an experimental laboratory, pet shop, veterinary clinic, or zoo?
33. Do you work with or around animals?
34. Do you work in a day-care center?
35. Do you garden or work in a yard to which cats and dogs have access?
36. Do you work in sanitation?
37. Can you trace the onset of symptoms (gastrointestinal disorders) to any of the above?
38. Do you engage in oral sex?
39. Do you practice anal intercourse without the use of a condom?
40. Have you had sexual relations with a foreign-born individual?
41. Can you trace the onset of symptoms (persistent reproductive organ problems) to any of the above?

MAJOR SYMPTOMS

Please note that although some or all of these major symptoms can occur in any adult, child, or infant with parasite-based illness, these symptoms might instead be the result of one of many other illnesses.

■ Adults

1. Do you have a bluish cast around your lips?
2. Is your abdomen distended no matter what you eat?
3. Are there dark circles around or under your eyes?
4. Do you have a history of allergy?

5. Do you suffer from intermittent diarrhea and constipation, intermittent loose and hard stools, or chronic constipation?

6. Do you have persistent acne, anal itching, anemia, anorexia, bad breath, bloody stools, chronic fatigue, difficulty in breathing, edema, food sensitivities, itching, open ileocecal valve, pale skin, palpitations, premenstrual syndrome, puffy eyes, ringing of the ears, sinus congestion, skin eruptions, vague abdominal discomfort, or vertigo?

7. Do you grind your teeth?

8. Are you experiencing craving for sugar, depression, disorientation, insomnia, lethargy, loss of appetite, moodiness, or weight loss or gain?

■ Children

1. Does your child have dark circles under his or her eyes?
2. Is your child hyperactive?
3. Does your child grind or clench his teeth at night?
4. Does your child constantly pick her nose or scratch her behind?
5. Does your child have a habit of eating dirt?
6. Does your child wet his bed?
7. Is your child often restless at night?
8. Does your child cry often or for no reason?
9. Does your child tear her hair out?
10. Does your child have a limp that orthopedic treatment has not helped?
11. Does your child have a brassy, staccato-type cough?
12. Does your child have convulsions or an abnormal electroencephalogram (EEG)?
13. Does your child have recurring headaches?
14. Is your child unusually sensitive to light and prone to blinking frequently, eyelid twitching, or squinting?
15. Does your child have unusual tendencies to bleed in the gums, the nose, or the rectum?

■ Infants

1. Does your baby have severe intermittent colic?
2. Does your baby persistently bang his or her head against the crib?
3. Is your baby a chronic crier?
4. Does your baby show a blotchy rash around the perianal area?

INTERPRETATION OF QUESTIONNAIRE

■ If you answered "yes" to more than 40 items, you are at high risk for parasites.

■ If you answered "yes" to more than 30 items, you are at moderate risk for parasites.

■ If you answered "yes" to more than 20 items, you are at risk.

■ If you are not exhibiting any overt symptoms now, remember that many parasitic infections can be dormant and then spring to life when you least expect them. Be aware that symptoms that come and go may still point to an underlying parasitic infection because of reproductive cycles. The various developmental stages of parasites often produce a variety of metabolic toxins and mechanical irritations in several areas of the body—for example, pinworms can stimulate asthmatic attacks because of their movement into the upper respiratory tract.

Source: Used with permission from Ann Louise Gittleman, *Guess What Came to Dinner?* Garden City Park, NY: Avery Publishing Group, 1993.

ORGANIC ACID TEST Q D I G I N

Organic acid urine testing provides a noninvasive window into how well your metabolism is working. Organic acids are formed as by-products of cellular metabolism, digestion of food, and by the metabolism of the gut microbes such as bacteria and yeast. I consider this test to be a general functional medicine screening and use it often. What comes out in our urine can give profound information about nutritional and immunological factors, including fatty acid metabolism, neurotransmitter metabolism, carbohydrate metabolism, oxidative damage, energy production, detoxification status, B-complex sufficiency, dysbiosis, methylation abilities, and inflammatory reactions. This is probably the best test for determining whether candidiasis is present. You can obtain this type of testing from Great Plains Lab, Genova Diagnostics Lab, Metametrix Lab, and others. It's a simple urine test, done at home and mailed back to the lab for analysis.

LEAKY GUT SYNDROME/INTESTINAL PERMEABILITY TESTING Q D I G I N

The method that is the recognized standard for intestinal permeability testing is the mannitol and lactulose test. Mannitol and lactulose are two types of water-soluble sugar molecules that our bodies cannot metabolize or use and are absorbed into the bloodstream at different rates due to their different sizes. Mannitol is easily absorbed into cells by people with healthy digestion, while lactulose has such a large molecular size that it is only slightly absorbed. A healthy test shows high levels of mannitol and low levels of lactulose. If large amounts of mannitol and lactulose are present, it indicates a leaky gut condition. If low levels of both sugars are found, it indicates general malabsorption of all nutrients. Low mannitol levels with high lactulose levels have been found in people with celiac disease, Crohn's disease, and ulcerative colitis. Your doctor can give you a test kit to collect urine samples. After collecting a random urine sample, you drink a mannitol/lactulose mixture and collect urine for six hours. The samples are then sent to the laboratory. This test is often done in conjunction with a stool or a parasitology test.

There are also newer tests to measure leaky gut/barrier function. These measure zonulin, zonulin antibodies, occludin, and levels of bacterial lipopolysaccharides (LPS). These tests are simpler to do and are rapidly replacing the lactulose /mannitol test.

SMALL INTESTINAL BACTERIAL OVERGROWTH ⌕ DIGIN

This test differs from the comprehensive digestive stool analysis in that it tests for dysbiosis of the small rather than the large intestine. According to Pimentel, 78 percent of people with IBS or fibromyalgia, and many with restless leg syndrome and chronic fatigue syndrome, have SIBO. The SIBO test measures breath levels of hydrogen or methane to determine whether there is a bacterial infection in the small intestine. Small bowel overgrowth occurs when bacteria in the large intestine travel to the small intestine. To perform the test, you drink either a lactulose or a glucose drink and collect breath samples. Hydrogen is produced when lactulose or glucose comes in contact with the gut flora. A significant rise in hydrogen levels indicates SIBO. This test is currently available at large teaching hospitals, from gastroenterologists, and through functional medicine labs.

AMINO ACID TESTING ⌕ DIGIN

Proteins are chains of amino acids put together. The average adult has about 22 pounds of protein in his or her body. These proteins are used structurally, as enzymes, and as neurotransmitters, and they are in every cell in our bodies. Using either blood or urine testing, you can determine whether your body is able to break down food and cellular proteins into usable amino acids. If levels are low, first look at food intake of protein. Are you actually eating enough of it? Typically we need about ½ gram of protein for each pound of our body weight. Surprisingly, I often discover low amino acids in people who have low energy, in children and adults who are "failing to thrive," and in people with emotional, behavioral, learning, and mood disorders, even in people who are eating enough protein. Correcting this requires a two-point approach: first, giving free amino acids and easy-to-digest proteins from foods or medical foods, and second, trying to find the underlying mechanism for the malabsorption.

FATTY ACID TESTING Q D I G I N

Often, we eat the wrong balance of fats, and fats can modulate mood and inflammation. Testing for essential and nonessential fatty acids can be done through either standard blood testing or by a finger-prick blood test. Surprisingly, in people who have been taking fish oils for a long time, we often see people who have terrific levels of omega-3 fatty acids but low levels of beneficial omega-6 fatty acids. It's the balance of total fats in our diet that creates health and reduces inflammation.

INDICAN TEST Q D I G I N

The indican test, or Obermeyer test, is a urine test that looks for the presence of indoles in your urine. The level of indican (a type of indole) found in urine gives information about how well you metabolize protein. People with poor digestive function, malabsorption, dysbiosis, gluten problems, and putrefaction of foods have high indican levels. Indican testing is an inexpensive, noninvasive way to screen for faulty digestion. The test won't identify where the problem begins, but it can be used to monitor whether digestion is an issue and how well the treatment plan is working. This test isn't done that often, even though it's a simple in-office test, because the chemicals are toxic.

LACTOSE, FRUCTOSE, AND SUCROSE INTOLERANCE TESTS Q D I G I N

There are two ways to test yourself for lactose intolerance: You can do a home elimination or you can do a breath test. Both are detailed in this section.

SELF-TESTING FOR LACTOSE, FRUCTOSE, AND SUCROSE INTOLERANCE ⌕ D I G I N

There are breath tests for lactose, fructose, and sucrose intolerance, yet you can typically figure out if you are having issues with any of these substances by using a simple home test. Symptoms of all of these overlap with those of IBS: diarrhea, constipation, gas, and bloating are the most common.

Self-Testing for Lactose Intolerance ⌕ D I G I N

Lactose intolerance affects about two-thirds of the global population. This self-test requires eliminating all dairy products from your diet for a minimum of 10 to 14 days. Obvious dairy sources are milk, yogurt, cheese, ice cream, creamed soups, frozen yogurt, powdered milk, and whipped cream. Less obvious sources are bakery items, cookies, hot dogs, lunch meats, milk chocolate, most nondairy creamers, pancakes, protein-powder drinks, ranch dressing, milk solids, milk curd, lactose, and anything containing casein, such as caseinate, lactose, sodium caseinate, potassium casein, casein hydrolysate, rennet, or whey. If you're not sure what's in a food, avoid it during the testing period. There can be foods that are labelled as non-dairy that still contain casein or lactose. It's probably easiest to prepare your food at home and go to work or school with a bag lunch during the test. If you eat at a restaurant or at a friend's home for a meal, be conscientious about what you eat.

If lactose intolerance is causing your problems, you will probably notice that your symptoms have changed significantly and that reintroduction of dairy products triggers a return of symptoms. Most people with lactose intolerance can tolerate small amounts of dairy products or specific dairy products. You may discover that you tolerate kefir but not yogurt, yogurt but not kefir; or that you tolerate raw milk cheese, goat's or sheep's milk cheese, but not regular cheese.

Self-Testing for Fructose Intolerance ⌕ D I G I N

Fructose malabsorption has symptoms that overlap with IBS. Hereditary fructose intolerance is rare, affecting 1 in 20,000 to 30,000 people. Yet it's now thought that about a third of us don't absorb fructose well. It's no wonder. We are eating significantly less high-fructose corn syrup than we did in 2000 (62.5 pounds per year), but we still consumed 39.8 pounds in 2017. That equals 6.8 teaspoons, 28.35 grams, or just over 1 ounce per day. Yet when given 25 grams, half of healthy adults had positive fructose malabsorption, and at 50 grams, two-thirds had fructose malabsorption. It's just too much fructose all at once. One-third of people who had IBS tested positive for fructose malabsorption, and 61 percent of people with Crohn's disease did the same.

Eliminate all fructose from your diet for 12 to 14 days. If fructose malabsorption is the key to your symptoms, you will notice significant improvement and that reintroduction of fruit, high-fructose corn syrup, and other high fructose-containing foods triggers a return of symptoms. If this is the case, limit consumption to one small serving of berries or fruit daily.

Self-Testing for Sucrose Insufficiency ⌕ D I G I N

Several years ago, while teaching a class on nutrition, one of the students stated that she was going to stop eating all refined sugar during the 8-week course. She invited the rest of us to join her. The results were stunning. People reported better energy and moods, lifting of depression, better sleep, weight loss, better blood sugar control, clearing of acne, and one woman reported that her migraines of 12 years had completely disappeared.

Genetic sucrase-isomaltase deficiencies are rare, and yet many people acquire sucrase insufficiency simply from overeating it. According to the U.S. Department of Agriculture, in 2017, we each ate 60.2 pounds of sucrose. That's 11.8 teaspoons, 49 grams, or nearly 2 ounces each day.

To do a self-test, stop eating all white sugar, brown sugar, high-fructose corn syrup, and food products that contain any of these sugars, including soda, cookies, candy, pastries, sweetened yogurt, juices, and others. Read labels carefully. Do this for at least 2 weeks, and preferably 4 to 8 weeks. If sucrose malabsorption is the key to your symptoms, you will notice significant improvement. A return to eating sugar will trigger a return of symptoms. If you find that you can tolerate a bit of sugar, experiment with the amount to find your "sweet spot."

LABORATORY BREATH TESTING FOR:

- ### SMALL INTESTINAL BACTERIAL OVERGROWTH (SIBO)

- ### SUGAR INTOLERANCES:

  - #### Lactose

  - #### Fructose

  - #### Sucrose

Breath Testing Overview

Breath testing is utilized for people who have IBS-like symptoms and helps to determine the underlying root cause. The technology for breath testing was developed by QuinTron and is widely utilized by gastroenterologists and other clinicians. These tests are performed either in office or with home kits. To perform these tests, you drink one or more sugar solutions and collect breath samples over a period of 2 to 3 hours. The concept of this is that if you have SIBO or sucrose, lactose, or fructose intolerance, the bacteria in your gut ferment and produce gases that are absorbed into your blood and released into your breath. Significant increases in gas provide the diagnosis.

Preparing for Your Breath Test

To get a good result from breath testing, follow these instructions or the instructions included from your doctor or kit. These recommendations are typical:

- If you have taken antibiotics or antimicrobial herbs, wait 4 weeks before doing the testing.
- Stop laxatives 1 week prior to testing.
- Stop taking motility agents 2 days prior to the test.
- Exposure to cigarette smoke, even secondhand, can falsify the test results. Avoid exposure to smoke at least 1 hour prior to the test, as well as during the test.
- Stay awake during the test.
- Wait at least 1 hour following exercise to do the test.
- 24 hours before the test, you can have only the following: water, coffee or tea (plain), baked or broiled fish, turkey, or chicken with salt and pepper, plain, steamed white rice, eggs, chicken or beef broth, and white bread.
- 12 hours before the test, begin fasting. Drink water only.
- Fast during the test.

Hydrogen and Methane Breath Testing for SIBO

Hydrogen and methane breath testing differs from comprehensive digestive stool analysis in that it tests for dysbiosis of the small rather than the large intestine. The SIBO test measures breath levels of hydrogen or methane, which rise after ingestion of a lactulose or glucose solution, to determine whether there is a bacterial infection in the small intestine. It's a 3-hour test that can be done either in a doctor's office or as a home test.

Breath Testing for Lactose Intolerance

Breath testing is used to officially determine lactose intolerance, which has symptoms that overlap with IBS. A lactose solution is drunk. A normal hydrogen level is

10 parts per million (ppm), whereas levels of 20 ppm or more are commonly found in people with lactose intolerance. Normal methane levels are 0–7 ppm, and an increase of 12 ppm or more between the two samples indicates lactose intolerance, even if hydrogen production is normal. Measuring both methane and hydrogen considerably decreases the likelihood of a false result.

Breath Testing for Fructose Malabsorption

A detailed explanation of fructose intolerance is given in the "Self-Testing for Fructose Insufficiency" section a few pages earlier in this chapter. Fructose insufficiency is common in people who have IBS, Crohn's disease, and who just don't feel well when they eat fruit or eat a lot of food with high fructose-corn syrup.

A fructose solution is given in a breath test to measure elevations in hydrogen levels. This will determine whether fructose insufficiency is a problem.

Breath Testing for Sucrase Insufficiency

As with fructose, we eat too much sucrose, or table sugar and brown sugar. Genetic sucrase-isomaltase deficiencies are rare, yet many people acquire sucrase insufficiency. Breath testing can uncover it.

Breath testing for sucrase insufficiency can also be utilized to determine whether there is damage to the brush borders in the small intestine, which results in fewer sucrase enzymes. In other words, this is another way to test for intestinal permeability. A sucrose solution is drunk, and carbon dioxide or hydrogen levels are measured over 3 hours from breath testing to determine brush border health.

The sucrase breath test can also be used to monitor brush border health in people with celiac disease and cystic fibrosis, and/or brush border damage from taking nonsteroidal anti-inflammatory drugs (NSAIDs), after cancer therapies, parenteral nutrition, or other causes.

FOOD ALLERGY AND FOOD SENSITIVITY TESTING

Allergy Testing

Testing for true IgE allergies is straightforward. It is most often done with scratch testing, but it can also be done with a simple blood test called modified RAST (radioallergosorbent test). Most allergists use scratch testing, and yet research indicates that blood testing obtains equivalent results. These tests are useful to determine reactivity to dust, pollen, animal dander, and foods. Research on the six-food elimination diet for Eosinophilic esophagitis demonstrates that the elimination diet provides a more accurate way to test for common food allergies than blood or scratch testing.

Food Sensitivity Testing

Testing for food and environmental sensitivities is less clear cut. These tests are useful for finding specific foods that you might be reacting to. They also are useful for determining increased intestinal permeability if many foods are reactive or if the foods that you eat every day are positive. If you haven't been eating eggs, dairy, gluten, or other foods for a long time (4 months or longer), it's possible that you won't see reactions to those foods because your body has settled and isn't currently reacting to them. Why bother checking for them if you don't eat them? If you get a negative test for a food that you don't eat, it's not possible to know if that's because you haven't eaten it or because it's been long enough that you can safely eat it. With wheat, dairy, and eggs, these are typically more fixed and don't improve much.

There is little standardization of food sensitivity laboratory testing. That means that labs use a variety of methodologies, and results don't compare well among methods; however, they can compare well when the same methods are used. Some labs test for generalized inflammation, such as Alcat or MRT/Leap to various foods by measuring inflammatory markers. Other labs test for specific antibodies (mainly IgG), while some labs test for IgA, IgM, or IgG4 antibodies. Some of these labs also test for IgE and true allergies, such as Genova and US Biotek. The Elisa Act test explores antibody reactions through white blood cell (WBC) activation. KMBO provides IgG testing combined with complement testing. Many integrative physicians are utilizing in their offices provocative sublingual and intradermal testing to explore sensitivities.

Some of the labs include environmental screening panels that measure antibody reaction to common chemicals. Several laboratories perform antibody testing for foods, candida, dusts, environmental chemicals, heavy metals, molds, and pollens.

What I find is that although they differ, all labs provide results that will give a pretty good indication of which and how many substances you are reacting to, and whether you have leaky gut. No labs can find all sensitivities, but they all find enough to lower your overall load to help you feel better.

SECRETORY IgA TESTING DIG IN

Secretory IgA (sIgA) levels can be found stool, saliva, and blood; sIgA is an immunoglobulin antibody found in saliva, throughout the digestive tract, and in mucous secretions throughout the body. It provides our first line of defense against bacteria, food residue, fungus, parasites, and viruses. (It is explained more fully in Chapter 9.) By sitting on mucous membranes, sIgA prevents invaders from attaching to them and neutralizes them.

High levels indicate that your immune system is dealing with some stressor, such as an infection or high levels of stress. Low levels indicate that you've been fighting the stressor for such a long time that your body can't mount a response.

HEIDELBERG CAPSULE TEST AND SELF-TESTING FOR ADEQUACY OF GASTRIC ACID DIG IN

The Heidelberg capsule test is a radiotelemetry test for functional hydrochloric acid (HCl) levels. It is a simple, effective technique to determine how much HCl your stomach is producing.

In this test, you swallow an encapsulated radio transmitter that's about the size of a B-complex vitamin; the device measures the resting pH of the stomach and also the stomach's pH when administered baking soda, which is very alkaline. Then, by observing how quickly the stomach returns to an acidic condition after the baking soda challenges, the physician can determine whether or not your stomach produces adequate HCl. Unfortunately, this test is not widely available.

Self-Testing for Low HCl/Achlorhydria

Many of us have low HCl levels. High or low levels of HCl can be expressed as heartburn or gastroesophageal reflux disease (GERD). This opens us up to SIBO, fungal and parasitic infections, poor digestion of protein, and poor absorption of minerals. There are several simple ways to test to see whether you have enough stomach acid. There is no research that documents their effectiveness, but many clinicians find them to be helpful. If you are currently taking proton pump inhibitors or acid-blockers, do not try any of these self-tests. *(Please read the section on Gastro-Esophageal Reflux Disease in Chapter 19 to see what your long-term strategies might be.)*

Self-Testing with Vinegar and Baking Soda

Some people find that they can determine whether they have too much or too little acid. This two-part test is simple to do. Follow these steps when you have heartburn or GERD to see if you notice any improvement or worsening of symptoms:

1. Dilute 1 tablespoon of vinegar in 2 ounces of water. If you have a lessening of your symptoms, it may suggest that you have low stomach acid. If you feel worse, it may indicate that the acidic environment is irritating your esophagus. If you experience any discomfort, you can neutralize it with milk or baking soda in water. Always dilute vinegar to prevent damage to your esophagus. Some people like to dilute it with apple juice or another sweet juice to make it more palatable. Bragg and other companies make delicious vinegar drinks.

2. Mix ¼ teaspoon of baking soda in 4 ounces of water. Drink the mixture on an empty stomach and see if you have a worsening or lessening of your heartburn/GERD. If you do, it suggests that you may have excess stomach acid. If you feel worse, you can neutralize this effect by drinking a couple of teaspoons of vinegar or lemon juice diluted in water.

If baking soda eases your digestive issues, you can continue to add baking soda to your water or other beverages. Limit your use to ½ tsp daily. If you keep having heartburn, look for the root issues. (See Chapter 19.)

There are cases in the literature where people have over-utilized baking soda. Each teaspoon of baking soda has about 1300 mg of sodium in it. A low-sodium diet is considered 1500 to 2500 mg daily, so this would be most of your daily allowance. Problems can be severe for people who have Zollinger-Ellison syndrome or pyloric stenosis (narrowing of the stomach where it meets the duodenum) due to losses of chloride. People with kidney disease can go into alkalosis. Others have experienced depletions of potassium or calcium.

Self-Testing with Alka-Seltzer Gold

Alka-Seltzer is very alkalizing, which is why it has been used for decades for heartburn. Alka-Seltzer Gold contains baking soda (sodium bicarbonate), potassium carbonate, and citric acid which gives it the fizz. You can also take Alka-Seltzer Gold with a meal that contains protein. If you experience any burping, it suggests that you have adequate stomach acid production.

Alka-Seltzer is meant for occasional use of up to 14 days. If you keep having heartburn or dyspepsia, look for the root issues. (See Chapter 19), Each Alka-Seltzer tablet contains about 309 mg of sodium; if you are on a restricted sodium diet, this needs to be taken into account.

Self-Testing with Betaine HCl

Betaine HCl testing has not been rigorously tested to see how valid it is, and yet is used widely in the integrative and functional medicine communities. In my own practice, I have seen many people benefit from doing this self-test. Many people have also found that taking Betaine HCl supplements reduces burping, belching, and heartburn; and improves mineral absorption. Be careful though: You are taking acid, so if you feel any discomfort or atypical symptoms, stop.

Precautions
- You are taking acid. Too much will burn your stomach. *Stop* taking if you are experiencing any discomfort.
- Administration of HCl/pepsin is contraindicated in peptic ulcer disease.
- HCl can irritate sensitive tissue and can be corrosive to teeth; therefore, capsules should not be emptied into food or dissolved in beverages.

Self-Test Instructions
1. Begin by taking one 350 to 750 mg capsule of betaine HCl with a protein-containing meal. A normal response in a healthy person would be discomfort—basically heartburn. If you do not feel a burning sensation, at the next protein-containing meal, take two capsules.
2. If there are no reactions after two days, increase the number of capsules with each meal to two capsules.
3. Continue increasing by one capsule every two days, slowly building up to eight capsules, for a maximum dosage of 2000 mg, if necessary, with each meal. You'll know you've taken too much if you experience tingling, heartburn, diarrhea, or any type of discomfort, including feelings of unease, digestive discomfort, neckache, backache, headache, fatigue, decreased energy, or any new, odd symptoms. If you experience tingling, burning, or any symptom that is uncomfortable, you can neutralize the acid with 1 teaspoon baking soda in water or milk.
4. When you reach a state of tingling, burning, or any other type of discomfort, cut back by one capsule per meal. If the discomfort continues, *discontinue* the HCl and consult your health care professional. These dosages may seem large, but a

normally functioning stomach manufactures considerably more, about 2000 mg per meal.

5. Once you have established a dose (either eight capsules or less, if warmth or heaviness occurs), continue this dose.

6. With smaller meals, you may require less HCl, so you may reduce the number of capsules taken.

Individuals with very moderate HCl deficiency generally show rapid improvement in symptoms and have early signs of intolerance to the acid. This typically indicates a return to normal acid secretion.

Individuals with low HCl/pepsin typically do not respond as well to supplements, so to maximize the absorption and benefits of the nutrients you take, it is important to be consistent with your HCl/pepsin supplementation.

Typically, I will try to wean people off of HCl supplementation over time by using digestive enzymes, bitters, umeboshi plums, acupuncture, and stress management techniques. (These are discussed more fully in Chapter 19 in the section on Gastroesophageal Reflux Disease.)

MICROBIOME TESTING

There are many labs that can check for diversity, density, phyla, and specific microbes using stool testing. These tests are developing fast. They can give some indication of what is going on in your microbiome, and yet the research validating the clinical benefits of the tests isn't strong at this moment. Expect that to change as the field expands. I've taken many of these tests and have found them to be useful and interesting.

GENOMIC TESTING

Our genes were believed to be set in stone. New research indicates that's not the case: Each cell in your body has exactly the same genes. Most are turned off, but some are turned on or are expressed. Our food, exposure to everyday chemicals, stress, mood, exercise, sleep, and our relationships all can change the expression of our genes, either moving us toward health or away from it.

One of the first studies demonstrating this was done by Dr. Dean Ornish in men with slow-growing prostate cancer. The Ornish program was 12 weeks in duration and included a low-fat, whole-foods diet; 1 hour daily of stress management;

a support group once a week; walking 30 minutes daily for 6 weeks; and a protein supplement, along with fish oil supplements, vitamin C, vitamin E, and selenium. The results demonstrated that 48 cancer protective genes were turned on and 453 oncogenes were turned off. A subsequent study reported that telomere length was greater in a person after the Ornish program.

This represents the fields of epigenetics and nutritional genomics, which are too broad to include in this book.

A good clinician can discover much about your genomic strengths and weaknesses by taking a good medical and family history, doing a nutritionally oriented physical, and looking at lab tests that reflect your nutritional status. For people who have complex health issues that are not resolving, genomic testing can be revealing. I compare our unique genomes to a dam that has thicker and thinner places. Genomic testing tells us where and how to patch those thin areas so that the ocean doesn't break through the dam. I've done several of these tests on myself, and by doing so, I have discovered areas that I can shore up.

There are many direct-to-consumer and physician-ordered gene tests that can help you determine places in your genome that can support optimal gene function. These tests give information about specific gene variations that may or may not affect your health. For example, if you have pathways that demonstrate that you'll need more folate than the average person, you may already be compensating by eating more green leafy vegetables. For me, this is true: I crave more vegetables than most other people do. Yet, if you discover this for yourself and are not eating many green leafy vegetables, eating more is an actionable step to normalize the function of your folate genes. These genes and their variances work as part of a symphony of genes. The significance of having one gene impairment for methylation needs to be placed in the context of the music that is being played: your life. A good clinician will look at your genomic results in the light of you, your life, and your health goals and concerns.

We are in the very early stages of learning about this epigenetics and nutrigenomics, and the interpretation of these tests is complex. Companies that provide a clinical interpretation of your test results choose SNPs (single nucleotide polymorphisms) such as APO-E and MTHFR-677, which have known health implications. There is money to be made and the amount of new testing companies are mushrooming. With no standardization or agreement on which SNPs are most actionable, each company has its own unique and marketable product, often with a line of nutritional supplements.

This will become the future of medicine, but the science is still developing. Nonetheless, I've found very useful information from these tests for myself. Too young so far. Stay tuned!

ELECTRODERMAL TESTING

After much positive research, electrodermal testing, such as computerized electrodermal screening, electrical acupuncture voltage (EAV), Voll testing, and many other devices, is being widely used in Europe. Although this test has met with resistance from the U.S. Food and Drug Administration (FDA), there are many skillful professionals who use it to diagnose and determine appropriate therapies.

The test measures the electrical activity of your skin at designated acupuncture points. You hold a negative rod in one hand, the practitioner places a positively charged pointer on a variety of points on your skin, and a meter measures the voltage reading between the points. The test can determine which organs are strong or weak, which foods help or hurt you, which nutrients you need or have excessive levels of, and how old patterns are contributing to your health today. It is a fast, noninvasive screening test that you do by simply holding onto a metal bar while being gently touched with a probe.

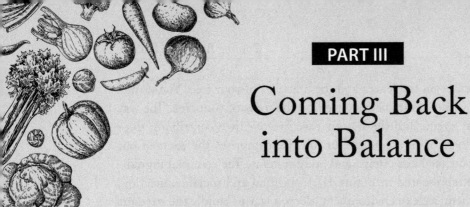

PART III

Coming Back
into Balance

In this part of the book, we delve into lifestyle. On this journey toward wellness, it may behoove you to work with a practitioner who is familiar with what you are trying to do. This could be a functional medicine, integrative, or naturopathic physician, nutritionist (CNS or CCN) or registered dietitian (RD), acupuncturist, chiropractor, coach, therapist, biological dentist, energy worker, shaman, or other professional in this field.

As with a tree, much of the roots are hidden. Working with emotional and spiritual blocks enhances healing and can help you move through plateaus. You may discover that one practitioner takes you so far, and then you will need to find another to take you through the next steps.

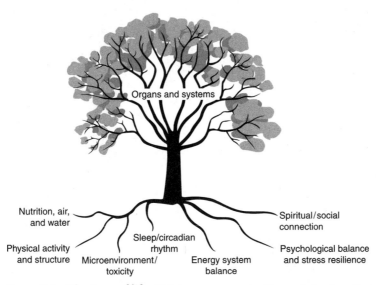

Figure III.1 **The tree of life.** (This image was used with permission from Paula J. Nemm MD. Optimal health and prevention research foundation.)

Most medicine focuses on the leaves and the branches of your tree. You want a team that can do that while simultaneously feeding the roots of your tree. The way we respond to everyday events and the way that we live our lives contributes to or detracts from our wellness bank account. Our lifestyle comprises the roots of our wellness tree. These roots feed our organs and body systems. The essential ingredients to build upon are represented in Figure III.1: spiritual and social connection, food, air, water, movement, a clean environment, sleep, a way to handle the stressors of daily life, and ways to balance our energetic output.

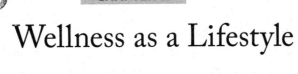

CHAPTER 12

Wellness as a Lifestyle

"The role of the practitioner—the doctor, nurse, or other medical professional—is to become a therapeutic tool for healing."

—David Rakel

So often we seek a doctor's care because of signs or symptoms. We feel more tired than we think we ought to; we have more gas than we think we ought to; we just feel more poorly than we think we ought to. Our doctors begin looking for disease and problems. We know that 75 percent of our health issues today have a basis in the way we eat and live. Yet medicine focuses on medication and surgery first, rather than lifestyle change. Medication stops the symptoms but not the underlying issue.

I once sold a minivan I'd had for a 15 years. It had a lot of small things wrong with it: I held up the back tailgate with a 2 × 4; the radio didn't work; the electric window on the driver's side of the car didn't work. These small issues happened over time and none of them were huge, so I learned to live with them. After all, the minivan drove well and got me where I wanted to go. This is a metaphor for our own lives. Our physical changes happen over time, and we learn to live with our headaches, bloating, heartburn, and so on.

When I was in practice, one of the biggest ways I helped people was to give them hope that their health could improve. The big question is this: Are you willing to change your life to change your health step by step?

Self-care is something we innately do. If you get a headache, you probably know what to do to make it better without going to see a doctor. If you get a cold, you also have a routine that works for you. I spend a lot of time in my own life practicing self-care: I exercise regularly and make sleep a priority; I shop for and cook healthy food; I use cooking as a creative outlet; I spend leisure time gardening, with friends and family, and by myself; I brush my teeth twice daily and have a routine to improve my gum health; I meditate sometimes; I read for pleasure every night before bed; I massage areas of my body if they ache; I get professional massages; I see a chiropractor for preventive care. This self-nurturing takes time, but it's worth it because it improves my well-being and health. It's also a demonstration that I'm worth it! You are too!

What does your self-care look like today? Take a few minutes to think about it or write it down.

When I first began studying health and nutrition, I was influenced by the vision of Don Ardell, PhD and John Travis MD, MPH, who coined the term *wellness*. Some of their ideas rang out to me then and still do today:

- Staying healthy takes less work than digging ourselves out of an illness. Strive for prevention.
- What if, rather than avoiding illness, I strive toward feeling my very best?
- What if I look at signs, symptoms and diseases as teachers, urging me to make changes?
- What if I have the resiliency of body, mind, and spirit that would allow me to achieve my goals and dreams more easily?
- What if, when I am ill, I take it in stride, knowing that I am more than my illness?

I can feel empowered by giving myself the gift of self-care. There have been times in my life when I've had the realization that I need an entire extra day a week for self-care. That, despite my best efforts, I have been focusing outward too much and not on my own physical well-being.

The word *wellness* is an important one; it implies that wherever we are beginning, we can feel better than we do right now. Our health on all levels is on a continuum, as demonstrated in John Travis's Illness-Wellness Continuum, shown in Figure 12.1.

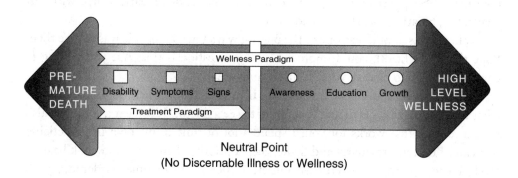

Figure 12.1 **The Illness-Wellness Continuum.**

This book can be used to keep you healthy and to help you return to your optimal state of wellness.

We can have a physical illness and still be well in mind and spirit. We can be hearty of body and yet have illness in our minds or spirits. Rather than feeling like a victim of your body-mind-spirit trichotomy, move toward feeling like a victor by empowering yourself. Decades ago, I heard Dr. Michael Lerner, founder of Commonweal, discuss going to nontraditional cancer centers around the globe. He found that every clinic saw medical successes but also people who died from cancer. Yet whether people lived or died from their cancer, they felt successful because they felt empowered. Even if we cannot change our physical condition as much as we would like, we can feel well.

Admittedly, there are many domains of wellness: relationships, finances, spirit, food, movement, and sleep, among others. Living life in balance is not all that possible. Imagine standing on one leg, balancing. Can you do that indefinitely? I can't! My life gets out of balance often. When it does, it's time to reassess and make changes.

John Travis's book *The Wellness Workbook* is an excellent place to begin. If this is an area that you'd like to delve into with tools and coaching support, check out www .wellnessworkbook.com. What follows is an exercise to see how well your wheel rolls.

WELLNESS WHEEL SELF-ASSESSMENT

Wellness Wheel Instructions
This exercise is a way to discover and prioritize which areas of your life need attention. You may feel that your relationships have little or nothing to do with the fact that you have chronic diarrhea, but until you find balance, you can't know for sure. The mind is not separate from the body. It is well documented that our thoughts influence our physical condition. All domains of wellness affect our sense of well-being.

Filling in Your Wellness Wheel
How satisfied are you today in each of these areas of your life? Rate them on a scale from 1 to 10, with 1 being the most dissatisfied and 10 being the most satisfied. On the Wellness Wheel, 10 would be at the outer edge of the circle, 1 in the center, and the other numbers in between.

Evaluating Your Responses
Now look at your Wellness Wheel. Would it roll? Which spokes are the shortest? The short spokes are the areas that you've paid less attention to recently, so they offer

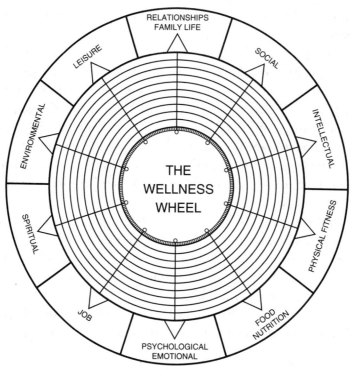

Figure 12.2   **The Wellness Wheel.**

the greatest areas of discovery and opportunity. They help you prioritize which areas you need to pay attention to the most today.

Next, study the overall look of your wheel. Are you generally satisfied or dissatisfied with your life? People with 8s, 9s, and 10s generally feel pretty good about themselves; their lives are moving in the right direction. People with 0s, 1s, 2s, and 3s may be feeling a lack of confidence and low self-esteem. If you have many short spokes on your wheel, you may want to boost your support systems. Find a friend to talk to or get a professional counselor to help you sort out your priorities. My Wellness Wheel changes each time I do this exercise, depending on what's going on in my life at that time. It is a dynamic, ever-changing wheel.

Now that you have looked at the spokes, choose one or two areas in which you see an opportunity for growth and change. Make a small, achievable goal, like "I will eat dessert only one time this week" or " I will begin exercising by taking three 20-minute walks this week" or "I will call my sister, whom I haven't spoken to since we had a misunderstanding a couple of months ago." Be reasonable and easy on yourself. Small, attainable goals lead to success, which leads to more goal-setting and more success. If you've never exercised, begin by walking or biking 20 minutes once or twice a week. If you'd like to cut out coffee, you can quit altogether or cut back gradually. Some people find they only "need" the first cup of the day; other people switch to decaf, while others combine regular coffee and decaf, half and half. Remember that the journey toward wellness is as important as the destination. Don't worry about "getting there"—enjoy the scenery!

When you work consistently on a wellness lifestyle, you'll feel the effects now and build health for your future. Of course, we do age, and we may meet with an unexpected illness, but in general, people who pay attention to how they feel have a greater sense of well-being. They also feel more empowered and in control of their lives.

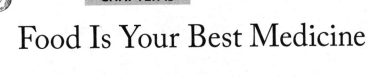

CHAPTER 13

Food Is Your Best Medicine

"Many of the things we claim to cherish—family relationships, cultural identity, ethnic diversity—were all intimately linked to the making and eating of food and now are changing as we outsource more and more of our food preparation to restaurants and industrial kitchens. Not only do we cook less than we used to, but more of us eat alone—at our desks, in our cars, standing at our kitchen counters. In America, the average family shares a meal fewer than five times a week."

—Paul Roberts, *The End of Food*

"Apprentices have asked me, what is the most exalted peak of cuisine? Is it the freshest ingredients, the most complex flavors? Is it the rustic, or the rare? It is none of these. The peak is neither eating nor cooking, but the giving and sharing of food."

—Nicole Mones, *The Last Chinese Chef*

Food is our most intimate contact with our external environment. What we eat, digest, absorb, assimilate, and excrete becomes us. You may already be eating a whole-foods, organic diet. If so, then the information in this chapter may be old news. Most people think they eat well. According to a Pew report, 73 percent of people report that they are "very or fairly focused" on eating healthy foods. There's a disconnect with how we feel about our diet and what we actually eat. We're getting fatter and sicker as a nation. Most of us are overfed and undernourished, getting over half of our calories in highly processed, nutrient-depleted foods. We eat more than half of our meals at restaurants or as takeout. According to the U.S. Department of Agriculture (USDA), in 2017 Americans, including children, each ate 115.8 pounds of sugar a year. We have increased our consumption of fructose by eating nearly 40 pounds a year of high-fructose corn syrup, and now a third of us have an acquired fructose intolerance. It's like fixing your home with the poorest materials possible. No wonder we are getting sicker and sicker as a nation.

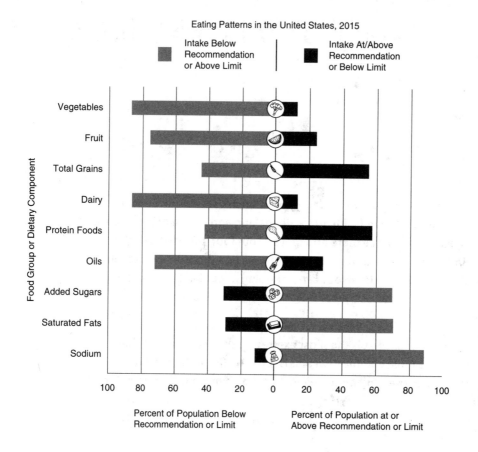

Eating Patterns in the United States, 2015

Intake Below Recommendation or Above Limit

Intake At/Above Recommendation or Below Limit

Percent of Population Below Recommendation or Limit

Percent of Population at or Above Recommendation or Limit

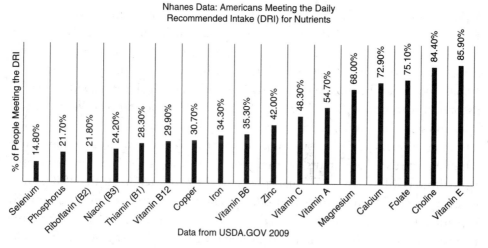

Nhanes Data: Americans Meeting the Daily Recommended Intake (DRI) for Nutrients

Data from USDA.GOV 2009

The energetics of food and the way that food talks to our cells provides an additional way of looking at food. Food is information. Food interacts with our genes, regulating or disrupting normal biological pathways. Each time we eat, we produce neurotransmitters that regulate mood and behavior; polyphenols in foods send messages to our immune system telling it to sooth and calm; from the soil where our food is grown, to the factory where it is packaged, to our kitchen counters where we prepare it, the foods we eat are filled with microbes and thus change our microbiome. Food also contains chemical messengers that tell our cells to replicate, excrete wastes, accept nutrients, and more. When we eat nutrient-dense, health-supportive foods, these messages are healthful and appropriate. But when we eat what Dr. Jeffrey Bland, the co-founder of the Institute for Functional Medicine, calls "new-to-nature" foods, foods laden with chemicals, pesticides, and synthesized ingredients (such as food colorings and restructured fats), we aren't giving our cells the right messages. Our bodies are familiar with foods that have been eaten for centuries. Manufactured foods and genetically engineered foods bring different types of messages. A 2019 paper by Abigail Baldrige and her associates report that 71 percent of packaged food is ultraprocessed. Another new study published on the JAMA Internal Medicine Network reports that eating "ultraprocessed foods" is associated with a shorter lifespan. However, the report also notes that people who eat the most ultraprocessed foods also have lower levels of income and education, live alone, are fatter, and work out less. So, there are socioeconomic reasons why people who eat the most ultraprocessed food have shorter lifespans.

Once you make the decision to rely on natural foods, your body and mind will adjust so that natural foods taste more delicious than manufactured derivatives. Once your sugar taste buds calm down, fresh fruit will taste sweet again.

I use a 90/10 rule: 90 percent of your food should be excellent for your body, and 10 percent just to goof off and let loose.

Old Nutrition: Fuel
Protein
Fats
Carbs
Vitamins
Minerals
Water

New Nutrition: Food is Information and Fuel
Old style, plus:
Polyphenols
Probiotic-rich foods
Prebiotic-rich foods
Antioxidants
Sustainability
Nutrigenomics
Organic
Gastrointestinal (GI) health

DIET = A WAY OF LIVING

The word *diet* comes from Greek and means "a manner of living" or "way of life"; the Latin root means "a day's journey." It's about everything that we ingest: our food, our thoughts, our pattern of movement, the TV shows we watch, the music we listen to, the news. Changing our food begins a process of nourishing ourselves and our families that may be the catalyst for even deeper changes.

I am less concerned about whether you are a vegetarian or a meat eater, on an Atkin's or Zone Diet, macrobiotic diet, Ayurvedic diet, Body Ecology Diet, kosher diet, or whatever your particular style of eating is. I am more concerned about whether you eat *whole foods, organically grown,* as often as possible. Good diets rely on natural, home-cooked, whole-food meals; they are devoid of artificial colors and flavors, trans-fatty acids, and refined sugar; and they are loaded with phytonutrients (health-protective substances found in plant foods such as fruits, vegetables, grains, beans, nuts, and seeds), fiber, and good-quality fats. The Mediterranean Diet has been shown to be an excellent place to begin with diet. It's a mostly whole-foods diet and is based on fresh, local food, olive oil, nuts and seeds, grains that are preferably whole, seafood, dairy, eggs, fresh herbs and spices, and many vegetables and fruits.

Table 13.1 **Mediterranean Diet Benefits**

Reductions in:	Improvements in and Prevention of:
■ Alzheimer's risk and cognitive decline	■ Alcoholic liver disease
■ Cancer: reduced death rate, reductions in colon cancer, breast cancer, gastric cancer, prostate cancer, liver cancer, head and neck cancers, pancreatic cancer, and respiratory cancers	■ Blood pressure
	■ Depression
	■ Diabetes and insulin sensitivity
	■ Digestive: prevents inflammatory bowel disease (IBD), benefits the microbiome
	■ Genomic benefits
	■ Immune function
■ Cardiovascular disease: heart attacks, stroke, heart failure, disability from cardiac problems, and death from heart disease	■ Inflammation and pain: Rheumatoid arthritis
	■ Kidney function
	■ Longevity
	■ Metabolic syndrome
	■ Neurodegenerative conditions: Parkinson's disease, Alzheimer's disease, cognitive decline
	■ Serum lipids (cholesterol, triglycerides)
	■ Weight control/obesity

While olive oil and nuts seem to supply a lot of the benefits in this diet, there are other important factors, including lifestyle and the environment. Traditionally, meals have been eaten in the community. Preparation of food is nurturing. For me, cooking at the end of a day is self-love. Eating with others strengthens relationships; and eating at home makes a hearth. The Mediterranean Diet also includes physical activity, adequate rest, and spending time socially with others.

The diet also benefits sustainability in several ways. It provides a nutrient-dense way of eating that is high in phytonutrients, it enhances biodiversity, it has a low environmental impact, and it an economic benefit to local economies.

There is a wealth of research that supports the Mediterranean Diet as an excellent preventive diet for chronic health conditions and metabolism.

Finding a digestion-enhancing, health-supportive diet that works for you and your family is what's important. The key is to make real changes—changes you can live with successfully on a long-term basis—in the way you approach food and your lifestyle in general.

Your Food Diary

Write down everything you eat and drink in a food diary (Table 13.1). If you experience symptoms, your energy drops, or your mood changes, write it down. See whether you can correlate specific foods to the way you feel mentally and physically.

A sample food diary shown in Table 13.2 looks like this:

Table 13.2 **Sample Food Diary**

DAY 1			
Time of day	*What did I eat?*	*Where was I?* *Who was I with?* *What was my mood?*	*Any change in how* *I feel, positive or* *negative?*

Keep the food diary for at least 7 to 14 days. Then examine it and answer the following questions to gain insight into your eating habits—good and bad:

- Did you eat breakfast every day? "Breaking the fast" provides much-needed fuel.
- Is your digestion better or worse at specific times of the day? Timing can be a clue to causes of indigestion (what, when, where, how fast, how much, and the like).
- How often do you eat? Some of us feel best on two or three meals a day, others with smaller, more frequent meals and snacks.
- Do certain foods and/or beverages provoke symptoms? Eliminate suspicious foods for at least two weeks and note any differences in how you feel. (See Chapter 14 for more on elimination diets.)
- Are your mealtimes relaxed or rushed? It's important to schedule meals with enough time so you don't feel rushed.
- Do you eat at least five servings of vegetables and fruits each day? What constitutes a serving is ½ cup of fruit and most vegetables. A serving of salad greens is 1 cup. Some studies report that eating eight or more servings of vegetables and fruits can lower all-cause mortality, cancer, cardiovascular disease, and stroke.
- What percentage of your food and drinks are high sugar, low fiber, or highly processed? Replace these with fresh, wholesome foods.
- Do you consume enough high-fiber foods? Fiber is consumed in whole grains, fruits, vegetables, and legumes.
- Are you hydrated? One simple way to figure out your daily need is to take your body weight, divide it by two, and drink that many ounces. For example, if you weigh 150 pounds, divide by two and drink 75 ounces of fluids. Most adults require 2 to 3 quarts of fluids each day. This can be from coffee*, tea, soup, foods such as steamed vegetables, and other fluids. Make sure that you choose healthful options, not soft drinks.

EATING PRINCIPLES TO LIVE BY

Eat Real Food

At least 80 to 90 percent of your food ought to be whole foods, as opposed to the average Western diet, which is over two-thirds processed and striped foods. Instead, transition to real food: high-quality protein from animal and legume sources, nuts,

---

* Coffee adds to your hydration but was formerly believed to be dehydrating.

seeds, vegetables, fruit, whole grains, organic dairy products, olive oil, and herbs, spices, teas, coffee, and water.

Food Is Information

Each bite we eat gives our genes and microbiome a set of directions. It can tell us to repair, replenish, and nourish, or it can increase inflammation systemically.

When you eat a meal or prepare one, consider the following questions:

- Is this food moving me toward health or away from it?
- What information is this food giving to my cells and genes?

The Life in Food Gives Us Life

When we eat junk, our immune system acts like junk!

Eat enzyme-rich, probiotic-rich, and prebiotic-rich foods. Eat fresh foods, grown locally when possible. If you've grown your own food or gone to farmer's markets, you know the vibrancy of that food. That vibrancy translates to your own vitality and health.

Eat a Rainbow Every Day

Eat 7 to 12 servings daily of colorful foods: green, orange, yellow, red, white/tan, and purple/blue. Eating more vegetables, fruit, nuts, seeds, and beans reduces inflammation, lowers risk of chronic disease, and enhances overall energy and well-being. These foods are loaded with vitamins, minerals, fiber, prebiotics, phytochemicals, and other substances that protect us from cardiovascular disease, cancer, diabetes, and other health issues.

Learn to Cook

OK, don't give me with the deer in the headlights look! Cooking expresses self-love and self-nurture. It also gives you control over the quality of the food that you eat. Cooking is easy, results in delicious food, and saves you money. When you cook your own food, you can plan to have leftovers that will tide you over at work or when you are pressed for time and can't cook. Taking cooking lessons on your own, or with friends or family can be a great way to learn new cooking skills and recipes and have fun!

Eat Local Foods in Season

Local produce is the freshest and has the highest level of nutrients. Ask your supermarket's produce manager and neighborhood restaurants to purchase locally grown products whenever possible. Put farm stands, community-support agriculture (CSA) markets, and farmer's markets into your food-shopping routine. This has the added benefits of supporting the local economy and helping the environment by cutting food transportation costs and consumption of fossil fuels. Act locally; think globally!

Knowing your farmers, fisheries, and what food is available locally helps the food supply become more transparent. The quality, freshness, and enzymes are most abundant in local foods eaten in season. Eating foods in season also reduces the amount of pesticides and herbicides we consume.

If You Are Tired in the Afternoons, Eat a Mini-Meal

Many of us have low blood sugar levels in the middle to late afternoon. This translates into fatigue, inability to focus, desire to nap, and/or grabbing the sweetest food we can find to bring up our blood sugar. Be certain to include protein and fat in your mini-meals.

If this sounds like you, have a healthy mini-meal or two in the afternoon. I call it a mini-meal to remind you to eat something healthful. Some possibilities include:

- Saving part of your lunch for later
- Leftovers
- A piece of chicken or fish with some carrots
- A protein smoothie or green drink
- Fruit with a handful of nuts
- Vegetables with hummus, baba ghanoush, or nut butter
- Pears or apples with hummus or nut butter
- A bowl of soup
- Popcorn with nutritional yeast
- Trail mix
- A few sushi rolls

Eat High-Quality Protein and High-EPA/DHA
Seafood, Organically and Sustainably Produced

If you choose to eat animal protein, such as poultry, beef, lamb, pork, bison, goat, dairy products, eggs, and/or seafood, try to make sure that it is of the best quality possible.

Poultry and meat animals are raised mostly in concentrated agricultural feeding operations (CAFOs), where at the end of their lives they receive cooked food that isn't natural for them and they live in conditions that are not conducive to their nature or optimal health. On the other hand, pasture-raised meat animals and poultry that run around on grass and soil have a healthier nutrient content. Environmentally, CAFOs are a disaster. Most water pollution is runoff from animal farming. The antibiotics given to farmed animals go into our rivers, streams, fields, crops, and bodies. The hormones they receive affect us after we eat their meat. Countries that switch from a grain-based to a meat-based economy become poorer, have more hunger and starvation, and strip their land of its natural resources.

When purchasing red meat, look for labels that tell you it has been grass fed or grass finished. If you are eating poultry, look for organic poultry. We are the food that our food eats. So, if I buy "natural" poultry in the market, probably that chicken was fed genetically engineered corn and soy products. The only way I can ensure that I am not taking in genetically engineered products is by purchasing organic meats and dairy products. Some of the best products can be purchased at your local farmer's markets or directly from the producer directly at the farm.

Eat wild-caught fish that is sustainably harvested. Personally, I buy only wild-caught fish. At a restaurant, I always ask what type of salmon it is and whether it is wild caught or farmed. If it's wild caught, the chef will give a specific type of salmon, such as sockeye, king, or Chinook. Most farm-raised fish has less healthful omega-3 fatty acid and more polychlorinated bromines than wild-caught fish.

Coldwater fish are also an excellent source of the omega-3 fatty acids that are essential to our good health and promote neurological development in babies and children—hence the old saying, "Fish is brain food." The fatty acids eicosapentaenoic acid (EPA) and docosahexaenoic acid (DHA), found in all of our cells, are especially critical for the eyes, brain, nervous system, heart, and glands. Although many of us can manufacture DHA in our bodies from other fats, like flaxseeds, others lack the enzymes and nutrients (zinc, magnesium, B_6) necessary for this conversion and must obtain DHA through diet. The fish richest in EPA and DHA are salmon, halibut, tuna, mackerel, trout, sardines, eel, and herring. Lower-fat fish or fish from tropical waters are still healthful to eat, but they do not contain significant levels of EPA and DHA. Eating low-mercury and low-toxin fish such as sardines is also beneficial. To get more information on which fish are healthiest, go to the Monterey Bay Aquarium for their Seafood Watch Guides: http://www.montereybayaquarium.org/cr/seafoodwatch.aspx.

Studies show that people who eat coldwater fish twice a week have a reduced risk of heart disease and stroke. Other studies have found fish oils to be protective against, or therapeutic for, allergy, Alzheimer's disease, angina, asthma, attention deficit disorder, cancer, depression, eczema, high blood pressure, high serum cholesterol, hyperactivity, inflammatory disorders, kidney disease, lupus, migraine, multiple sclerosis, psoriasis, rheumatoid arthritis, and schizophrenia. Although supplementation with fish-oil capsules is beneficial, the best way to get these oils is to eat the fish itself.

If you like them, eat organically raised or pastured eggs. Eggs got a bad rap when they were linked to high cholesterol levels, but many researchers now believe that eating eggs has little or no effect on normal serum cholesterol. Recent studies show no significant change in the cholesterol of healthy people after six weeks of consuming two hard-boiled eggs daily, and other studies show that eating eggs can actually raise levels of "good" cholesterol (high-density lipoprotein, or HDL; "bad" cholesterol is low-density lipoprotein, or LDL). Eggs also contain high amounts of phospholipids that are integral to our cell membranes and are a precursor to the important neurotransmitter acetylcholine.

Eat More High-Fiber Foods

Researcher Dennis Burkitt, MD, noticed in the 1970s that rural Africans eating a traditional diet had almost no colon cancer, constipation, diabetes, diverticular disease, heart disease, or irritable bowel syndrome (IBS), whereas Africans consuming a Western diet had a heightened incidence of these problems. In a hospital in India, he found that the incidence of appendicitis was only 2 percent of that in a similar American hospital, and that there was virtually no hiatal hernia, which affects nearly 30 percent of Americans over 50 years old. After examining many factors, Dr. Burkitt concluded that the large amount of fiber in traditional diets was crucial for health maintenance.

We have since learned much more about fiber and its contributions to health:

- Diets high in soluble fiber help with Crohn's disease, hiatal hernia, IBS, and peptic ulcer.
- High-fiber diets reduce the risk of heart disease, high blood pressure, and certain types of cancer, including colon cancer.
- Fiber has been shown to normalize serum cholesterol levels.
- High-fiber diets reduce the incidence of colon polyps and bowel disease.
- Dietary fiber helps prevent obesity by slowing digestion and the release of insulin and stored glucose into the bloodstream.
- Improving bowel function can help prevent diverticulosis, appendicitis, hemorrhoids, and varicose veins.

We also know that low-fiber diets lead to the digestive disorders suffered by one out of four Americans. We eat an average of 14 to 15 grams of fiber per day, when adults should actually eat 25 to 30 grams of fiber daily (the same amount that Americans ate in 1850). Soluble fibers are equivalent to prebiotics. They provide food for the microbiota. (See Chapter 6 for more information.)

The richest food sources of fiber are also the four food groups that make up the bulk of a healthful eating plan: whole grains, legumes (all beans except string beans), vegetables, and fruits. (See Table 13.3.) Soluble and insoluble fibers, which work differently inside the body, are mixed in foods, so if you eat a wide variety of high-fiber foods, you will get both types of fiber. As a group, beans and legumes have the highest fiber content.

Eating whole-grain products is an excellent way to increase your fiber intake. Think of using non-gluten-containing grains (and grainlike seeds) such as quinoa, millet, rice, wild rice, amaranth, sorghum, tapioca, corn, risotto, teff, and buckwheat. Unfortunately, many people with dysbiosis cannot tolerate gluten-containing grains (wheat, barley, rye, spelt, kamut, triticale), and some people with digestive issues cannot tolerate *any* grains. Soaking grains and beans before cooking will release minerals and make them more digestible.

Table 13.3 **Amount of Fiber in Selected Foods**

Food	Amount of Fiber	Food	Amount of Fiber
Fruits (raw)		**Legumes/Starchy Vegetables (cooked)**	
Apple with skin	1 medium = 4 g	Baked beans, canned	½ cup = 6.5 g
Peach	1 medium = 2 g	Kidney beans, fresh	½ cup = 8 g
Pear	1 medium = 4 g	Lima beans, fresh	½ cup = 6.5 g
Tangerine	1 medium = 2 g	Potato, fresh	1 = 3 g
Vegetables (fresh)		**Grains**	
Asparagus, cooked	4 spears = 1 g	Bread, whole wheat	1 slice = 2 g
Broccoli, cooked	½ cup = 2.5 g	Brown rice, cooked	1 cup = 2.5 g
Brussels sprouts, cooked	½ cup = 2 g	Cereal, bran flake	¾ cup = 5 g
Cabbage, cooked	½ cup = 1.5 g	Oatmeal, cooked	¾ cup = 3 g
Carrot, cooked	½ cup = 2.5 g	White rice, cooked	1 cup = 1 g
Cauliflower, cooked	½ cup = 1.5 g		
Romaine lettuce, raw	1 cup = 1 g		
Spinach, cooked	½ cup = 2 g		
Summer squash, cooked	1 cup = 3 g		
Tomato, raw	1 = 1 g		
Winter squash, cooked	1 cup = 6 g		

Plan Ahead and Carry Food with You

Planning ahead and carrying your own food are great tools for healthful eating. Planning helps you create balanced meals and saves shopping time. Carrying snacks for yourself and your kids helps keep your moods and blood sugar levels even. It also saves you money and time, and you can ensure that the snacks are healthful.

An extension of this rule is to make bag lunches. That way you have some control (or at least the illusion of control!) about what you eat at work and what your children eat at school. Just put in some leftovers or a sandwich with a salad and/or a piece of fruit, add a beverage, and you've got lunch. Lidded containers simplify the process. (To save time, I often begin making the next day's bag lunch while putting away leftovers from dinner.)

Eat Regular Meals and Fast 12 or More Hours Nearly Every Day

A developing body of research indicates that intermittent fasting has regenerative effects on most tissues and organs in our bodies. The brain cleanses itself at night while we sleep; cells clean house of damaged proteins and perform maintenance. Studies show that intermittent fasting helps lowers risk of developing type 2 diabetes and a variety of cancers, supports weight reduction, and protects brain and cardiovascular function. Research indicates that a minimum of 12 hours of fasting, such as finishing dinner by 7 PM and not eating breakfast until at least 7 AM optimizes this function. Fasting for longer—13, 14, 16, or up to 18 hours—may provide even better health benefits. See what works best for your own body.

Listen to Your Body: Respect Your Own Biochemical Uniqueness

Don't listen to me or anyone else. Okay, listen to me a little! Experts are just that, experts, but they don't live in your body, you do! Your body is wise. If you listen, it will tell you what makes you feel more vibrant and energetic and which foods drag you down.

The foods that are best for any person are those that agree with that person's body and unique biochemistry at a particular moment in time. You will probably need to experiment with your own diet and your family's diet to discover what works best for you. Furthermore, these needs will change over time. Pay attention!

Eat When You Are Hungry and Stop When You Are Satisfied

From the time babies are born, they let us know when they're hungry; they drink as much formula or breast milk as they want, and then they stop sucking when they're satisfied. As they begin eating solid foods and thereon through childhood, children know when they are hungry or full, but then we start encouraging them to just eat a little bit more or to taste something because "it's yummy," or we treat them with cookies or ice cream to reward them for eating their meals. We get a cookie or sweet when we experience pain. We quickly learn that food is love. So we learn to eat when we aren't hungry.

Emotional overeating is one of the reasons for obesity in this country. If you are eating when you aren't hungry, try to figure out what's going on in your life that's triggering the desire to eat. It can be nearly anything: procrastination, fatigue, stress, need to feel appreciated, to celebrate, to socialize, loneliness, anger, and so on. Don't eat if you aren't hungry, but also don't wait until you are overhungry because that's when our blood sugar levels drop, we lose control and eat the sweetest, fastest foods in sight.

Relax While Eating

Many times we don't even stop what we're doing long enough to sit down when we eat. Remember that eating is a time for rejuvenation of body and spirit and a time to connect with yourself and with those you are eating with. Focus on your food by eating mindfully and chewing your food well. One way I've found to encourage peace of mind during meals is to say grace. It puts me in touch with the bounty of our earth, directs my attention to the people I am with and to my gratitude for their presence in my life, helps me thank the people who produced the food, and reminds me that we all depend on each other and community. Family meals are important. Turn the television off and have a family dinner almost every night.

Choose Organically Grown Foods Whenever Possible

Organic foods generally have higher nutrient levels because farmers who use organic methods add more nutrients to the soil, knowing that healthy plants can better fend off pests and that the nutrients end up in the crops. Organic plants create higher levels of antioxidants and protective polyphenols. A study from Doctor's Data reports that mineral levels in organically grown apples, pears, potatoes, wheat, and wheat berries are twice as high as in their commercially grown counterparts. Italian researchers found that levels of polyphenols, which are active antioxidant nutrients, are about a third higher in organic peaches and about three times higher in organic pears. Another recent study found that wild berries had twice the antioxidant level as commercially grown berries. As consumer awareness of such benefits increases, organically grown foods are becoming more plentiful and are now stocked in many supermarkets. Refer to the Clean 15 and Dirty Dozen list from the Environmental Working Group (www.ewg.org) to see which foods have the highest and lowest pesticide residues.

Eating organically produced foods is your *only* way to avoid the genetically engineered ingredients that are found in about 80 percent of packaged foods.

Organic food production also protects soils and water, treats animals more humanely, and helps prevent antibiotic resistance. Conventionally (nonorganically) raised animals are routinely given growth-promoting antibiotics and hormones, and animal production accounts for an estimated 70 percent, or 25 million pounds, of the antibiotics used annually in the United States. When we eat nonorganic dairy, poultry, eggs, and meats, we ingest small amounts of these drugs. Antibiotics in animal feed also create the perfect environment for bacteria to develop resistance; as stronger and newer antibiotics are developed, some bacteria survive by adaptation, and these strains can then pass to humans in our food and through contact with farm animals. Conventional animal production thereby lessens the effectiveness of drugs that we so rely on.

Drink Lots of Clean Water

Our bodies are 70 percent water. If we don't adequately hydrate our cells, they cannot function properly. Moreover, the water we drink and consume in food is an essential carrier, bringing in nutrients and taking away wastes. In *Your Body's Many Cries for Water*, Fereydoon Batmanghelidj, MD, describes the numerous, even fantastic roles that water plays in the body. Good hydration can help prevent many health problems, from gout to asthma; for example, Dr. Batmanghelidj believes water is the best cure for ulcers. Drinking plenty of clean, pure water every day is one of the most promising routes to digestive wellness.

Unfortunately, any chemical we use will show up in our water supply, as groundwater is easily contaminated by runoff. The U.S. Environmental Protection Agency estimates that 1.5 *trillion* gallons of pollutants leak into the ground each year, with the highest incidence of contamination by lead, radon, and nitrates (from fertilizers). More than 700 chemicals have been found in tap water, but testing is commonly done for fewer than 200 of these, and the significance of chemicals in such low concentrations as parts per trillion is often unknown.

It's essential that water be treated with chlorine or chloramine to kill microbes that can make us ill. Yet, if they stay in our water, they also affect our microbiomes. Inexpensive charcoal filters can remove chlorine and many pollutants from tap water. A pitcher with a simple carbon filter such as Brita or Pur can help purify your drinking water at little cost.

In Europe, bottled water is preferred for its high mineral content. Bottled water isn't always better than tap water, however, especially if it's just tap water that's been filtered. Water from plastic containers may also contain small amounts of plastics that are known to have hormone-disrupting effects. If you regularly buy bottled water, ask the manufacturer for information on water source, type of plastics used, mineral content per glass, and levels of toxic substances. If you rely on local tap water, find out where it originates, how it's processed, and what's been added to it, and ask your water department for an analysis. If you have a well, get a water sample tested for bacterial content and pollutants.

Therapeutic Elimination Diets for GI Healing

If we had a drug that worked as effectively as elimination diets do, it would be the best-selling drug of all time. If we can find the "right" diet for the "right" person at the "right" time, that person can feel remarkably better in two weeks. Healing will take longer, and yet the effects happen fast for most people.

Since writing the fourth edition of *Digestive Wellness,* we have obtained more experience and research on using therapeutic elimination diets. Although it would be lovely, there isn't one specific protocol yet that helps us to determine exactly which dietary approach will work best for a person at a given moment. Yet we have ways that we can think about the person and their needs and come up with a pretty good idea.

First, consider the person. The Mediterranean Diet is a great diet that will work for most people who are healthy. Moving to an 80 percent whole foods diet will be a radical shift in itself, which can have profound effects on health, enhancing people's energy, mood, sleep, digestive issues, pain relief, and more. It may be also as much as your patient or you are willing to consider.

Second, the Elimination Diet is an excellent overall diet to rebalance the DIGIN variables. In my own experience, and from the clinical experience of the faculty at the Institute for Functional Medicine, the first therapeutic intervention to try is the Comprehensive Elimination Diet. This is considered to be the gold standard for figuring out whether someone has food reactions and for reducing inflammation systemically. It removes of the main allergens and problematic foods and is a whole foods diet. (A Comprehensive Elimination Diet plan is available at www.digestivewellnessbook.com.)

Third, if dysbiosis is the main issue, look at a diet that focuses on that condition. Consider using such a diet first if someone's main issues resemble irritable bowel syndrome (IBS): gas, bloating, abdominal pain, constipation, diarrhea, or alternating diarrhea and constipation.

Fourth, consider which of the DIGIN areas have the most urgent need for a decision about which plan to use. Also, there may be foods that make us feel better or worse, which helps health care professionals to match someone with a specific dietary approach. For example, if carbohydrates make a person feel worse, that points to dysbiosis or enzyme insufficiencies. People with neurological or psychological issues often benefit from a gluten-free food plan. The foods that we are hooked on are often the foods that make us sick. Often when someone says, "I just couldn't live without dairy (or wheat, or sugar)," it is likely that this food or food group is triggering reactions. Occasionally, someone's digestive function is so impaired that she or he is eating only a few foods, indicating that it's time to do some repair and gently broaden the diet. Conversely, sometimes people feel better or energized after eating foods, and this can also help guide which plan to choose.

Often, people are eating well and still don't feel well. In this case, people benefit from a therapeutic diet as part of a healing protocol. *Such a food plan is meant to be temporary, not as a lifestyle, although there may be some specific foods or groups of foods that are permanently problematic for a specific person. The ultimate goal is to heal the gut and then broaden what people can eat with the goal of them being able to eat nearly all foods and thrive.*

There is a dizzying number of plans being promoted and a lot of overlap in mechanisms that help these plans work, so if you don't see an exact match, look for one that's similar. No matter which of these you choose, you may get benefits. The lists below are to help you optimize the benefits.

The ones that work have this in common:

- They emphasize eating vegetables, protein, and healthful fats.
- They remove the most common allergens: eggs, dairy, wheat/gluten, sugar, alcohol, and refined and packaged foods.
- They reduce inflammation, help to heal intestinal permeability, and modulate the microbiome.
- They encourage drinking 3 or more quarts of water daily.
- Dysbiosis plans limit carbohydrates; some plans limit all grains.
  - Once your gut is back in balance, you begin reintroducing healthful foods back into your diet one at a time. This allows you to watch for signs to determine if and what foods you may safely add and which you need to continue to avoid.

THE DIGIN WAY OF THINKING

Consider the DIGIN Model when determining which diet to try first. Which of the following issues is likely to be the one that needs to be addressed first? Begin there. Take that approach and see how far it takes you. If it fails or you plateau, try a different one. Here's an overview of my current thought process based on clinical experience and research.

Each of these diets begins with eliminating categories of foods, seeing whether you improve, and then adding them back in slowly in order to determine which one(s) may be provoking your symptoms/issues.

Digestion/Absorption

Enzyme Insufficiencies: Lactase, Fructase, Sucrase Q D I G I N

Symptoms of lactase, fructose, and sucrase insufficiencies overlap with those of IBS and include gas, bloating, diarrhea, constipation, and alternating diarrhea and constipation.

(See the relevant sections in Chapter 11 on each substance specifically for more details.)

- Lactose-free diet: Eliminates all lactose; best used in people with lactose insufficiency.
- Low-fructose diet: Significantly limits fructose; best used in people with genetic fructose insufficiency, people who have acquired fructose intolerance, and people who feel worse after eating fruit.
- Low-sucrose diet: Significantly limits sucrose; best used in people with sucrase insufficiency.

Note: There is often an overlap between these sugar intolerances and histamine intolerance (discussed later in this chapter).

Malabsorption and Maldigestion Q D I G I N

- **Restorative foods:** Best used in people who are malnourished, frail, debilitated, or who have low digestive fire/chi. (*See Chapter 15.*)
- **Elemental Diet:** This diet is essentially a fast; it has been used for decades and has excellent research. In this plan, only medical food is eaten for 2 to 3 weeks. (*See later in this chapter for more details.*)

Microbiome

Dysbiosis Plus Enzyme Insufficiencies: Diamine Oxidase and N-methyltransferase Q ᴅ ɪ ɢ ɪ ɴ

■ **Low-histamine/low-bioactive amine diet:** Although we associate histamines with allergies, histamine intolerance actually is due to enzyme insufficiencies of diamine oxidase (DAO) and/or N-methyltransferase (HMT), dysbiosis in the gut, or a combination of the two. If fermented foods, leftovers, and probiotics don't agree with you are probably affected by histamines. Symptoms can be the same as allergy symptoms or may involve itching; hives; swelling of the face, throat, and mouth; a drop in blood pressure; racing heartbeat (tachycardia); anxiety and/or panic attacks; chest pain; conjunctivitis; headaches; fatigue; confusion; irritability; digestive issues, especially heartburn, indigestion, and reflux; and rarely brief loss of consciousness for 1 to 2 seconds. In children, histamine intolerance often presents as diarrhea, abdominal pain, headache, and chronic, intermittent vomiting. This can be done by removing high histamine foods or by removing high histamine foods from any of the other food plans.

Resources: Dr. Janice Jonega, *A Beginner's Guide to Histamine Intolerance* and *Histamine Intolerance: The Comprehensive Guide for Healthcare Professionals*. Websites: https://histamine-sensitivity.com. Dr. Jill Carnahan: https://www.jillcarnahan.com /downloads/HistamineRestrictedDiet.pdf.

Dysbiosis Diets: Restrict Prebiotics and Carbohydrates Q ᴅ ɪ ɢ ɪ ɴ

Consider this type of eating plan when dysbiosis is the main issue. These diets provide only selected carbohydrates to starve out low-grade infection, reduce inflammation, and rebalance the microbiome. These are not meant to be long-term diets but rather to be used therapeutically for months.

People with the following conditions may benefit: IBS, gas, bloating, diarrhea, constipation, Crohn's disease, and ulcerative colitis. The microbiota feed on sugars, so there could also be sugar craving or the perception that sugar makes you feel worse.

■ **FODMAP DIET:** The FODMAP eating plan was theorized and researched initially by Drs. Peter Gibson and Sue Shepherd. It restricts all high prebiotic-rich foods: fructans, oligosaccharides, disaccharides, monosaccharides, and polyols. There is a large body of research on this plan. The best research to date concerns IBS and small intestinal bacterial overgrowth (SIBO). In addition, it can be used when you suspect that gluten is an issue but a gluten-free diet doesn't help.

Resources: *The Complete Low-Fodmap Diet* by Sue Shepherd and Peter Gibson; FODMAP APP and *The Monash University Low Fodmap Diet:* Best phone app and guide to the FODMAP Diet. Sue Shepherd: shepherdworks.com.au; Kate Scarlata: https://www.katescarlata.com; Patsy Castos: https://www.ibsfree.net; Allison Siebecker: https://www.siboinfo.com.

- **Specific Carbohydrate Diet (SCD):** This is a grain-free, low-disaccharide, and low-lactose food plan. Dr. Elaine Gotschall's daughter was prescribed this eating plan by Dr. Sidney Hass because she had ulcerative colitis, and it was cured. The best research to date is in pediatric Crohn's disease and disaccharide deficiency, and to a lesser degree on ulcerative colitis and Crohn's disease in adults, and also in people for whom the basic elimination diet has failed. Currently, there is a multicentered study in 184 people who have active Crohn's disease, comparing the Mediterranean Diet and the Specific Carbohydrate Diet (SCD). This research was funded in 2016 and will conclude in 2020. The impetus is due to the many people with Crohn's disease who report benefit from the SCD.

Resources: *Breaking the Vicious Cycle*, by Elaine Gotschall. Websites: Breaking the Vicious Cycle: http://www.breakingtheviciouscycle.info; Pecan Bread: pecanbread.com; Nutrition in Immune Balance: https://www.nimbal.org/. Cookbooks: *Grain-Free Gourmet* and *Everyday Grain-Free Gourmet* by Jodi Bager and Jenny Lass. Comparative Effectiveness of Specific Carbohydrate Diet and Mediterranean Diet to Induce Remission in Patients with Crohn's Disease: https://www.pcori.org/research-results/2016/comparative-effectiveness-specific-carbohydrate-and-mediterranean-diets-induce.

- **Antifungal Diets/Anti-candida diets:** Although clinicians have been using antifungal diets with success since the late 1980s, we have little published research on them. These are low-carbohydrate diets that modulate the microbiota and reduce inflammation. Research reports that antifungal diets may be of benefit in people with psoriasis, people who have taken a lot of antibiotics, people who have taken a lot of prednisone or cortisone, and people with sugar cravings. It's possible that some people who benefit have SIBO or a combination of fungal and bacterial dysbiosis. (See more on the Candida Questionnaire and testing information in Chapter 11, and in Chapter 23.)

Resources: Donna Gates, *Body Ecology Diet* and https://bodyecology.com; Elizabeth Larsen, "Kicking Candida," https://experiencelife.com/article/kicking-candida/.

- Elemental Diet: This diet is essentially a fast; it has been used for decades for people who need to rest their digestive tracts and has excellent research into its efficacy. It is currently used with people who have short bowel syndrome, eosinophilic esophagitis, inflammatory bowel disease, people with celiac disease who do not heal better without gluten in their diet, SIBO, pancreatitis, and radiation-induced GI damage.

In this plan, people "fast," eating only a medical food for 2 to 3 weeks. A "medical food" is one that is formulated specifically to help people who have a specific health need. Elemental food formulas have easy to digest carbohydrates and fats, free amino acids, and vitamins and minerals.

According to Dr. Allison Siebecker, if necessary, people may add broiled, plain chicken breast without skin; weak black tea, herbal tea, or coffee; magnesium for constipation; and small amounts of stevia to sweeten the medical food.

Caution: Because this approach is extreme, follow it under the care of a qualified clinician. Also, note that medical foods used for GI issues typically taste bad, so have low expectations. With the use of the Elemental Diet, there is the potential for a lot of weight loss, so be wary about using it in someone who would be harmed by losing weight. In addition, use with caution with someone with a history of eating disorders and people who have diabetes. It may cause fungal overgrowth in some people. Insurance may or may not cover these medical foods.

Resources: Allison Siebecker: Information and homemade formula: https://www.siboinfo.com. Integrative Therapeutics: https://data.integrativepro.com/product-literature/info/physicians-elemental-diet-original-dextrose-free-info-sheet.pdf. Other products used in the Elemental Diet include Peptamin, Neocate Jr., Splash and Vivonex.

INTESTINAL PERMEABILITY/GUT MICROBIOME/ 🔍 DIGIN

INFLAMMATION/IMMUNE:

These diets are great all-around eating plans to help heal a leaky gut, balance the microbiome, and lower inflammation. Typically, these are the first approaches considered. Yet, if someone has obvious dysbiosis, begin with a dysbiosis plan. Consider when someone has leaky gut, known food allergies, eczema, asthma, food sensitivities, pain and inflammation, IBS, IBD, migraine headaches, arthritis, mood and attention issues, autoimmune issues, and other conditions.

- **Elimination Diet:** This is considered the gold standard for determining whether food is a main factor in systemic inflammation and health. It covers both innate and adaptive (antibody) immune reactions. Consider using this plan for someone has known or suspected food reactions, allergies, intolerances, or sensitivities. This is a low-antigen and low-inflammatory diet. In my own practice, I have seen people with digestive issues, autoimmune conditions including lupus and celiac disease, allergies, eczema, fatigue, food reactions, autism, IBS, Crohn's disease, arthritis, migraine headaches, depression/anxiety, focus, sleep issues, and other conditions see benefits quickly.

Resources: See Elimination Diet, posted at www.digestivewellnessbook.com; Tom Malterre and Alissa Segersten's book, *The Elimination Diet,* and website, https://wholelifenutrition.net/articles/elimination-diet/free-elimination-diet-resources; and Institute for Functional Medicine/Elimination Diet at *Experience Life Magazine*: https://experiencelife.com/article/the-institute-for-functional-medicines-elimination-diet-comprehensive-guide-and-food-plan/.

- **6-Food Elimination Diet:** This eating plan is most researched for people with eosinophilic esophagitis, with over 20 studies. This therapeutic food plan removes fewer foods and food groups than the Elimination Diet. Lucedo, et al., in 2013 were the first to explore this dietary approach. The 6-food elimination diet was effective in 72 percent of people who tried it for eosinophilic esophagitis. After 3 months on the diet, they remained disease free for a year. Foods that are eliminated include dairy, eggs, wheat (by that term, I include all gluten-containing grains), soy, peanuts legumes, and tree nuts. Since then, additional studies have been done in adults and children that demonstrate the benefits of this food plan.

Resources: University of Wisconsin, https://www.uwhealth.org/healthfacts/nutrition/553.pdf; American Academy of Allergy Asthma and Immunology: https://www.aaaai.org/global/latest-research-summaries/Current-JACI-Research/diet-eoe.

- **Gluten-Free/Casein-Free/Egg-Free Diet:** Consider this option when someone is willing to remove only the top three problematic food groups.
- **Gluten-Free/Casein-Free Diet:** We have little published research on this plan, although it is widely used in the autism community. There is some research on benefits in people with schizophrenia. Consider when someone is willing to make some change, but not too much.
- **Gluten-Free Diet:** This eating plan is necessary in someone with diagnosed celiac disease and a good trial for someone who has diagnosed or suspected non-celiac gluten intolerance or wheat intolerance.

- **Casein-Free Diet:** This should be utilized in people with known or suspected milk-protein allergies. (See more details in Chapter 11 to learn more about hidden sources of casein.)
- **Paleo Diet, also called the Hunter-Gatherer Diet, the Autoimmune Protocol Diet, or Paleo-Immune Diet:** First explored by Loren Cordain PhD, the Paleolithic diet has been found to reduce all-cause mortality, improve insulin sensitivity and glucose levels in people with type 2 diabetes, reduce inflammation and oxidative damage, and slow or reverse the effects of autoimmune disease. Papers discuss the Paleo Diet in people with GI issues and demonstrated reductions in fatty liver, and one paper explores the benefits in people with inflammatory bowel disease, demonstrating drops in calprotectin and improvements seen on endoscopy. The Paleo Diet includes foods that our ancestors might have eaten, including all meats, poultry, fish, eggs, nuts, seeds, vegetables, fruit herbs, spices, healthy fats, and oils like olive and coconut oil. What it doesn't include is processed foods, grains of all kinds, dairy products, processed sugar, beans, lentils, soy, or peanuts. I've found that many people with GI issues benefit from a grain-free and dairy-free diet. Some people thrive on this diet. I think of this as a therapeutic diet to be used until a person feels better. Once that occurs and the root issues have been resolved as well as possible, begin a therapeutic challenge of foods to see which foods can be added back into the diet.

Resources:

- Loren Cordain PhD, *The Paleo Diet.* https://thepaleodiet.com/
- Datis Kharazzian PhD, DHSc, DC, MS, MMSc, FACN, Dr. K News: http://drknews.com/autoimmune-gut-repair-diet
- **IFM ReNew Food Plan:** ReNew Food Plan (which is similar to the Paleo Diet) was developed by the Cleveland Clinic's Institute for Functional Medicine and the Institute for Functional Medicine. Consider this as a 2-week "reboot" for people who have autoimmune, GI, neurological, dysbiosis, and other complex chronic issues. This approach eliminates common allergens and pro-inflammatory foods, helps to identify foods and food groups which may be triggering symptoms, and helps support detoxification pathways. It has low-histamine options built into the plan. There are no grains and no packaged foods. This plan is based upon research, yet so far there is no published research on this specific plan.

Resources: Institute for Functional Medicine: https://www.ifm.org/news-insights/renew-food-plan-stabilizes-blood-sugar-insulin/

- **Oligoantigenic Diet:** This diet typically has only foods that are not commonly eaten by an individual (often limited to 5–10 foods). The diet that was utilized in research included lamb, chicken, potatoes, rice, bananas, apples, cabbage, sprouts, cauliflower, broccoli, cucumber, celery, carrots, parsnips, water, salt, and pepper, plus calcium supplements. In the 1980s, research was done on this diet and its effects on migraine headaches and children with seizure disorders who also had additional complications. The findings demonstrated benefits; of 45 children with seizures, 25 were seizure free on the diet, and 11 others saw reduced seizure episodes.
- **Wahls Diet:** Dr. Terry Wahls cured her own multiple sclerosis and has published clinical studies with her patients who have used this nearly ketogenic food plan and demonstrated improvement in motor function, energy, mood, and quality of life. This approach is a low-carbohydrate plan that restricts many foods, eliminates common allergens and pro-inflammatory foods, and helps to identify foods and food groups that may be triggering symptoms. At this time, this diet is recommended for people with multiple sclerosis. In a personal communication with Dr. Wahls, she states that has seen regression of symptoms in people with IBD and a number of autoimmune conditions, including diabetes, rheumatoid arthritis, lupus, psoriatic arthritis, and fibromyalgia. Dr. Wahls also hopes to do research on the diet in people with amyotrophic lateral sclerosis (ALS), also known as Lou Gehrig's disease.

Resources: Terry Wahls: https://terrywahls.com.

- **Gut and Psychology Syndrome Diet (GAPS Diet):** We have no published research on this plan. Dr. Campbell McBride healed her son's autism by using this food plan that combines the Specific Carbohydrate Diet and the principles of the Weston Price Foundation of traditional eating into one.

Resources: *Gut and Psychology Syndrome* by Natasha Campbell-McBride, www.gapsdiet.com.

- **Low-Lectin Diet:** We have no published human research on the low-lectin diet at this time; weak animal research links wheat germ agglutinin and soybean agglutinin to increased permeability. There are no indications at present to recommend this plan, although anecdotally many people benefit.

ENTERIC NERVOUS SYSTEM: Q D I G I N

For someone who has depression, neurological symptoms and conditions, anxiety, or issues with attention or cognitive decline, consider the Elimination Diet first. Based on current research and understanding of mechanisms, plans that may be the most helpful include the following (described in more detail earlier in this section):

- Comprehensive Elimination Diet
- 6-Food Elimination Diet
- Gluten-Free/Casein-Free Diet
- IFM ReNew Food Plan
- Autoimmune Paleo Diet
- Wahls Diet

Detoxify: While doing the Elimination Diet or the Gluten-Free, Casein-Free, Gluten-Free/Casein Free, Gluten/Casein/Egg Free, or 6-Food Elimination diets, you may want to gain an extra advantage by adding a protein powder that upregulates Phase 1 and Phase 2 liver detoxification pathways. Using a rice-based medical food (such as UltraClear/Rice or UltraClear Plus/Rice by Metagenics), begin slowly, with 1 to 2 scoops daily. Virtually all other supplement companies also have medical foods that enhance liver detoxification, and any of these can be used, so long as all the ingredients are allowed on the plan. Therefore, rice-based or hemp-based products are best in this instance. Adding a medical food allows the diets to work more deeply and effectively.

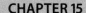

CHAPTER 15

Restorative Foods for Healing

Sometimes we are so debilitated, raw, inflamed, or compromised that we have to go back to eating basics and heal deeply before we can eat normally. I call this the "Restoration Diet." This plan is a temporary plan to help build vitality in someone who is ill or weak. I've utilized it with clients who tell me that they are have been able to eat only a limited amount of foods over the last months or year. I have utilized it with someone who is elderly and not able to easily digest; and I've utilized this with people who are having issues from chemotherapy for cancer.

When you've had the flu, your natural instinct is to choose a temporary diet that looks much like this restoration diet, one that includes soups and easy to digest foods and fluids.

Eating well-cooked food lessens the digestive burden to leave more energy for healing. In previous chapters, we've discussed the use of digestive enzymes, umeboshi plums, and other tools to help increase the fire in your belly. In this chapter we'll be talking about specific foods and specific diets that can accelerate healing.

HEALING FOODS DIET: NOURISH THE BELLY'S FLAME WHILE SOOTHING THE MEMBRANES

When working with clients, who are debilitated or only able to eat a few foods. I find myself recommending the same diet over and over for people whose digestive system is weak. You may or may not tolerate or like all of these foods. Eat what you like. Eat what works. This will be different for each person. When healing, our body thrives on foods that are simple to digest. You may want to think like a sick person or like a baby when it comes to food. Yes, a baby. I've worked with many people who need to puree foods in order to utilize them. You may need to stay on this type of diet for a week or two, or even a couple of months, before your body can handle more. As you get stronger, you'll begin to want to try new foods and explore. The more success you get, the more adventurous you'll become.

Cooked Foods

You'll find that warm, well-cooked foods are easier to digest than raw and cold foods. You may love salads, but they may not love you at this moment in time. Even if you choose to eat your food at room temperature, it will be more healing if you have cooked it previously. You may want to invest in a slow cooker, pressure cooker, or an Instant Pot, which combines the best of both. With a slow cooker, you simply toss food in and it cooks all day or at night while you are sleeping.

You can also put grains and beans in a slow cooker to let them soak for a few hours before cooking. This releases the phytic acid, which binds minerals and makes the food not only more nutritious but easier to digest as well.

Eat Frequently and in Small Amounts

You'll digest and use your foods best if you eat small meals and snacks throughout the day and evening. Eat something every one to three hours.

Protein

Your body needs protein to heal. I typically don't eat any red meat, but after major surgery I ate brisket several times a day for the first six weeks. I was like a junkie who couldn't get enough. Red meat is a protein similar to my own muscle protein. My body needed it to heal. The following list offers great ways to get protein into your diet:

- Bone broths, vegetable broths, miso broth.
- Soups: Lentil soup, bean soup, vegetable or chicken soup. You can add sea vegetables to add minerals.
- Well-cooked meats, such as brisket, stews, or chicken that was boiled.
- Bone marrow: You can take beef bones and roast them to eat the marrow. This is very nourishing.
- Stews: Vegetables plus protein, perhaps some grain, potatoes, or yams.
- Eggs: poached, soft-boiled. Buy organic eggs, fresh, and local if possible.

- Dairy: You may or may not thrive on dairy. Try goat's milk kefir to begin with. You can also try homemade yogurt, either with sheep's or goat's milk. If raw (fresh) milk is available in your area, you may want to try drinking it or making yogurt or kefir from it. You can also make kefir or yogurt with coconut water, coconut milk, or soy milk.
- Protein powder: You can use this for snacks or to add nutrients and calories at mealtime. There are many good protein powders. Look for rice protein, pea protein, hemp protein, or whey protein. Whey is dairy based, so if you have problems with dairy products, whey may or may not work well for you. You can drink them with water or diluted juice, or use as the base for a smoothie with fruit.
- Dahl: Made with red lentils, this is typically an easy bean to digest.

Fats

Your body also needs fats. They burn slowly and also nourish and soothe your nervous and immune systems.

- Healing fats: Butter, ghee, coconut oil, olive oil, hemp seed, flaxseed, avocados, coconut milk, coconut water.
- Some people tolerate nuts and seeds, or seed and nut butters. Use these minimally at first. Nut butters, such as almond butter, cashew butter, and macadamia nut butter, are often tolerated in small amounts. These can even be added to a smoothie or mixed with water to make a sauce to put on vegetables. Tahini, sesame butter, can be used the same way. If you tolerate nuts well, eat them. If you soak them first, you will make them more digestible. Roasting nuts also makes them easier to digest.

Grains

Eat non-gluten-containing grains such as rice, quinoa, millet, amaranth, teff, and buckwheat. Make these well cooked, like gruel, or put them into soups. This is common in Oriental medicine where congee, soaked and well-cooked grains, is used as part of a regular diet as well as for restoration. You will digest these best if you soak the grains first and if you use more water than you typically would. Most grains require two parts water to one part grain. To make grains easier to digest, I recommend three or four parts water to one part grain. Let the grain soak in the water for a few hours before you cook it. Soaking tricks the grains; they "think" that it's spring and time to sprout, and they release precious minerals and nutrients that you'll be able to use. You'll find that the grain is easier to digest, plus the cooking time is cut in half.

Vegetables

If you look at your plate, at least half of what you eat each day ought to be vegetables. Cook these well, culture them, juice them, or eat in soups or stews. Fruits and vegetables contain excellent fibers and prebiotics, protein, minerals, vitamins, polyphenols, and carbohydrate. Here are some suggestions on what to choose:

- Well-cooked vegetables, including *all* non-starchy vegetables and root vegetables. Root vegetables have more starch in them and can be more filling and satisfying. Be brave and try new vegetables: artichoke (boiled soft), arugula, asparagus, bamboo shoots, beets, broccoli, Brussels sprouts, cabbage, carrots, cauliflower, celery, celery root (great in soup), chard, collard greens, cucumber, eggplant, fennel bulb (in soup or roasted), garlic, green beans, kale, leeks, mushrooms, mustard greens, okra, parsley, peas, potatoes (best boiled or in soup or stew), spinach, sweet potatoes, onions, winter squash, turnips, turnip greens, watercress, yams, zucchini.
- Cultured vegetables, such as sauerkraut.
- Sea vegetables: Common sea vegetables include kombu, arame, dulse, and nori. These foods provide minerals and easy-to-utilize proteins. Drop some kombu or other sea vegetable in soup while it's cooking. Use sheets of nori to wrap vegetables or grains in; buy them flaked to use instead of salt in cooking and at the table. Soak some dulse and add it to your vegetables. Add some kelp flakes to your protein powder. You typically find these in the Asian section of a health food store or in an Asian market.
- Fresh vegetable juices prepared and used the same day. Try carrot, ginger, beet, kale, parsley, apple, watercress, cabbage, or sauerkraut.

Fruit

The amount of fruit that people can tolerate when in a weakened condition varies. Use your body to discover the right amount for you. Start with these suggestions:

- Very ripe fruit
- Cooked fruit
- Applesauce
- Diluted fruit juices

Beverages

It's important that you stay hydrated. Your body is two-thirds water. You may find that drinking teas or warm water is most soothing. Here is a list of beverages to try:

- Water, water with a bit of juice, water with lemon, water with raw apple cider vinegar
- Teas, such as mint, slippery elm, fennel, fenugreek, ginger, umeboshi, roobios, green tea
- Fresh vegetable juices
- Broths

Herbs and Spices

Use fresh or dried herbs and spices in cooking: salt, pepper, basil, oregano, dill, caraway, fenugreek, fennel, cumin, coriander, cinnamon, nutmeg, allspice, and so on. Try to avoid "hot" spices such as cayenne and chili powder unless they call out to you!

MEDICAL FOODS

If you are wasting away and cannot eat much at all, you may want to consider eating a medical food. I've found that medical foods can be lifesaving for people who are literally starving. These are hypoallergenic "foods" that are composed of nutrients that are already fully digested. Proteins are presented as free amino acids. Fats are presented as fatty acids. Carbohydrates are simple. Vitamins and minerals are in basic forms that are easily utilized. Typically you would want to drink these one to six times daily to either replace or supplement your diet. There are many of these on the market today; your physician or nutritionist may recommend Pepta-men or Vivonex or other products. Supplement companies, including Metagenics, Integrative Therapeutics, Thorne, Xymogen, and others, also manufacture these products. For advanced conditions, you may even want to explore the Elemental Diet (discussed in Chapter 13). Specialized diets for gut healing are also discussed more fully in Chapter 13. Depending on what state you live in and what your doctor writes as a diagnosis, medical foods may or may not be reimbursable through your health care plan.

RECIPES

Here are a few basic recipes you may want to try. They are all nutrient laden and gut healing. For more recipes and cooking videos, go to www.digestivewellnessbook .com/resources

Four-Minute Chicken Stock

Yield: 1 gallon

Bones from poultry, fish, beef, lamb,
shellfish, or whole chicken or whole
carcass (remove meat when cooked—
about 1 hour)
8–10 cups water
1–2 tablespoons lemon juice or vinegar
1–2 teaspoons salt
½ teaspoon pepper
2 carrots
1 onion

2 stalks celery
½ cup chopped fresh parsley, or 2
tablespoons dried parsley
1–2 teaspoons sage
1–2 teaspoons rosemary
1–2 teaspoons thyme
2–3 bay leaves
2 tablespoons raw apple cider vinegar or
juice from 1 lemon

Put all ingredients into a large pot. Bring to a boil. Let simmer over low heat for several
hours (4–24) or in a slow cooker on low. Remove bones and vegetables. Let sit until
cool, then skim off fat.

This will keep about 5–6 days in your refrigerator. You can easily freeze this and use it
when you are ready for it.

Uses for Broth

- Use as stock for soup.
- Drink as a warm beverage.
- Use as the cooking liquid for vegetables and grains.
- Make gravy from the fats.

Magic Mineral Broth

Yield: 6 to 7 quarts

*Inner Cook notes: If you don't have time to make this from scratch, substitute Pacific
or Imagine brand vegetable stock, add equal parts water, a piece of kombu, and one
potato. Boil 20 minutes and strain.*

Cut the following four ingredients into
large chunks:
6 unpeeled carrots, including 3 with tops
2 unpeeled medium yellow onions
1 leek, both white and green parts
1 stalk celery, including the heart
4 unpeeled garlic cloves, halved
½ bunch flat-leaf Italian parsley
4 medium red potatoes, quartered with
skins on

2 Japanese or Hannah yams or 2 sweet
potatoes, quartered with skins on
1 garnet yam, quartered with skin on
1 tablespoon sea salt
1 6-inch-by-1-inch strip of kombu
2 bay leaves
12 peppercorns
4 whole allspice or juniper berries

In a 12-quart stockpot, combine all ingredients. Fill the pot with water to two inches below the rim, cover, and bring to a boil. Remove the lid, decrease heat to low, and simmer a minimum of 2 hours. As the stock simmers, some water will evaporate; add more if vegetables begin to peek out. Simmer until the full richness of the vegetables can be tasted. Strain the stock using a large-mesh strainer. (Be sure to have a heat-resistant container underneath.)

Bring to room temperature before refrigerating or freezing.

Magic Mineral Broth can be frozen up to six months in a variety of airtight container sizes for every use.

Used with permission from Rebecca Katz. Recipe from *One Bite at a Time* by Rebecca Katz, founder of The Inner Cook. Berkeley, CA: Celestial Arts Publishing, 2008.

Melody's Dahl
This serves 4 hungry people.

Serve this dish with rice and steamed vegetables. Use chutney and/or cultured vegetables as a condiment.

1 cup red lentils (they are actually orange)

4 cups water

1 teaspoon salt

1 teaspoon turmeric powder

1–3 teaspoons grated fresh ginger

2 tablespoons oil or butter or ghee or coconut oil

1 teaspoon powdered cumin

1 teaspoon powdered coriander

Wash red lentils and soak for 2–12 hours. Bring water and salt to a boil and add red lentils. Add turmeric powder and ginger. Turn down heat to a low simmer and cook about 30 minutes (or about an hour if you didn't have time to soak the lentils first). Stir occasionally so that dahl doesn't stick to the bottom of the pot.

Just before serving, take a small frying pan and heat oil, butter, or ghee on medium to medium-low heat. When oil is hot, add cumin and coriander. Cook 1 minute and then add to the dahl. Stir the dahl. Cook a couple more minutes and serve with rice and steamed vegetables.

Bone Marrow Three Ways
1. Add marrow bones to soups and stews. The marrow will "melt" into the dish.

2. Ask the butcher to cut the bones into two- to three-inch sections. Soak these in cold water for 12 to 24 hours. Change the water a few times to keep the pinkish color. Boil for 20 minutes. Scoop out the marrow with a spoon. You can sprinkle this with salt and eat it or use it in soup or as a garnish.

3. Roasted marrow: Take two- to three-inch pieces of marrow bones. Place in an ovenproof frying pan or on a cookie sheet standing upright. Roast at 450°F for 20 minutes. The marrow is ready when loose and giving. If you cook it for too long, it will simply melt away.

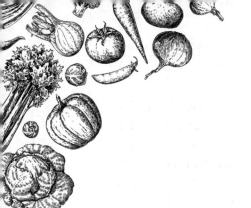

CHAPTER 16

Balancing Stress on All Levels

"In Sri Lanka, we often compare human life to a river. When river water falls down the hills, it creates a beautiful waterfall. When it crashes on rocks, white foam is created, expressing its incredible hidden beauty. When the river silently flows through the valleys, it becomes mysterious and magical. These different things that happen to the river water along its path are all manifestations of its beauty. So, too, if we are to make meaning out of our odyssey as human beings on this planet, we have to accept that whatever happens on our way adds to life's beauty."

—Bhante Wimala, *Lessons of the Lotus: Practical Spiritual Teachings of a Travelling Buddhist Monk*

It is the meaning we attach to our experiences that makes them stressful or stress-free. Last week we had heavy rains. I loved the rain. The sound of it reminded me of the heavy rains of my childhood in the Chicago suburbs. The creek below my house grew, and I could hear it in the mornings from my bedroom. I settled in and took life a bit more slowly. The foliage developed a deep green hue that felt nurturing and satisfying. The land needed the rain. All of this fit my mood. But when I mentioned this to two people, the responses that I got were: "I hated the rain. I'm sensitive to mold and couldn't breathe" and "It's a good thing it stopped raining; otherwise, we would have had flooding in a few days." It is our perspective and beliefs that shape whether something is stressful or pleasurable. To me, the rain was a delicious treat. To others, something dreaded. What is true and real for one person is different from another's true and real. One is no truer than the other.

Adverse Childhood Experiences (ACEs)

Research surveys looking at adverse childhood experiences (ACEs) have found that the more of these that a person has, the greater the risk for poorer outcomes in life and increased risk for adult diseases. Questions on these surveys focus on emotional, physical, or sexual abuse; whether there was substance abuse or mental illness in the family; whether the mother was mistreated; whether a family member was in prison; and whether there was emotional or physical neglect. Nearly two-thirds of the participants answered yes to one of these categories.

As ACEs increase, so does the risk of developing mental health issues, drug and alcohol dependency, abusive relationships, and other risky behavior; there is also an increased risk of heart attack, diabetes, stroke, asthma, depression, disability, and other diseases. Both the risk and the severity for inflammatory bowel syndrome (IBS) rise as the ACEs increase. IBS was specifically associated with a history of emotional abuse and having a mentally ill or imprisoned household member.

(Resource: Questionnaires and more data on ACEs can be found at the Centers for Disease Control and Prevention: https://www.cdc.gov/violenceprevention/acestudy /about.html.)

Chronic Stress, Risk, and Digestive Disorders

It has been said that 80 percent of the reason people seek medical attention is ultimately stress. Stress disrupts the gut barrier and the microbiome. It also changes our hormonal balance and enteric nervous system and leads to chronic, low-grade inflammation. Chronic stress has also been associated with inflammatory bowel disease (IBD), ulcers, diarrhea, other digestive issues, plus cardiovascular disease, fibromyalgia, asthma, eczema, arthritis, posttraumatic stress disorder (PTSD), chronic pelvic and abdominal pain, increased infections, headaches, slow wound healing, neurological disease, Alzheimer's disease, cancer, anxiety and depression, and chronic fatigue syndrome.

Emotional and Spiritual Release

From the time we are small, we attach meaning to events. When you first spilled milk from your glass and got yelled at for it, you attached: "not good enough" or "less than" to that spill. This happens to all of us; we carry these meanings and conditioning around as adults, and they are deeply held entities, even though we aren't even aware of it. In my clients, I often find that I can go only so far by trying to balance biochemistry. It's easy to focus on what we can see, which is the physiology and biochemistry of the body. Yet, what can be seen often feels to me like the tip of the iceberg.

Often, emotional and spiritual blockages prevent healing from occurring on a deep level. Once these are released, more healing takes place. Working with a therapist, a co-counselor, a coach, an energetic healer, an acupuncturist, a body-worker who incorporates emotional release, a shaman, someone who works with either emotional freedom technique (EFT) or eye movement desensitization and reprocessing (EMDR), a homeopathy specialist, or other professionals can help to facilitate the release of emotional issues that keep your healing stuck. I recall being at a meeting of the Crohn's and Colitis Foundation. Attendees were talking about their healing from IBD. Changing their diets played an enormous role, but they all also attributed their healing to working with a therapist, a shaman, or an acupuncturist.

THE ONLY CONSTANT IS CHANGE

From the moment we are born, we begin to change, and this continues until we take our last breath. Our body changes; our ideas change; our desires change. This is the nature of life. And all changes around us, too. People come and go; jobs come and go; babies are born; loved ones die; we travel; we move houses; we leave for college; we retire; and so on.

Fear of change motivates behavior in some people. To keep life steady and predictable, we often box ourselves in so that we have control. But this is an illusion. No matter how hard we try to protect ourselves from change, change happens. (See Figure 16.1.) No matter how hard we try to control our lives, change happens. We'd be just as likely to control the seasons.

When I was younger, I took a self-defense course to become more streetwise living in Chicago. My instructor said a very wise thing: "If you have enough time to be

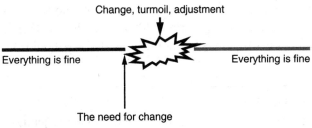

Figure 16.1   **How transitions happen.**

afraid, you have enough time to think about solutions." This statement has rung true for me many times in my life. Rather than spending my thoughts on fear or worry, I can be creative and try to see what solutions are available.

Change typically happens in an instant. We're moving along and suddenly our life gets derailed by losing our job, falling in love, realizing that we want to go back to school, getting sick, finding out our spouse is having an affair, an earthquake, planes crashing into the World Trade Towers, finding out that we'll be doing another tour of duty in the military, having a traffic accident, finding out that company is coming, and so forth. When we live in the present moment and accept what is, we are relieved of a great burden. Think of yourself flowing down a river toward the ocean. Sometimes you'll meander; sometimes you'll work hard to keep your head above water because the flow is so quick. Other times you'll be stuck in an eddy, going nowhere. Our lives are exactly this way. We are just flowing down the river of life. We don't control the river's flow. We just bob along, trying to keep our head above water and enjoying the scenery.

STRESS OR OPPORTUNITY?

Though we mainly think of stress as a negative thing, it does have a positive side. The stress of going to college, being in the military, getting married, having children, or earning a promotion provides opportunities and challenges that force us to change, grow, and strive to fulfill our potential.

But even positive stress can overwhelm us, causing distress. When we bite off more than we can chew, we feel stressed out. In many instances, we have little control over stressors, like illness, loss of a job, financial worries, and death. But even in these circumstances, we have control over our thoughts and behavior. This is where stress management offers many benefits. Studies have shown that people who have emotional hardiness handle distress more easily than people with less resilience. Hardy people take on a challenge, make a commitment, take control, and see what happens. If success comes their way, it encourages them to try new things. If they fail, they pick themselves up and try again, recognizing that experience gained from

ANYTIME ABDOMINAL BREATHING EXERCISE

Take 10 deep breaths through your nose. As you inhale, feel your belly expand; feel the inhalation spread until it fills your lungs to the top. Exhale by letting your lungs gently deflate. Notice how you feel. If you're calmer, remember this tool and use it as needed.

"failure" adds to life's perspective. Fortunately, it's possible for anyone to learn hardiness skills.

Mental stress is one of the greatest challenges to our immune systems, putting pressure on nearly every organ and system in the body. When we feel stressed out, our bodies react with an increased heartbeat, shallow and rapid breathing, a release of adrenaline, and raised blood sugar levels and oxygen rates. Our muscles tense so we can move quickly. An increased blood supply is sent to our brain and major muscles, with decreased blood flow to our extremities. Even our pupils dilate and we sweat more. Our bodies react this way because our minds tell us there is a dangerous situation that requires quick thinking and movement. Historically, this might have been a bear on our path, a forest fire, or the exhilaration of the hunt. Today, it can be anything from a near car collision, to three phone lines ringing at once, to burned toast! Because our first reaction is to unconsciously hold our breath and breathe shallowly, deep-breathing exercises are an excellent stress-management tool. Breathing deeply brings more oxygen to our tissues while waste products are excreted. It slows us down, so we feel more balanced and centered and can make clearer decisions. Deep abdominal breathing is something you can do anywhere, and no one can tell!

How do we know when we're under too much stress? Our body will usually tell us before our mind does. We may get a neck ache, backache, or headache, a sick feeling in our stomach, hives, fatigue, or a myriad of other symptoms. But even though our body is telling us to stop, we keep on going. Our culture rewards this type of behavior. But we owe it to ourselves to listen to our own needs more carefully and to respond to them in kind. Pain and discomfort are our body's way of asking us to pay attention, now!

SIGNALS OF STRESS

Emotional	*Physical*	*Behavioral*
Moodiness	Muscle tension	Overuse of drugs/alcohol
Worry	Aches and pains	Overeating
Irritability	Fatigue	Forgetfulness
Hostility/anger	Sleep disturbances	Clumsiness
Bad dreams	Diarrhea	Depression
Lassitude	Digestive symptoms	Tension
Defensiveness	Headaches	Poor eating
Difficulty concentrating		

We can tune into these signals, or we can choose to ignore the messages and carry on with our activities. If we ignore them, the symptoms may go away, or they may blast louder and louder until we are forced to pay attention or our bodies break down. Being attentive to small signals allows us to gently get back on track without experiencing major upheavals in our lives.

The most important component of a good stress-management program is to have a plan with reasonable and realistic goals. If you need to, get a buddy or professional who will support you. Think of the ways in which you might slip or lose your way and prepare for them. Once your goals and support system are in place, you can spring into action.

SELF-RENEWAL

Do you take time each day for self-renewal and nurturing yourself? Getting restful sleep, taking time to exercise, spending time doing things you enjoy, and eating healthful foods are the foundation of a healthy lifestyle. How do you nurture yourself? How do you renew?

Exercise

The best stress-management tool is exercise. When I ask people to describe the benefits of their exercise program, they tell me they have more energy, have higher self-esteem, and feel more relaxed. Exercise makes us stronger and more flexible and increases our balance, which helps keep us injury free. Regular exercise helps control blood sugar levels so our energy is more sustained, and being fit lowers the risk of heart disease. In addition, our bodies release endorphins, morphine-like molecules in the brain, which make us feel happy and reduce pain!

Positive Thoughts

Positive thinking is an important part of stress management. If you could tape the conversation in your brain for an hour or two, you might find you had a lot of self-criticism or self-doubts. With practice we can easily learn to "flip" these negative images and turn criticism into a positive thought or plan of action. When we catch ourselves playing a negative tape, we need to eject it and put in a new tape. Instead of thinking "My ulcerative colitis will get worse and worse until I need surgery," you can flip the image and say, "So far I haven't licked this problem, but if I am persistent, I can improve my health."

Get Restorative Sleep

Essential to healing is getting enough sleep. As a culture, we are sleep deprived. Set your schedule so that you get at least seven to nine hours of sleep every night. This is where your body heals and recenters. Without adequate sleep, it is nearly impossible to heal. It is beyond the boundaries of this book to discuss sleep hygiene and tips and tools for sleeping better, but here are just a few tips:

- At least one hour before bed, turn off your computer. Now it's time for a bath or reading, listening to calming ideas, or relaxing with some music.
- Go to bed at the same time each night; wake up at the same time each day. Our parents knew something when they regulated our bedtime!
- Take calcium and magnesium before bed. This helps to relax your nerves and muscles.
- You may find teas that contain chamomile, hops, valerian, and/or passionflower to be calming and restful.
- I keep a spray bottle of water with a bit of lavender oil mixed into it beside my bed. If I find that I'm not falling asleep, I give myself a couple of spritzes on my forehead. Works, for me, like a charm.
- Some people find that taking 1 to 3 mg melatonin, or 5-hydroxy-tryptophan (5HTP) at doses of 50 to 200 mg, helps with sleep.

Remember to rest when your body is tired. It is not culturally normal to nap unless we are in preschool or are elderly. Yet in many cultures, napping is an essential habit. Rather than pushing yourself when you've run out of steam, take time to rest or nap. You'll find that this is restorative.

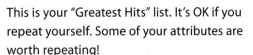

"THE GREATEST HITS" OF YOURSELF

Close your eyes for a minute and think of all your most wonderful attributes. Compliment yourself freely. Take some time to appreciate your good points and achievements. Think about times in your life when you helped someone, fell in love, were in a beautiful place, made someone happy, and really felt good about yourself. Now quickly write down all of your best attributes. Don't be shy: overstate!

This is your "Greatest Hits" list. It's OK if you repeat yourself. Some of your attributes are worth repeating!

If you'd like to, keep this list somewhere so you'll be reminded of how terrific you are and how many blessings fill your life. Liking ourselves also helps our view of others and the world around us.

FINDING BALANCE

Prioritizing helps us find the balance point in our lives. Balance is hard to achieve and maintain, but it is an honorable goal. Like many people, if something really interests me, I take on new responsibilities and enjoyable events until I become overwhelmed. Then I make a list of all of my commitments and prioritize them to see what I can let go of responsibly. Soon my life is back in balance—until the next exciting possibility comes along and I'm overcommitted again. To be honest, I'm the queen of overcommitment, but when I say ouch, I reevaluate and let go. Be assertive: Learn to say no!

Many years ago, I read *The Goddess Within Us* by Dr. Jean Shinoda Bolen. My big aha was that we expect ourselves to play many roles perfectly—wife/husband/mate, daughter/son, mother/father, businessperson, athlete, spiritual being, homemaker, cook, artist, and civically dedicated citizen, both locally and globally. Yet the Greek and Roman gods and goddesses were excellent at only one thing. So why do we put such unreasonable and unrealistic demands on ourselves? A Buddhist saying is: "Expectation is the root of all suffering." If we can be easier on ourselves and in our relationships, we can find more love, contentment, and peace.

Most of us invest a lot of energy in our work, home, family, and friends. We begin with a barrel filled with apples. If we keep giving our apples away, soon our barrel is empty. We all need time to fill back up to rejuvenate. Sometimes I ask my clients to take two hours during the middle of the day to rejuvenate themselves. The usual response is: "That sounds terrific, but you know it's never going to happen." But inside they know they really need to do this, so they figure out a way to make it happen.

Your prescription: Take an hour or two every day to recharge your batteries. It's not important what you do. Each of us finds renewal in different things. Here are some ideas: read something for fun, play a musical instrument, listen to music, garden, exercise, be outdoors, build something, have a date with a friend, write a letter, keep a journal, enjoy a hobby, take a class, go to church/temple, read holy scriptures,

COMPARTMENTALIZATION EXERCISE

Imagine you are sitting before a rolltop desk with pigeonholes in it. In each hole is a scroll tied neatly with a ribbon. See yourself opening one scroll at a time, examining it, putting it back in its proper place, selecting another, and repeating the process. Do this for several minutes. Find a way to use these pigeonholes in your daily life to help you accomplish tasks step by step. Practice this exercise to help you create closure between tasks and events in your life.

or meditate. Vacations are an important way to put our lives in perspective, to value what is truly important. When was the last time you took a vacation? If it's been more than a year, see if you can create the space to take one . . . even if it's just for a few days.

On the other hand, many people never grab for the ring, and they watch the world go by because they're worried about taking a risk. Because we are afraid, we box ourselves into worlds that are small, hoping to gain control of the chaos "out there." Fear is also stressful. Break out of your box. Act! Oh, to have loved and lost is way better than never to have loved at all.

OVERCOMING OVERWHELM

Compartmentalizing thoughts is a useful tool. Since we can think about or act upon only one responsibility at a time, it helps to put each one in a "compartment." The pearl here is to be able to be 100 percent present and focused on each task while you are doing it. This frees the mind and calms the spirit.

Quick Ideas for Stress Management

- Eat healthy foods.
- Develop better communication skills; learn to really listen.
- Exercise regularly.
- Spend time outdoors.
- Make time for yourself each day for pleasure or relaxation.
- Meditate or learn self-hypnosis or visualization techniques.
- Realize that you don't have to be perfect.
- Think creatively.
- Go at your own pace.
- Think of solutions, not problems.
- Prioritize.
- Keep journals.
- Live one day at a time.
- Play and laugh.
- Spend time with friends and family.
- Be flexible.
- View your problems as an opportunity for growth.
- Plan for chaos in your daily schedule.
- Set clear priorities and stick to them.

- Breathe deeply.
- Plan ahead: Wake up 15 minutes earlier each morning, keep your car in good working order, put a duplicate car key in your wallet, and so on.
- Learn to say "No!"
- Turn off your phone or let your voice mail pick up the calls.
- Take a bath, shower, steam, or Jacuzzi.
- Make lists.
- Keep a calendar or appointment book.
- Reduce your driving speed by 10 miles per hour.
- Take one day a week to relax.
- Honor the Sabbath.
- Believe that people have good intentions and are doing the best job they can.
- See the world through a "loving" filter.

If you begin with just one or two of these stress-management techniques, you'll find more peace and balance in your life. Find what works for you and make each one into a habit. If you want to truly heal your body, you will find that exploring your emotional and spiritual self speeds up the process.

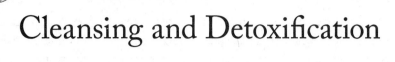

CHAPTER 17

Cleansing and Detoxification

"It can be strongly said that the health of an individual is largely determined by the ability of the body to detoxify."

—Joseph Pizzorno, ND, and Michael Murray, ND,
Encyclopedia of Natural Health

"Brushing, clipping, combing, cutting, shampooing, picking, scratching, shaving, washing, scrubbing, sweating, blowing, breathing, coughing, sneezing, clearing, burping, defecating, flatulating, discharging, dripping, draining, menstruating, spitting, sweating, urinating, vomiting, wiping, methylating, acetylating, glucuronidating, sulfating, glutathionylating, glycinating. . . . Ridding oneself of unwanted stuff is a lot of work. The serious part of this work is synthetic, and unlike the items in the first part of my list, requires the lion's share of daily energy requirements involved in making new molecules."

—Sidney Baker McDonald, MD

We are exposed to toxins everywhere—from the air we breathe to the foods we eat, even as a result of metabolism. These toxins affect our nervous system and cause irritation and inflammation throughout our bodies. People have always been exposed to toxic substances, but today's exposure to contaminants far exceeds that of previous times. Increased exposure began during the Industrial Revolution and blossomed after World War II. Baby boomers grew up with the slogan "Better Living Through Chemistry," and we believed it! In 2018, the American Chemical Society's *Chemical Abstracts* index listed 1.44 million chemicals, and 85,000 of those are used in commerce. The U.S. Department of Health reports 2,000 new chemicals each year.

While it would be lovely to believe that the U.S. government screens every new compound thoroughly for safety before it's put into the marketplace, that doesn't happen. It lacks the resources to do so. The Toxic Substances Control Act was first created in 1976, and it was not updated until 2016.

The Environmental Working Group (https://www.ewg.org) estimates that on average, each adult uses nine personal care products daily, with 126 different chemical ingredients. Women use more products than men, so the tally for women goes up to 168 chemicals from personal care products alone. One day I counted, and I'd used eight products before leaving the bathroom in the morning: shampoo, conditioner, soap, toothpaste, eye cream, face cream, hand lotion, and floss—and that's not even counting makeup.

This doesn't include the small amounts of gasoline that we take in when we fill up our tank; or the outgassing of flame retardants and stain protection from furniture, carpets, dust, and treated clothing; nonstick pots and pans; paint and flooring in our homes; endocrine-disrupting plastics; bisphenol A (BPA) and phthalates from fragrances we take in through candles, air fresheners, and personal care products; or chemicals from foods, pesticides, herbicides, medications, and cleaning products.

There are thousands of food additives used in processing that are not listed on labels. Hundreds of inert ingredients are used in cleaning products, home herbicides, and pesticides, as well as heavy metals in fertilizers. The long-term effects of the wireless technologies that we utilize daily and that surround us are still an unknown factor.

We assume that each chemical has been demonstrated to be individually safe but our assumption is also that these chemicals are safe in combination. No one has yet tested chemicals in combination. We may be consuming dozens of food additives in a single meal. Even as a kid, I knew from my neighbor's chemistry set that adding several substances together got a different reaction than using each one alone. We are all involved in an uncontrolled experiment, and small amounts of each of these might not be an issue; however, when combined, many of us are canaries in a coal mine with bodies that cannot handle it.

The first step: Stop bringing these chemicals into our homes. The Environmental Working Group has excellent resources, including a healthy living app for your phone. The "Dirty Dozen" and "Clean 15" foods lists, published each year inform us about pesticide residues in food. They also have an app called "Healthy Living" that allows people to scan or enter food and personal care products to determine how healthful or unhealthful they may be. For more resources from the Environmental Working group, go to www.ewg.org

The World Health Organization also has some exellent resoures on environmental exposures, which can be found at:
(https://www.who.int/topics/environmental_health/factsheets/en/;
https://www.who.int/ceh/risks/cehchemicals/en/).

Annually, we consume, on average, 6 to 9 pounds of food additives, including colorings, preservatives, flavorings, emulsifiers, humectants, and antimicrobials. More than 1 billion tons of pesticides are used in the United States every year.

Resources:

- *The Toxin Solution* by Joseph Pizzorno
- *Fateful Harvest* by Duff Wilson; this is a must-read book!
- *Unsafe at Any Meal* by Renee Joy Dufault
- Environmental Working Group (https://www.EWG.org)
- "National Report on Human Exposure to Environmental Chemicals" by The Center for Disease Control's Agency for Toxic Substances and Disease Registry (ASTDR): https://www.atsdr.cdc.gov/substances/index.asp
- The US Department of Health has a listing of more resources on environmental exposure and risk at: https://www.hhs.gov/programs/prevention-and-wellness/the-environment-your-health/index.html
- *Our Stolen Future* by Theo Colburn, Dianne Dumanoski, and John Peterson Myers

By assisting your body in removal of stored toxins through detoxification programs, your body can more easily heal itself.

As the quote at the start of this chapter from Dr. Sidney Baker McDonald says, our bodies spend a lot of energy getting rid of unwanted wastes from our bodies. When we take in more than our liver, skin, sweat, and bile can handle, we store fat-soluble chemicals in tissues throughout the body.

TRADITIONAL CLEANSING

Throughout time, and in various cultures, people have seen the need for periodic internal cleansing. Native Americans and Mexicans use sweat lodges. Ancient Roman bathhouses had rooms for bathing in steam, warm water, and cold water. Jewish women have used ritual mikvah baths to cleanse both body and spirit. Most Scandinavian people have home saunas, and our own health clubs have saunas, steam baths, hot tubs, and Jacuzzis. The Japanese use Waon dry heath treatments. The Turkish have Hammam-style bathhouses, and the Russian's Banya is a combination of a sauna and steam bath. People "take the waters" in Europe and parts of the United States. Hawaiians use steam and a form of massage, called lomilomi, where they scrub people clean with sterilized red Hawaiian dirt and sea salt. In fact, mud and clay have been used worldwide to draw toxins from the body while simultaneously providing essential nutrients.

Fasting is an important part of many religious holidays and customs. Both Jesus and John the Baptist fasted to gain mental and spiritual clarity. During the month of Ramadan, an important Muslim holiday, people fast during daylight hours. Jewish people fast on Yom Kippur. Indigenous people of many cultures use fasting as a way to clarify thought and provoke visions.

INTERMITTENT FASTING, FASTING, AND FASTING-MIMICKING DIETS

Recent research on intermittent fasting and fasting-mimicking diets shows that they are beneficial stressors that can reduce inflammation, balance immunity, and prevent and treat chronic disease. Studies have shown benefits in pain reduction in people with osteoarthritis, rheumatoid arthritis, and multiple sclerosis; improvements in energy; weight reduction; lowering of high blood pressure; fewer headaches; and decreased depression. Fasting is helpful in the prevention and treatment in people with diabetes, cardiovascular risk, and metabolic syndrome and provides improved effectiveness of chemotherapy in cancer treatment and enhanced triglycerides and inflammatory markers.

Giving the digestive system and body a rest from food allows autophagy (cellular assessment and maintenance). When you have a couple of days off, you might use that time to renew yourself, clean your house, and get your life organized. Your body renews when you rest. Taking it easy on food for a few days each month or fasting 12 to 14 hours between dinner and breakfast can have profound overall benefits.

Resources:

- *The Longevity Diet*, by Valter Longo
- *The Alternate Day Diet*, by James B. Johnson, MD and Donald R. Laub, MD

Removal of waste material—detoxification—is essential to the healthy functioning of our bodies. This is shown in the many ways the body cleanses itself. Skin is our body's largest organ. In addition to being a protective organ, it is an organ of elimination through perspiration. Sneezes clear our sinuses. Lungs breathe out carbon dioxide, and even the breath allows for removal of some wastes. Kidneys filter wastes from the bloodstream. Stool is the residue from the digestive process. The liver filters the substances that are absorbed through the digestive barrier into the bloodstream. White blood cells gobble up bacteria and foreign substances, and the lymphatic system clears the debris from circulation. During a cleansing program, your body more rapidly recycles materials to build new cells, take apart aged cells, and repair damaged cells.

HOW YOUR LIVER DETOXIFIES

Some of the many functions of the liver are to act as a filter, to let nutrients pass, and to transform toxins into safe substances that can be eliminated via urine and stool. When the liver gets overloaded, these toxins are stored in the liver and released into tissues throughout our bodies.

Your liver detoxifies chemicals in a two-phase system, which is a lot like washing our clothes. First we wash, and then we rinse out the dirt so that our clothes are clean. In phase I, the Cytochrome P-450 enzyme system, your body pulls stored fat-soluble toxins from tissues throughout your body. In phase II, these substances are prepared so that they can exit the body. Adding a water-soluble molecule to each of these fat-soluble chemicals allows them to be excreted through bile, stool, and urine. Between phase I and phase II comes an intermediary stage. Just as when we wash clothes and the water gets really dirty before the clothes are rinsed and spun, if we pull out intermediary metabolites for disposal too quickly, the substances that were stored in the tissues enter the bloodstream. If phase II enzyme systems are slow, which is common, we end up in a more toxic state than before we began. This is why some people feel worse on a cleanse or detoxification program. Phase III detoxification occurs when the wastes are moved from the cell into the bloodstream and stool to be finally removed from your body.

How well the liver detoxification system works is determined by your genetics, how well nourished you are, and how toxic you are. This process demands energy and requires many nutrients to function properly. In Figure 17.1, you can see the many nutrients that are required in phase I, phase II, and the intermediary phase. Because many of us lack antioxidants, micronutrients, amino acids, and other nutrients, this process doesn't work optimally.

All medications pass through the cytochrome P450 enzyme pathway. Common medications can inhibit the liver's ability to process toxins adequately. For example, acetaminophen (Tylenol) causes liver damage when used in combination with alcoholic beverages. Cimetidine, an ulcer medication, limits the liver's ability to detoxify foreign substances. Our genetic predisposition makes it easier or harder for us to metabolize drugs and move them out of our body. I have had clients who are poor phase II detoxifiers. When they take a drug or supplement or are exposed to a chemical, they are slow to convert it. It stays in their system longer than for most people, so the doses they need for supplements and medications are typically smaller. I recognize this because when they try to cleanse or take medications or supplements, they are extremely sensitive to them. On the other hand, there are people who need to

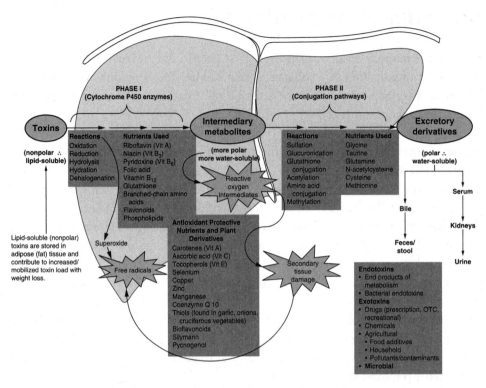

Figure 17.1 **Liver detoxification pathways and supportive nutrients.** (Used with permission of the Institute for Functional Medicine.)

take a larger dose of a supplement or medication because their phase I and II systems work superfast, metabolizing the substances quickly.

FOOD AND DETOXIFICATION

Food can affect the way our liver detoxifies, too. Naringenin and other molecules in grapefruit juice slow down phase I detoxification pathways. Many people are told not to drink grapefruit juice because it changes the dosages of medication they need. The catechins in red wine and the piperine in black pepper also slow the metabolism of drugs. Several studies indicate that eating a diet high in animal protein increases the level of intermediary metabolites. This is not seen in people eating a vegetarian diet. Eating more fruits and vegetables helps the liver to detoxify better. Polyphenols in foods such as red wine, green tea, turmeric, ginger, and spices have been shown to reduce rates of cancer and most other illnesses. Glucosinolates in cruciferous vegetables also help us detoxify and lower cancer risk.

Research demonstrates that changing to an organic diet quickly reduces solvents and chemicals from our bodies. Children who ate a diet comprised solely of organically grown food for one week experienced a 60.5 percent drop in pesticide and pesticide metabolite levels of 13 pesticides, insecticides, and herbicide 2,4-D, according to a study published in *Environmental Research in* 2019.

Consuming more vegetables, fruits, herbs, and spices, getting enough protein, and taking a good multivitamin with minerals can upregulate these pathways.

WHO BENEFITS FROM A CLEANSE OR DETOX?

Complete the following questionnaire to compare your "before and after" results. See what symptoms improved.

MEDICAL SYMPTOMS QUESTIONNAIRE (MSQ)

Name: _____   Date: _____

Rate each of the following symptoms based on your typical health profile for:

☐ Past 30 days   ☐ Past 48 hours

Point Scale

0: *Never* or *almost never* have the symptom
1: *Occasionally* have it, effect is *not severe*
2: *Occasionally* have it, effect is *severe*
3: *Frequently* have it, effect is *not severe*
4: *Frequently* have it, effect is *severe*

Head

_____ Headaches
_____ Faintness
_____ Dizziness
_____ Insomnia
Total _____

Eyes

_____ Watery or itchy eyes
_____ Swollen, reddened/sticky eyelids
_____ Bags, dark circles
_____ Blurred or tunnel vision *(does not include near- or far-sightedness)*
Total _____

Ears

_____ Itchy ears
_____ Earaches, ear infections
_____ Drainage from ear
_____ Ringing/hearing loss
Total _____

Nose

_____ Stuffy nose
_____ Sinus problems
_____ Hay fever
_____ Sneezing attacks
_____ Excessive mucus
Total _____

Mouth/Throat

_____ Chronic coughing
_____ Gagging, throat clearing
_____ Sore throat, hoarseness
_____ Swollen/discolored tongue,
        gums, lips
_____ Canker sores
Total _____

Heart

_____ Irregular/skipped beats
_____ Rapid/pounding beats
_____ Chest pain
Total _____

Skin

_____ Acne
_____ Hives, rashes, dry skin
_____ Hair loss
_____ Flushing, hot flashes
_____ Excessive sweating
Total _____

Lungs

_____ Chest congestion
_____ Asthma, bronchitis
_____ Shortness of breath
_____ Difficulty breathing
Total _____

Digestive Tract

_____ Nausea, vomiting
_____ Diarrhea
_____ Constipation
_____ Bloated feeling
_____ Belching, passing gas
_____ Heartburn
_____ Intestinal/stomach pain
Total _____

Joints/Muscle

_____ Pain or aches in joints
_____ Arthritis
_____ Stiffness/limited movement
_____ Pain or aches in muscles
_____ Feeling of weakness or
        tiredness
Total _____

Weight

_____ Binge eating/drinking
_____ Craving certain foods
_____ Excessive weight
_____ Compulsive eating
_____ Water retention
_____ Underweight
Total _____

Energy/Activity

_____ Fatigue, sluggishness

_____ Apathy, lethargy

_____ Hyperactivity

_____ Restless leg

_____ Jet lag

Total _____

Mind

_____ Poor memory

_____ Confusion, poor comprehension

_____ Poor concentration

_____ Poor physical coordination

_____ Difficulty making decisions

_____ Stuttering or stammering

_____ Slurred speech

_____ Learning disabilities

Total _____

Emotions

_____ Mood swings

_____ Anxiety, fear, nervousness

_____ Anger, irritability, aggressiveness

_____ Depression

Total _____

Other

_____ Frequent illness

_____ Frequent or urgent urination

_____ Genital itch or discharge

_____ Bone pain

Total _____

Grand total _____

©2009 Institute for Functional Medicine

DETOXIFICATION AND CLEANSING PROGRAMS

Most detoxification programs focus on the liver or colon. The liver is, in my opinion, the most overworked organ of the body. It has responsibility for manufacturing 13,000 enzymes, producing cholesterol, breaking down estrogen, regulating blood sugar, filtering blood, manufacturing bile, breaking down old red blood cells, and detoxifying harmful substances.

Detoxification techniques such as fasting, modified fasting, metabolic cleansing, colonic irrigation, steaming, mud packs, saunas, herbal detoxification programs, and hot tubs all have therapeutic benefits. When choosing a detoxification program, it must meet specific criteria: it needs to (1) work with your life and your values, (2) be thorough, and (3) be gentle and nurturing to your body.

I have personally and professionally relied on three main detoxification programs that are effective and gentle: fruit and vegetable cleansing, metabolic cleansing, and low-temperature steams and saunas. I also recommend vitamin C flushes between cleansings. Other professionals may prefer fasting programs or colonic irrigation, which in the right hands can be powerful tools for healing. Because there are many fine books on fasting and colonic irrigation, I have not included information about them here.

ELIMINATION DIETS

You can use virtually any of the elimination diets outlined in Chapter 13. The elimination diets and the ReNew and Autoimmune Paleo protocols work well to cleanse and reduce inflammation in most people.

FRUIT AND VEGETABLE CLEANSING

The first cleanse that I ever used consisted of eating just fruits and vegetables, 8 to 12 cups daily, 7 to 10 days.

I used this cleanse as a jump-start for many of the weight control groups I facilitated. While this works amazingly well, some may not feel that it provides enough food to keep blood sugar levels even. This worked well for me when I was younger, yet as I age, I feel the need for more protein. Occasionally, I eat fruits and vegetables with lean proteins and some oils for 1 to 3 weeks as a gentle cleanse.

In this gentle cleanse, you may eat all you want of fruits and vegetables, and use olive and sunflower oils, salt and pepper, and other herbs for 7 to 10 days. Fresh fruit and vegetable juices are an excellent source of easily assimilated nutrients and alkalizing minerals and can enhance the detoxification pathways. You can have raw, steamed, juiced, grilled, stir-fried, and cultured vegetables. You can have raw, juiced, cooked, frozen, or dried fruit. You can use canned fruit if it's packed in its own juice. You can make smoothies. Eat large salads every day. Make salad dressings with lemon or lime and olive oil, salt, pepper, and fresh herbs. Make pots of vegetable soup. Make a batch of roasted or baked root vegetables for something hearty to eat.

It's important to eat every two to three hours to keep your blood sugar levels normal. The major benefit of this detox method is that you can do this on your own, without professional supervision. Of course, if you are under a doctor's care or taking medication of any kind, you'll need to let your physician know of your plans. The first few days may require mental and physical adjustments to your new regimen, but most people feel a sense of general well-being. You may notice that many of your outstanding symptoms disappear or become less aggravated.

You may also experience some discomfort during the first three or four days. Headaches, bad breath, skin breakouts, and changes in bowel habits are fairly common and may be the result of withdrawal from caffeine, sugar, alcohol, or other substances. They are an indicator that toxins are being flushed out or that your body is going through withdrawal. To facilitate this, drink a lot of water, diluted juices, and all herbal teas except those containing caffeine. Dandelion tea is especially useful.

Some people develop rashes or pimples as the skin works hard to eliminate toxins. Taking saunas, steam bathing, and massaging your skin with a soft, dry brush or loofa can help your skin. If you are constipated, make sure you eat enough fiber-rich fruits and vegetables (apples, broccoli, pears, sweet potatoes, peas, brussels sprouts, corn, potatoes, carrots, greens, blackberries, bananas, strawberries, raspberries, and spinach). Constipation opens up a chance for toxins to be reabsorbed into your bloodstream, causing symptoms such as headaches and nausea, so add a fiber supplement if needed; psyllium seeds or psyllium seed husks work well. Begin with 1 teaspoon in water, and drink quickly before it turns into a gel. Aloe vera juice may also help regulate your bowels.

After the cleansing, slowly reintroduce healthful foods such as beans, tofu, chicken, and fish. Then add healthful grains, nuts, seeds, and cultured dairy products.

METABOLIC CLEANSING

Metabolic cleansing is a gentle yet deep method of detoxification, and it is the best, most thorough program I have used. The foundation of this program is a hypoallergenic-sensitive, rice-based protein and nutrient drink that is designed specifically to assist with phase I and phase II liver detoxification*. There are many companies that make this type of product. You can find them in the resource directory at http://www.digestivewellnessbook.com.

---

* Many people who have used previous editions of this book have written to ask, so I'm putting in the details here. I typically use UltraClear Plus Rice or Renew by Metagenics. Originally, I used this product because it was backed by research demonstrating a reduction of signs and symptoms in a variety of conditions by 50 percent in 3 weeks. Then I discovered that it matched my body's needs well. Metagenics has an entire line of UltraClear products that are whey, rice, or soy-based. Most of the other supplement lines have similar products. Other products I recommend include MediClear by Thorne, Core Support by Ortho Molecular, Metabolic Detox Complete by Metabolic Maintenance, DetoxiCleanse by BioClinic Naturals, VegeCleanse or PaleoCleanse by Designs for Health, Comprehensive Detox Kit or Vital Clear by Vital Nutrients, Clear Change by Metagenics, BioCleanse Powder by NutraBioGenesis, and Purification Process by Standard Process.

These can be mixed with water or another beverages. You can also create a quick smoothie by adding green vegetables and berries. Often I add a small piece of fresh ginger and turmeric and a sprinkle of cinnamon to taste.

The use of liver detoxification protein drinks has been researched for its health benefits. These drinks have been reported to be of enormous benefit in people with fibromyalgia, chronic fatigue syndrome, arthritis, weight loss, and other conditions.

I use this product along with the Elimination Diet that is outlined in Chapter 13. If you know that you are sensitive to bananas, melons, or other foods that are allowed on the plan, avoid them as well. It is possible for people to continue their normal daily routine while on this program.

Typically, I begin people with two scoops of the detoxification drink once daily for several days; then I have them increase to two scoops twice daily for several days; finally, take two scoops three times daily until they are ready to complete the cleanse.

This program is administered only through health professionals who can monitor your progress, determine when you should quit, and help you adjust if you have any difficulties. If you take any medications, this program can metabolize them out of your body more quickly, negating the effects. Do discuss this with your clinician if you have any negative signs or symptoms. Most people find a dramatic alleviation of symptoms and a distinct improvement in energy levels. The high levels of nutrients found in the rice protein drink and in the fruits and vegetables help the liver activate its detoxification pathways and move unwanted materials out of the body. The intention here is to allow your digestive system to rest, relax, and heal itself.

Once you have completed the cleansing, it is important to slowly reintroduce foods back into your diet. Being a food sleuth takes a lot of patience; it's not always apparent which foods cause adverse symptoms. But with persistent detective work you can discover many of them. Keep a running record of everything you eat and of your symptoms. Food sensitivities often display delayed reactions, so it may take up to 48 hours to feel the effect of a newly introduced food.

You may want to have testing done for food allergies and sensitivities at this time. If you have uncovered a problem, these tests can further pinpoint which foods and substances are making you ill.

VITAMIN C FLUSH

I learned the vitamin C flush technique from Russell Jaffe, MD, and am indebted to him for this protocol and many other things. It's something that I personally have used, and I have used it with my children. Over the past 20 years, I've also used this flush with many clients. Although it's a bit harsh on some people, others say that after the first or second time, they feel better than they've felt in years. This is especially true in people with chronic fatigue and autoimmune conditions. A good-quality ascorbate can be utilized by the body to produce energy. Because of that, I often hear that energy levels dramatically improve after a vitamin C flush.

Vitamin C has been well researched for its ability to help detoxify bacterial toxins, drugs, environmental toxins, and heavy metals from our bodies. Its gentle and potent detoxification counteracts and neutralizes the harmful effects of manufactured poisons.

High levels of vitamin C help detoxify the body, rebalance intestinal flora, and strengthen the immune system. The vitamin C flush can be used between metabolic cleansing therapies or at the first sign of a cold or infection. If your immune system is weak or you've been exposed to a lot of toxins, you may want to do a vitamin C flush once a week for a month or two. On days when you are not doing a vitamin C flush, take a minimum of 2,000 to 3,000 mg. Humans are one of the only animals that do not produce their own vitamin C, so we need to replenish our supply daily.

For a vitamin C flush, take vitamin C to the level of tissue saturation. You'll know you've reached it because you will have watery diarrhea. You'll need to purchase powdered mineral ascorbate C, which is more easily tolerated by most people because it doesn't change your pH balance. The amount you take varies depending on your personal needs that day. Many of us require about 5,000 mg; others optimally need a lot more or a lot less. For instance, if you're coming down with a cold, have chronic fatigue syndrome, or are under excessive stress, you'll probably need a lot more.

To begin, take ½ teaspoon, about 1,500 mg, of vitamin C powder or a mineral ascorbate or pure ascorbic acid, mix with water or fruit juice, and drink. You will get gas but don't stop there. Repeat every 15 minutes until you have watery diarrhea. It will seem as if you are urinating out of your backside. It will have a brown, green, or yellow color. As soon as this starts, stop taking the ascorbate.

Rapidly adding vitamin C helps prevent bloating and cramping. Keep track of how much vitamin C you take. This will help you determine your optimal dosage. In divided amounts, take daily one-half to three-quarters of the amount it takes to produce a vitamin C flush.

Over time, your needs may increase but then substantially decrease as repair occurs.

SAUNAS: MANY HEALTH BENEFITS

Saunas are useful to eliminate fat-soluble chemicals from our systems. They are commonly used to help detoxify those who have had high exposure to pesticides, solvents, pharmaceutical drugs, and petrochemicals. Although we have little research in this area, it's believed that slow, steady sweat encourages the release of fat-soluble toxins through the skin from their storage sites in our tissue at rates 2 to 10 times higher than by filtering blood for urine.

There are many health benefits of saunas, including relaxation and socialization. Although more studies need to be done to demonstrate this ancient practice, it's compelling, with much new research being published between 2017 and 2018. Most of the work to date has been done on the use of Finnish dry saunas. A recent analysis of 2,682 Finnish middle-aged men reported the following benefits on the circulatory system: temporary lowering of diastolic and overall blood pressure, prevention of hypertension, temporary lowering of heart rate, and lowering of low-density lipoprotein (LDL) cholesterol. Other researchers have seen benefits in people with stable heart disease: More frequent use of saunas (1–7 times weekly) correlated with a decrease in risk from sudden death, ischemic heart disease, strokes, and other cardiovascular events. Sauna research also demonstrates improvements in pain reduction in arthritis and headaches; less flu; improvements in people with heart failure; decreased risk of developing Alzheimer's disease and other neurocognitive issues; improvements in people with respiratory issues, including asthma and chronic obstructive pulmonary disease (COPD); and a reduction in acute and chronic infections, including pneumonia. There is even a paper in the works exploring the possibility of using saunas to remove uremic wastes in people with end-stage kidney disease.

Research using infrared saunas is less available. There is some evidence that it increases quality of life in people with type 2 diabetes, normalizes blood pressure, and offers improvement in people with congestive heart failure. There is also some evidence on pain reduction and improvements in chronic fatigue. One study found that patients with rheumatoid arthritis and ankylosing spondylitis saw improvements in pain, stiffness, and fatigue, but the experiment was only 4 weeks long and didn't reach statistical significance. Nonetheless, it reported no adverse effects.

During the sauna process, we lose sodium, potassium, zinc, and chloride via our sweat, so remember to rehydrate and replenish yourself by drinking water and vegetable juice or diluted fruit juice. Saunas upregulate the parasympathic nervous system, activating our relaxation response. Taking saunas increases hormones such as cortisol, adrenaline, noradrenaline, growth hormone, thyroid-stimulating hormone, the renin-angiotensin-aldosterone system, and prolactin. It also has been demonstrated to increase nitric oxide (NO), improve insulin sensitivity, and reduce oxidative stress and inflammation. It ultimately opens our lungs, relaxes our muscles, makes us more flexible, and thins synovial fluid in our joints. It also gives us a good cardiovascular workout, similar to doing moderate to vigorous walking.

Who Should Not Use Saunas?

While the side effects of saunas are mainly low, there are some risks. Make sure that you hydrate well and replace trace minerals with juices or a good multivitamin/mineral supplement. Use common sense, too—if you feel faint or weak, get out at once.

If you have high blood pressure, low blood pressure, a history of heart issues, are pregnant, or want to become pregnant, check with your doctor before embarking on a sauna program. Saunas in young men do lower sperm counts. And deaths, while infrequent, have occurred, mostly involved with drinking alcoholic beverages during a sauna.

Saunas help us to release xenobiotic toxins from our fat cells. Many compounds have been reported to be released, including minerals, urea, drugs, and polychlorinated bromines (PCBs). In addition, hyperthermia is well known to help with cancer treatment and is being used in some oncology centers in the United States and Europe.

After you are done sweating, you ought to take a cool shower with soap and then towel off. Wash all towels you've used in the sauna and after your shower—do not use them a second time. It will wash away the toxins and keep you from reabsorbing them.

Precautions

Saunas are contraindicated in women who are pregnant and for people with aortic stenosis, unstable angina, and recent heart attack. If you have extreme toxicity from environmental chemicals, you'll need to detox under the supervision of a physician. The temporary release of toxins into your circulation can be quite severe and debilitating. Some clinics specialize in using saunas for medical detoxification. In her excellent book *Poisoning Our Children*, Nancy Sokol Green describes her experience in a detox clinic in depth: "On the fourteenth day of detox, I started experiencing allergic symptoms, such as eyelid swelling, while I was in the sauna! . . . I was actually beginning to reek of the pesticides that had been sprayed in my home. . . .

Several of the patients at the clinic who were sensitive to pesticides had to stay away from me as I triggered adverse reactions in them."

Saunas are a useful detoxification therapy when used preventively and therapeutically. If you are using a sauna therapeutically, do so under the supervision of a physician who can guide you through the process. And next time you get into your car that's been warmed by the sun, spend a few minutes basking in the glory of the heat. You have your own infrared sauna!

Natural Therapies for Common Digestive Problems

"Hope cannot be said to exist, nor can it be said not to exist.
It is just like the roads across the earth.
For actually there were no roads to begin with,
But when many people pass one way a road is made."

—Lu Hsun, 1921

Maya Angelou said, "I did then what I knew how to do. Now that I know better, I do better." I hope that these pages will help you to know better so that you can do better.

Part IV provides a comprehensive list of self-care ideas for the most common digestive problems. We start our journey at the mouth and move south. Some of the following ideas alleviate symptoms, while others work to help your body heal the underlying cause. The remedies are mostly nutritional and herbal because those are the fields I know best; I have included other modalities whenever possible.

The most important ones are listed first. Read each section that applies to you, find the remedies for your symptoms, and see which ideas come up frequently and try those first. Also try the remedies that make the most sense intuitively.

In all cases begin with the DIGIN model for optimal healing then look for specifics in these chapters.

Each herb or nutrient is listed separately, but often they can be found in combination supplements. You'll notice that specific recommendations are repeated for many problems. Although each health condition has its own unique properties, many have similar characteristics that respond to similar treatment programs. You'll probably want to work with a health professional to tailor a program that will best suit your needs, yet hundreds of people have let me know that they've implemented ideas from this book and dramatically improved their health.

Health care is both a science and an art. You may need the science in the form of lab testing, diagnosis, and evaluation of your needs. Your clinician will order the customary lab work. I have included information about functional lab tests that are most likely to reveal new information; these tests will probably be unfamiliar to your physician. You will find a resource directory of suggested laboratories and supplement companies online at http://www.digestivewellnessbook.com.

The art of healing comes into play when determining which paths to follow, which ideas have the most merit, and which dosages are appropriate. Healing often happens in layers. Sometimes you try the right thing at the wrong time. Later, you try it again with great results because the initial obstacle has been removed. If the first program you try doesn't work or works only partially, try another. You can feel better when you are persistent and patient. Remember, our symptoms are our body's way of telling us to pay attention, that something is out of balance. By listening, we often have the inner wisdom to know exactly what we need.

Begin your program by taking a multivitamin and mineral supplement. Think of a multivitamin with minerals as inexpensive health insurance, and arm yourself with an excellent supplement. Your diet is likely to be deficient in several nutrients that supplements can provide. Because minerals are bulky, you'll find yourself taking anywhere from two to nine pills daily. Or you may find a multivitamin and take your calcium and magnesium separately. Read the ingredients on the label carefully. If a product contains artificial colors, preservatives, shellac, or carnauba wax, put it back on the shelf and keep looking. Also, look for an expiration date and batch number. Although I love food-based supplements, if you have a lot of food sensitivities or allergies, think twice about taking one. It's likely that one of the foods that's in the supplement may be one that you react to. Look for a multivitamin and mineral supplement that contains at least the following.

Recommended Multivitamin with Minerals

- 1,000 mg of calcium
- 400 to 600 mg of magnesium
- 400 IU of vitamin D
- At least 100 IU of vitamin E
- At least 250 mg of vitamin C
- 200 mcg of chromium
- 200 mcg of selenium
- 5–10 mg of manganese
- At least 15 mg of zinc
- At least 200 mcg of folic acid
- At least 10 mg of each B vitamin

If you do this, the rest of the nutrients will be in line.

The Mouth: Bad Breath/ Halitosis, Cheilosis, Gingivitis and Periodontal Disease, Nutrients and Teeth, Mouth Ulcers/Canker Sores, Thrush, Tongue Problems, and Burning Tongue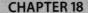

The health of our teeth, tongue, and gums is integral to the health of the rest of the digestive tract. Digestive enzymes in saliva begin the process of carbohydrate digestion, and chewing sends signals to the brain, which in turn sends signals to the stomach that food is on the way. Thorough chewing of food can help with indigestion.

Irritation and inflammation in the mouth can be signs of food or chemical sensitivities or allergies. The mouth is our first contact with ingested allergens. Careful investigation of the mouth area can give information about a person's nutritional status. Bleeding gums indicate the need for vitamin C and bioflavonoids. Receding gums indicate bone loss, so bone nutrients are needed. Deep pockets in gums increase our risk for periodontal disease and may indicate the need for vitamin C, bioflavonoids, and coenzyme Q10 (CoQ10).

BAD BREATH OR HALITOSIS

Using mouthwash for bad breath is like putting an adhesive bandage on a broken leg. First, consult a dentist to see if it is caused by poor dental hygiene, periodontal disease, or tooth infections. Halitosis is typically caused by dental issues. If you experience this, follow your dentist's advice, and also look in the section on gum and tooth health that follows. But also look deeper: Halitosis often signals digestive imbalances lower down in the digestive tract. Bad breath can signal an infection of some sort: *Helicobacter pylori*, chronic tonsillitis, chronic sinusitis, or digestive dysbiosis. Other contributors include low hydrochloric acid (HCl) levels in the stomach, gastroesophageal reflux disease (GERD), poor flora, liver disease, pancreatic or kidney disease, respiratory infections, and constipation.

Healing Options

- **Check for infection.** Halitosis has been associated with *H. pylori*, a bacteria involved in stomach infection. Ask your doctor to check you for *H. pylori*. *H. pylori* was found in 15 percent of people with periodontal disease. See the sections on GERD and gastric ulcers in Chapter 19 for treatment options.
- **Eliminate constipation.** See the section on stool transit time in Chapter 2 and do the self-test. See also the section on constipation in Chapter 24.
- **Try a probiotic supplement.** Take one or two capsules of acidophilus and bifidus between meals.
- **Consider possible lactose intolerance.** Lactose intolerance can cause bad breath, other digestive symptoms, and headaches. The simplest way to discover if you have lactose intolerance is to avoid all dairy products and dairy-containing food for two weeks, and see if your symptoms improve.
- **Look for other causes if the problem persists.** If you continue to have problems, you might be fermenting rather than digesting your food. First, check out your HCl levels. (See Chapter 11.) Second, ask your doctor to run a comprehensive digestive stool analysis (CDSA) with parasitology evaluation. You may have dysbiosis, parasites, or an *H. pylori* infection (the bacteria implicated in ulcers). A CDSA can help you find out what's amiss.

CHEILOSIS, OR CRACKS IN THE CORNERS OF THE MOUTH AND LIPS

Our skin is continuously replacing itself, and the places where our skin folds need to be replaced even more often. B-complex vitamins, particularly vitamins B_2 (riboflavin) and B_6 (pyridoxine), assist in formation of new skin. Cracks at the corners of our lips, called cheilosis, are most often associated with these nutrient deficiencies. They can easily become infected by yeast (*Candida albicans*). If they do not respond to nutritional therapy, have a physician look for other causes.

Healing Options
Take B-complex vitamins. Try 50 to 100 mg one to three times daily in trial for four weeks.

GINGIVITIS AND PERIODONTAL DISEASE

Gingivitis is inflammation of the gums that, if left alone, often progresses to periodontal disease, inflammation of the bone around the teeth. Although the inflammation is in the mouth, it's well established that people with inflammation in their gums have increased risk of heart disease and atherosclerosis, Alzheimer's disease, low-preterm birth weight from mothers with periodontal disease, cancer, and obesity. Because periodontal disease is a sign of infection and inflammation, there are bidirectional associations among all of these conditions, plus additional associations with metabolic syndrome, diabetes, and chronic kidney disease. A Scottish study with more than 11,000 participants demonstrated that people who brushed their teeth less than twice daily had a 70 percent higher risk of having heart disease than people who brush twice daily. This was also demonstrated with higher levels of inflammatory markers such as C-reactive protein and fibrinogen. Seems like a pretty easy thing to do: Brush twice a day and floss once a day.

Periodontal disease increases with plaque buildup, age, long-term use of steroid medications, and in diabetics, people with systemic disease, and smokers. The presence of silver fillings, which contain 50 percent mercury, has also been found to predispose people to periodontal disease. One study showed that when silver fillings were removed, 86 percent of the 125 oral cavity symptoms being studied were eliminated or improved.

Gingivitis and periodontal disease are complex problems that have complex solutions. Periodontal disease will affect 9 out of 10 Americans during their lifetimes, and 4 out of 10 will lose all their teeth. Regular dental care is essential. Again, follow your dentist's advice and practice consistent oral hygiene by brushing and flossing daily.

Nutrition plays a critical role in dental health. One recent study looked at gingivitis, plaque adhesion, and calculus deposit with regard to the eating habits of teenagers. They concluded that teenagers with diets adequate in nutrients had better oral health than teenagers with diets that contained fewer nutrients.

NUTRIENTS AND OUR TEETH

Teeth are made of bone material and need the same nutrients for rebuilding as other bones. It has long been considered that receding and inflamed gums were a sign that people brushed too hard, causing damage to the gums, but new theories propose that gums recede because bone throughout the body, including the teeth, is demineralizing. Bones need protein and 20 other micronutrients to remineralize; the same goes for teeth. Calcium alone cannot reverse the problem. Stress and fast-paced living can cause bone loss by making the body more acidic. To compensate, the body takes alkaline materials from bones and teeth.

Vitamin C deficiency causes bleeding gums and loose teeth and contributes to gingivitis. Bleeding gums is one symptom of scurvy, a vitamin-C-deficiency disease. We rarely see outright scurvy in our population, but we often see people with bleeding gums. Vitamin C is also important for bone formation and collagen synthesis and is essential for gum repair. Vitamin A is also necessary for collagen synthesis and formation of gum tissue.

Other researchers look to zinc deficiency or a low zinc-to-copper ratio as the culprit in gum disease. Zinc is integral to maintenance and repair of gum tissue, inhibits plaque formation, and reduces inflammation by inhibiting mast cell release of histamine. It also plays a role in immune function.

Vitamin E has been used clinically for periodontal disease. Bacterial plaque, long known to be a culprit in tooth decay and gingivitis, produces compounds that weaken and irritate the gum tissue. They include endotoxins and exotoxins, free radicals, connective tissue–destroying enzymes, white blood cell poisons, antigens, and waste products.

Antioxidant nutrients, vitamin D, and CoQ10 have been associated with improved gum health, reduced periodontal pocket depth, and decreased tooth movement. Bioflavonoids make the tissues stronger, reduce inflammation, and cross-link with collagen fibers, making them stronger. Because bioflavonoids work synergistically with vitamin C, bleeding gums often respond to vitamin C and bioflavonoid supplementation. My favorite bioflavonoid is quercetin.

Folic acid, a B-complex vitamin, is important for maintenance and repair of mucous membranes. The need for extra folic acid was first noted for pregnant women, while subsequent studies have shown that it plays an important role for gingival health in all people.

Healing Options

- **Brush your teeth twice daily.** Brush your teeth twice a day and floss once a day. Essential oils commonly found in toothpastes, such as peppermint, clove, cinnamon, rose, neem, tea tree oil, rosemary, and lavender, have anti-microbial properties. You can easily make your own toothpaste by using 3 tablespoons each of coconut oil and baking soda, and optionally adding 5 to 15 drops of essential oil; add 1 to 2 teaspoons of powdered myrrh if you'd like. Mix and use.

- **Floss daily.** Flossing helps to remove plaque.
- **Use an oral irrigator.** Using an oral irrigator such as a Waterpik or HydroFloss provides a mechanical way to deeply clean below the gumline, and reduce gum inflammation. In my own irrigator, I've often added hydrogen peroxide, liquid chlorophyll, liquid silver, or other dental products designed for irrigation to deepen the healing. Use your irrigator daily as directed.
- **Make dietary changes.** Focus on fresh fruits, vegetables, whole grains, and beans. Foods rich in flavonoids, such as blueberries, blackberries, and purple grapes, are beneficial.
- **Take a multivitamin with minerals.** Because you are depleted in many nutrients, arm yourself with an excellent multivitamin with minerals. Because minerals are bulky, you'll probably take anywhere from two to nine pills daily. In the introduction to Part IV, you'll find my recommendations on what to look for in a multi-vitamin with minerals.
- **Try coenzyme Q10.** Take 75 to 200 mg daily for three months.
- **Check your vitamin D levels.** Check 25-OH vitamin D levels. Although "normal" is considered to be above 30 to 32 ng/ml, optimal levels range from 50 to 100 ng/ml. Take 5,000 IU vitamin D3 daily and retest in three months. Work with your doctor on this.
- **Take antioxidants.** Vitamins C and E, selenium, glutathione, N-acetyl cysteine (NAC), superoxide dismutase (SOD), beta-carotene, and other antioxidant nutrients are depleted in diseased gum tissues. Supplementation can facilitate repair. For ease of use, purchase an antioxidant supplement. Use as directed for three months.
- **Take vitamin C.** Try 500 to 1,000 mg one to three times daily. For maximum benefits, use until your tissues are saturated. See Chapter 17 for information on a vitamin C flush.
- **Try bioflavonoids.** Use quercetin, bilberry (blueberry), grape seed extract, or Pycnogenol for their anti-inflammatory and antioxidant effects.
- **Try myrrh.** Myrrh has been used since biblical times. It has soothing and antiseptic properties for mucous membranes.
- **Use a folic acid mouthwash.** Use of a 0.1 percent folic acid mouthwash can be quite effective. Be sure to have your blood tested for pernicious anemia first, because folate supplementation can cause nerve damage in people with vitamin B_{12} deficiencies.
- **Try fish oil capsules.** In a controlled placebo trial, it was found that MaxEPA fish oil capsules significantly reduced gingival bleeding and reduced inflammatory factors. Take 2 to 4 g EPA/DHA daily.

MOUTH ULCERS OR CANKER SORES

Mouth sores are common. Most of us have experienced mouth ulcers, canker sores, or cold sores, but some have chronic problems. Usually found inside the mouth, canker sores, called aphthous stomatitis or aphthous ulcers, are the result of poor intestinal flora, food sensitivities or allergies, stress, hormonal changes, and nutritional deficiencies. High-sugar and high-acid foods, such as pineapples, citrus, and tomatoes, sometimes trigger canker sores.

If you have recurring canker sores, thoroughly investigate the possibility of food sensitivities. Also, make sure your toothpaste, mouthwash, and floss aren't causing the problem. A study showed that use of Piroxicam, a nonsteroidal anti-inflammatory drug (NSAID), caused mouth ulcers that resolved when the patient was taken off the medication. If you have mouth sores that don't resolve after several weeks, let your doctor or dentist examine you.

Healing Options

- **Investigate allergies and sensitivities.** Cigarettes, toothpaste, mouthwash, and flavored dental floss can cause irritation. Make sure they are not the source of your problem. Food sensitivities often are. Rule them out carefully with an elimination-provocation diet or food allergy or sensitivity blood testing.

- **Try a probiotic supplement.** Lactobacillus acidophilus is often beneficial in prevention and treatment of canker sores. Take capsules or powdered probiotic supplement as directed on the label. Products vary in dosage.

- **Take B-complex vitamins.** Deficiencies in vitamins B_1, B_2, B_6, B_{12}, and folic acid have been associated with recurrent canker sores. People with B-complex deficiencies showed significant improvement of mouth ulcers during three months of supplementation with B-complex vitamins.

- **Consider gluten sensitivity.** Gluten is a protein fraction found in wheat, rye, spelt, barley, and oats. A considerable amount of research has been done on the connection between gluten intolerance and mouth ulcers because people with celiac disease (also called sprue) often have recurring mouth sores. About 25 percent of people with chronic canker sores have elevated antibodies to gluten, which indicates a specific sensitivity. When they avoid gluten-containing grains, their mouth sores go away.

- **Address iron-deficiency anemia.** Iron deficiency is associated with canker sores. If you get recurrent canker sores and are anemic, you may respond to iron supplementation. People who are not anemic will not benefit. Ask your physician to test you for anemia. Take 30 to 75 mg of elemental iron daily. Because iron tends to be constipating, a slow-release iron, like Feosol or generic equivalents, may be helpful. Floradix, an herbal iron supplement, is gentle and works well. Cooking in cast-iron pots and pans is another way to gain iron from your diet.

- **Practice stress-management skills.** Ask yourself if stress plays a significant role in your canker sores. If so, work on your stress-management skills.
- **Take zinc.** Zinc deficiencies have been linked to mouth ulcers. Zinc plays an important role in healing wounds and immune system function. In one study, zinc supplementation helped heal canker sores 81 percent of the time in people with low zinc levels or a low zinc-to-copper ratio.

Topical Remedies

- **Use ice.** Ice compresses dry up canker sores quickly. Apply ice directly to the sore for either 45 minutes once a day or for 5 minutes several times a day. You'll still have a scab that needs to heal, but the sores won't be painful.
- **Try licorice root.** Licorice root is soothing to the mucous membranes of the digestive tract, and chewable licorice can help reduce inflammation and pain from mouth ulcers. Licorice promotes healing of mucous membranes by stimulating production of healing prostaglandins. Just be sure to buy deglycyrrhized licorice (DGL), which means it has had the glycyrrhizins removed. Glycyrrhizins can raise blood pressure and lower serum potassium levels. Chew two licorice tablets between meals as needed up to four times daily, or eat real licorice, such as Panda brand. Most licorice is made with anise, not licorice.
- **Try myrrh.** Myrrh is an herb that has been used since biblical times to soothe mucous membranes. It has antiseptic properties and can be used in a variety of ways. Chewing gum with myrrh can be temporarily soothing, and a glycerin tincture can be used topically to soothe the sores. It can be combined with the herb goldenseal in tea, paste, or tincture.
- **Try goldenseal.** Goldenseal is soothing to mucous membranes and also has antiseptic properties. It can be taken internally in a tincture, as a tea, in capsules, or dabbed directly on the sores.
- **Try castor oil.** An old Edgar Cayce remedy is to soak a cotton swab in castor oil and apply to the canker sore.

THRUSH

Thrush is a yeast infection in the mouth and throat. It has a white, cottage-cheesy look and is common after use of antibiotics. Thrush can be treated with either prescription or natural medicines. If it persists, you must treat yourself systemically. It is of primary importance to use probiotic supplements of acidophilus and bifido-bacteria to reestablish normal mouth-throat flora. Natural remedies such as garlic, grapefruit seed extract, pau d'arco, and mathake tea, along with dietary changes, can make your body inhospitable to candida. Follow the protocols for candida infections. In one study, one-third of people with thrush were found to have folic acid, vitamin B_6, or vitamin B_{12} anemia, so it's worth having your doctor check you for anemia and B-vitamin status.

TONGUE PROBLEMS

Tongue problems can arise from systemic illness, so celiac disease, diabetes, Behcet's disease, anemia, and syphilis should be ruled out by your physician. More often, tongue problems are indicators of nutritional needs or mouth irritants, such as smoking or other chemicals.

Glossitis is an inflammation of the tongue, which can make it extremely red and smooth, like a bald tire. Studies have found that glossitis is a sign of protein calorie malnourishment, nutritional deficiencies, or marginal nutritional deficiencies of several vitamins and minerals. Glossitis affects 5 percent of our elderly. It most often signals the need for increased B-complex vitamins and iron. You will often find a reddened tongue with pellagra, which is caused by a deficiency of niacin (vitamin B_3).

Other people may also develop what's called a geographic tongue, where the center of the tongue looks like a miniature Grand Canyon. Look in a mirror, look at your friend's and family's tongues, and you'll probably find one. Cracks down the center of the tongue are an indication of the need for increased B-complex vitamins, especially folic acid and B_{12}, and possibly zinc and iron. A bald or pale tongue may be associated with deficiencies of folic acid, B_{12}, B_2, or iron. A tongue with scalloped edges has been associated with grinding one's teeth (bruxism), temporomandibular joint issues (TMJ), a niacin or B_{12} deficiency, hypothyroidism, or having a tongue that's relatively large for your mouth.

BURNING TONGUE

I've worked with several people who have burning tongues. I've found that it's often associated with candida issues, although the research on it is mixed. Take a look at the section on candida and yeast overgrowth in Chapter 7 to find out if it can help you. Burning tongue is also associated with cadmium overload. Sources of cadmium include denture paste, cigarette smoke, and some white flour products. Research also reports that this can be associated with menopause and hypothyroid, so think about hormone therapies. Use of lipoic acid, a powerful antioxidant, can help. Stress, anxiety, and depression are all associated with burning tongue syndrome. I, too, would be anxious if my tongue burned all the time, but do look at stress factors in your life that may be contributing.

Healing Options

- **Take B-complex vitamins.** The most important B vitamins for tongue health are riboflavin (B_2), niacin (B_3), vitamin B_{12}, and folic acid. Choline is found in B-complex vitamins and also plays a vital role in tongue health. Take 50 to 100 mg of B complex one to three times daily for a trial period of four to six weeks.
- **Address iron-deficiency anemia.** Iron-deficiency anemia can also cause a sore and inflamed tongue. Have your physician check to make sure your iron status is normal. Thorough testing would include hematocrit, hemoglobin, ferritin, TIBC, and transferrin.
- **Take zinc.** Zinc is important for healing. Take 25 to 50 mg daily.
- **Investigate food sensitivities.** Check for food sensitivities using an elimination diet or another method found in Part III.
- **Take vitamin E.** One study of elderly people with glossitis found that they had lower serum levels of vitamin E. It is not known if vitamin E is just a marker or if it will help therapeutically, but vitamin E has low toxicity and is worth trying. You should take 400 IU every day.
- **Try lipoic acid.** In one study 26 percent of people benefited from lipoic acid. Begin with 100 to 300 mg daily.

The Esophagus and Stomach: Belching, Barrett's Esophagus, Eosinophilic Esophagitis, Dyspepsia, Gastritis, and Gastroparesis  DIGIN

The most common problems in the esophageal area are belching, medically called eructation; heartburn, also called gastric reflux; and Barrett's esophagus.

BELCHING OR ERUCTATION

Belching is a symptom of gas in the upper part of the digestive tract. Air trapped in the stomach can be painful, and belching is a safety valve that relieves the pressure. It is a release of trapped air from the stomach and usually comes from swallowed air. Just as a baby needs to be burped if she swallows air, we also burp if we swallow air—it's normal. Other than being culturally embarrassing, it's usually without problem.

Foods and drink that contain air contribute to belching. Without fail, when I have a carbonated drink, I burp. Whipped cream and egg whites can have the same effect on many people. Gulping drinks and food causes us to take in more air, while eating slowly prevents us from swallowing air. People also swallow air during exercise, while chewing gum, and while sucking on pipes, straws, or cigarettes. If you are overweight, you are more likely to belch from exercise.

On the other hand, if you are someone who belches a lot, figure out why. Often people who belch too much have issues with low hydrochloric acid (HCl) levels. Some have *Helicobacter pylori* infections.

Functional Laboratory Testing

- *H. pylori* **infection:** Sometimes *H. pylori* infection can cause belching, with or without other digestive symptoms. Ask your doctor to test for *H. pylori*.
- **The Heidelberg capsule:** This test measures your ability to produce gastric acid when challenged with alkaline substances. See Chapter 11 for complete details and for self-testing for gastric acid sufficiency.

Healing Options

- **Make lifestyle changes.** Eat slowly and chew your food well. Avoid carbonated beverages. If you smoke, stop. (Be glad you have such a benign reason to stop.) Reach and maintain ideal body weight. Stop chewing gum or sucking on candy. As an alternative, you can suck on or eat umeboshi plum, or you can make it into a tea. These salty, fermented plums are highly alkalizing and aid in digestion.
- **Do a self-test or do a Heidelberg capsule test to see if you have enough HCl.** I often find that taking betaine HCl capsules eliminates belching in my clients. (See Chapters 3 and 11 for more information.)
- **Try charcoal tablets.** These can absorb toxins, make breath smell better, and calm an overexcited digestive system.
- **Check your supplements.** Some supplements, such as fish oils, can cause belching. Try any of the remedies for heartburn, gastric reflux, and hiatal hernia.

HIATAL HERNIA

Hiatal hernia occurs when a portion of the stomach gets pushed through the diaphragm and into the thoracic cavity where it doesn't belong. Hiatal hernias may or may not cause symptoms, but the most common symptom is heartburn; they can also be a cause of gastroesophageal reflux disease (GERD). Hiatal hernias are found in about 20 percent of all middle-aged Americans. Dr. Dennis Burkitt, called the father of fiber, hypothesized that hiatal hernia was a contemporary problem and the result of a modernized diet. Straining with bowel movements is one cause. Chiropractic or osteopathic adjustments adjustment can gently put the stomach back in place, and in many cases only a single adjustment is necessary. If acupuncture and chiropractic care don't help with hiatal hernia, surgery may be needed.

HEARTBURN/GASTROESOPHAGEAL REFLUX DISEASE (GERD)

GERD, also known as heartburn, is caused by stomach acid backing up into your esophagus. It's not that you necessarily have too much acid, but rather acid that is in the wrong place. The esophageal sphincter is supposed to keep the stomach contents in place, but if the sphincter relaxes, acid can push up into the esophagus. Stress, alcohol, and some foods can keep the lower-esophageal sphincter from closing properly. The most common symptoms are burning regurgitation, pain, sense of fullness, gas, nausea, and trouble swallowing. Less common symptoms include coughing, chest pain, wheezing, excessive salivation, belching, and a sour taste in the mouth.

GERD is alarmingly common: 44 percent of us have heartburn monthly, 10 to 20 percent weekly, and 10 percent daily. Another 3 to 7 percent suffer from Barrett's esophagus, an esophageal illness caused by chronic acid reflux that results in scarring, constriction of the esophagus, swallowing disorders, and an increased risk for esophageal cancer.

For most people, heartburn is a mild, self-limiting problem, yet for 20 percent of us, it becomes a serious health problem. It's important to look for the root causes using the DIGIN model. Stress plays a huge role. A long time ago, a friend with GERD came to visit while he was on a life sabbatical. I was living in Hawaii at the time, and he spent his days on the beach walking and relaxing and then would come home for meals with my family. After a couple of weeks, his need for acid-suppressing medications completely resolved. Figuring out how you can simplify your life and relax more can go a long way to solving the problem. Sensitivities to gluten and other foods can also trigger symptoms. I have several clients whose GERD vanished after they stopped eating gluten-containing grains, eggs, or other foods. A 2017 paper reported that a Mediterranean diet plus alkaline water worked as well as, if not better than, proton pump inhibitors (PPIs). The Mediterranean diet has many other benefits as well, with none of the potential negative effects of PPIs. Another paper reported that people eating a Mediterranean diet reduced the incidence of GERD. There are a couple of small studies that report less GERD after low-carbohydrate containing meals than after high-carbohydrate meals.

Lifestyle plays a role in GERD. Other triggers include wearing tight-fitting clothes, lying down, bending over, and eating large meals or specific foods. If you experience heartburn in the middle of the night, be sure to eat your last meal at least four hours before going to bed. Heartburn is common among pregnant women, whose organs are squashed in a most peculiar way. Some drugs can also cause heartburn or reduce the tone of the lower esophageal sphincter. The most common are nonsteroidal anti-inflammatory drugs (NSAIDs), aspirin, steroids, birth control pills, diazepam, nicotine, nitroglycerine, progesterone, Provera, and theophylline.

GERD has been split into two categories: erosive and nonerosive reflux disease. The two types are distinguished by gastroenterologists doing endoscopy. Nonerosive reflux disease (NERD) is the most common type. No inflammation is seen during scoping, and it's less likely to be helped with acid-blocking medications. In 30 percent of cases, GERD is erosive and will respond better to antacids, H2 blockers, and PPIs. PPIs are only effective in about 30 to 40 percent of people with GERD.

There are several categories of medications that are used for heartburn and GERD. One option that works well and is not widely used is that of alginates. These create foamy rafts that provide a barrier for the lower-esophageal sphincter so that gastric acid doesn't back up into the esophagus. Alginates are available through all pharmacies and some health food stores. These are well tolerated and are safe to use. Heartburn sufferers commonly take antacids, such as Tums, Rolaids, Maalox, and Mylanta, for temporary relief. H2 acid blockers such as Tagamet, Pepcid, Axid, and Zantac have been used for a long time and partially block acid production. PPIs, such as Prilosec, Prevacid, and Nexium, are also used to block production of stomach acids completely. Most of these are sold over the counter, although some PPIs are prescription only.

According to Laura Targownik, MD, 8 to 10 percent of adults are taking PPIs. The best use of PPIs is in the short-term, for 3 to 4 months. This allows the inflammation to heal. After stopping PPIs, 60 percent of people stayed symptom free a year later. Yet many people continue to take PPIs long term; when they stop, they often have rebound symptoms, which encourages them to stay on the medication.

However, the longer you've been taking PPIs and the more often you take them, the harder it can be to wean yourself off them. Gerard E. Mullin, MD, gastroenterologist at Johns Hopkins Hospital, recommends trying the following by working with your physician:

- Do not stop taking the PPIs cold turkey. Begin by changing your diet, stress, and lifestyle and finding the triggers and root issues that contribute to your GERD. This could be hiatal hernia, gastroparesis, or another GI disorder.
- Work with a clinician to wean yourself off PPIs. Begin by alternating the PPI every other day with an H2 blocker or melatonin. Slowly wean off the PPI. Switch to an over-the-counter acid blocker, acupuncture, and other soothing supplements as needed.

There are other repercussions of taking acid blockers. People with Barrett's esophagus who take PPIs to prevent further development of cancer have high levels of leaky stomach (gastric hyperpermeability). People on PPIs have been shown to have decreased levels of calcium, magnesium, and zinc; iron deficiency; vitamin B_{12} deficiency; and increased risk of developing osteoporosis, depression, irritable bowel syndrome (IBS), pneumonia, and *Clostridium difficile* infectious diarrhea. Blocking stomach acid increases your risk of developing small intestinal bacterial overgrowth (SIBO). The parietal cells respond to these medications by making more acid. Eventually the parietal cells get exhausted, so over the long term, antacids cause the parietal cells to make less HCl and intrinsic factor, which is necessary for absorption of vitamin B_{12}. People who stay on PPIs long term have an increased risk of developing gastric polyps and atrophic gastritis, which both increase the risk of developing stomach cancer.

People on these medications often have poor digestion. There is also evidence that pancreatic enzymes aren't activated without proper stomach acid. HCl is needed for proper digestion of protein. Symptoms can present as bloating, pain, and diarrhea.

People on PPIs also have higher levels of IgE antibodies after three months of usage. Women over the age of 50 who take PPIs for more than a month increase the risk of hip fracture due to poor mineral absorption. The longer women take PPIs, the higher the risk of hip fracture. Use of the older H2 blockers does not increase risk.

Functional Laboratory Testing

- *H. pylori* test
- Heidelberg capsule test
- Food sensitivity testing
- Celiac testing

Healing Options

- **Try osteopathic care and chiropractic adjustment.** Seek chiropractic care for hiatal hernia. Cranial-sacral adjustments can often correct gastric reflux, especially in children. Chiropractic or osteopathic adjustment is often all the therapy you need for these problems.
- **Try acupuncture.** Acupuncture treatments can be effective for GERD.
- **Make dietary changes.** Late-night eating can trigger GERD. Offending foods are individual—you need to discover what yours are. I've seen people respond to a gluten-free diet and others respond to an egg-free diet. The National Institute of Diabetes and Digestive and Kidney Disease recommends eliminating the following foods and food groups to discover which ones contribute to your GERD: citrus fruits, chocolate, caffeinated drinks, fatty and fried foods, garlic, onions, mint flavorings, spicy foods, and tomato-based foods like spaghetti sauce, salsa, and pizza. Eating a whole-foods Mediterranean diet or a low-carbohydrate diet rich in vegetables and fruits can often help.
- **If you are overweight, lose weight.** One of the contributors to GERD is being overweight. Losing weight can help.
- **If you smoke, stop.** GERD is higher in people who smoke than in those who don't.
- **Drink plenty of water.** Some people find that increasing water consumption up to a gallon of water a day resolves acid reflux. Dr. F. Batmanghelidj

popularized the water cure for GERD and ulcers in his book *Your Body's Many Cries for Water.*

- **Place a six-inch beam under the head of your bed.** If you suffer from nighttime heartburn, raising the head of your bed can alleviate symptoms. Although you might think that raising your bed would feel strange, the difference is barely noticeable, and the heartburn improves.

- **Consider possible *H. pylori* infection.** *H. pylori* is a bacteria that has been implicated in gastric and duodenal ulcers. In some cases, it is also involved in gastric reflux. Treatment with antibiotics and bismuth-containing supplements or drugs can eradicate the bacteria.

- **Try HCl supplements.** Heartburn has traditionally been treated with antacid therapy, but often it responds well to supplementation with betaine HCl capsules. Often, the symptoms of excess stomach acid and decreased stomach acid are the same. (See sections in Chapter 3 and 11 for more information on HCl.)

- **Drink cabbage juice.** Cabbage juice is a long-standing remedy for heartburn. Its high glutamine content is probably the key to its success. Cabbage juice has a strong flavor, so dilute with other vegetable juices. The dosage is about 3 cups daily. The taste is strong, so when you are juicing it, add fruit to taste.

- **Try zinc carnosine.** Zinc carnosine can reduce inflammation and promote healing of the mucosal membranes in the esophagus and is the most widely studied type of zinc utilized in ulcer research. research. Best results occur after at least 8 weeks of use. Dosage: 150 mg total of zinc carnosine, taken in 2 doses of 75 mg or 3 of 50 mg. This provides 32 mg total of zinc.

- **Try Iberogast.** Iberogast is a combination herbal product that has been beneficial in people with GERD, IBS, and gastroparesis. It is soothing, anti-microbial, and regulates motility. Dosage: up to 20 drops 3 times daily, diluted in liquid before or with meals.

- **Try melatonin.** Melatonin is an antioxidant and hormone that lets our bodies know it's time to sleep. Melatonin also has effects of reducing gastric acid and strengthening the muscles of the lower esophageal sphincter (LES) by reducing nitric oxide production, which relaxes the LES. There have been several favorable papers demonstrating that melatonin supplementation can give relief to GERD. Several people reported being very sleepy, and a few had diarrhea, headache, and an increase in blood pressure. Another paper showed similar findings using 3 mg of melatonin. Papers have also reported that a combination of omeprazole twice daily at 20 mg, plus either melatonin at 4 mg twice daily or L-tryptophan at a dosage of 250 mg twice daily helped heal GERD and ulcers more effectively than with the omeprazole alone. Dosage: 3 to 8 mg daily of melatonin with or without omeprazole at 20 mg twice daily. Or 250 mg of L-tryptophan twice daily with omeprazole 20 mg twice daily.

- **Try slippery elm bark.** Slippery elm bark has demulcent properties, and it's gentle and soothing to mucous membranes. It has been a folk remedy for both heartburn and ulcers in European and Native American cultures and was used as a food by Native Americans. It can be used in large amounts without harm. Drink as a tea or chew on the bark. To make a tea, put 1 teaspoon of slippery elm bark in 2 cups of water. Simmer for 20 minutes and strain. Sweeten if you want, and drink freely. You can also purchase slippery elm lozenges at health food stores and some drugstores.
- **Use lobelia.** Massage tincture of lobelia externally onto the painful area and take two to three drops internally. This remedy is recommended by Dr. John Christopher, one of the greatest American herbalists of the 20th century.
- **Use ginger.** This root can provide temporary relief in tea. Steep ½ to 1 teaspoon of powdered ginger or a few slices of fresh ginger per cup of boiled water for 10 minutes and drink. If you like, sweeten it with honey. Use freely.
- **Try meadowsweet herb.** Also a demulcent, meadowsweet soothes inflamed mucous membranes. To make a tea, steep 1 to 2 teaspoons of the dried herb in 1 cup of boiled water for 10 minutes. Sweeten with honey if you like. Drink three cups daily.
- **Repair your gut with soothing nutrients.** Taking healing nutrients will repair the damage in your esophagus. Use zinc (especially carnosine), glutamine, fish oils, gamma oryzanol, turmeric, and ginger. Eat okra.

BARRETT'S ESOPHAGUS

Barrett's esophagus is an esophageal illness caused by long-term acid reflux (GERD) that results in scarring and constriction of the esophagus and swallowing disorders. It affects between 3 and 7 percent of adults in the United States. It's hard to know exactly how many because 25 percent of people who have Barrett's have no symptoms. In those who do, the common signs are frequent heartburn, difficulty swallowing food, and sometimes chest pain. It is more common in men than in women and in people who are white or Hispanic. Smoking, getting older, and obesity increase your risk.

Barrett's itself may or may not cause any symptoms. Barrett's does not cause cancer, but it often precedes it. The risk of developing esophageal cancer is 30 to 125 times higher in people who have Barrett's esophagus than those who don't, although the risk is still low, at 1 in 200. The incidence of Barrett's has risen more than 350 percent since the mid-1970s. People with known Barrett's esophagus should be frequently monitored for early detection of cancer. Only 5 percent of people who develop esophageal cancer knew that they had Barrett's prior to being diagnosed with cancer, so people who have chronic GERD ought to be seen by a gastroenterologist for an evaluation. Barrett's esophagus can occur in people without gastric reflux, but it is three to five times more common in people who do have it. Treatment with acid-blocking drugs sometimes improves the extent of Barrett's, but it doesn't correlate with a reduction in cancer rates. Still, people who have a diagnosis of Barrett's esophagitis have a protective benefit from taking PPIs long-term.

Production of peroxynitrite, a damaging free radical, contributes to Barrett's esophagus. Vitamin C, glutathione, and folic acid are known to help reduce the formation of damaging peroxynitrites. Barrett's is diagnosed by doing an upper-gastrointestinal (GI) endoscopy and biopsy.

The following healing options may help with the symptoms of Barrett's esophagus. They may also help prevent cancer of the esophagus, which is the long-term problem to be concerned about. Very little literature about this is available, but I am working with what is known in other areas of the digestive tract and personal experience with clients. It is necessary to continue to have medical testing and to be vigilant about this illness. You may also benefit from the many suggestions in the section on heartburn and gastric reflux.

Healing Options

- **Eat a diet high in folate.** Folic acid, found in a huge variety of foods, prevents esophageal cancer and colon cancers. Research on giving folic acid supplements, on the other hand, has been mixed. Giving folic acid supplementation *may* actually increase the risk of developing esophageal cancer. It remains to be seen how genetics play a role; people who have variations in the methylation genes gene have different needs for folic acid than people with normal methylation expression. Nonetheless, you will do well to eat high–folic acid foods, such as brewer's yeast, black-eyed peas, rice germ, soy flour, wheat germ, liver, soy beans, wheat bran, legumes of all types, asparagus, lentils, walnuts, spinach, kale, nuts, greens of all types, peanuts, broccoli, barley, brussels sprouts, and more.

- **Increase antioxidant nutrients.** Several studies indicate that free radical damage helps initiate Barrett's esophagus. Antioxidant nutrients are useful in nearly every condition. Selenium levels in people with Barrett's esophagus are lower than in controls. Glutathione levels are reduced, while malondialdehyde and NF-kappaB levels are increased. It is prudent to increase levels of antioxidant nutrients such as vitamin C, carotenoids, vitamin E, selenium, N-acetyl cysteine (NAC), lipoic acid, folic acid, and others. You can begin with a combination antioxidant supplement with 200 to 400 mcg selenium. Add an additional 1,000 IU of vitamin E, 1,000 to 2,000 mg NAC, and at least 1,000 mg vitamin C. You may want to use the vitamin C flush described in Chapter 17.

- **Try probiotics and digestive enzymes.** No published research on the use of probiotic bacteria or on the use of digestive enzymes in Barrett's is available, but it would make sense to give each a trial.
- **Try gut-healing herbs and nutrients.** The use of supplemental glutamine has not been studied in people with Barrett's esophagus, but it is the main fuel of the small intestine and may be of benefit in the esophagus as well.

DGL licorice, slippery elm, marshmallow, gamma oryzanol, turmeric or curcumin, fish oils, and other herbs and supplements that are used to reduce inflammation make sense to try. (See Chapter 10.)

EOSINOPHILIC ESOPHAGITIS

Eosinophilic esophagitis (EoE) is a chronic, allergen-based immune condition of the esophagus that is the most common cause of difficulty swallowing in children and adults. Food gets impacted in the esophagus, effecting the ability to swallow. Eosinophils are typically elevated when people have allergies or parasites. Officially identified in 1993, this disease has emerged with the highest prevalence in many developed countries, including the United States, the United Kingdom, Japan, Spain, Australia, Switzerland, and Italy. The incidence is 0.5 to 1 in 1,000 people, yet it is seen in 2 to 7 percent of people who get an endoscopy for any reason. Incidence is rising, and it's not fully understood why, but there are overlaps in people who have hay fever and/or food allergies, were born of C-section, have connective tissue disorders, and live in cold or arid climates. *H. pylori* bacteria seem to be protective. *H. pylori* has also been found to be protective from other allergic conditions, such as asthma and eczema. There is a small amount of research linking EoE to heavy metals. At the present time, the only way to monitor EoE is with biopsies done via endoscopy.

Symptoms of EoE can also include painful or difficult swallowing, regurgitation, nausea or vomiting, diarrhea, failure to thrive in children (poor growth or weight loss), stomach or chest pain, GERD, poor appetite, bloating, anemia, blood in the stool, malnutrition, and difficulty sleeping. People will often have food allergies, eczema, or asthma. Children may not want to eat because it hurts. In addition, scarring from untreated EoE can make it difficult to swallow, so some of these children are shorter and weigh less than they should because they fail to eat enough. Many children with EoE have white specks or plaques in the esophagus, which tend to occur when the condition is severe.

One study found asthma in one-third of children with EoE; EoE is being called "asthma of the esophagus" because allergic reactions to foods and also environment allergens such as mold, dust, and pollen appear to play a big role. People with EoE are advised to go on a diet that eliminates all foods to which they are allergic. Physicians also encourage the use of an elemental diet, using medical foods that are hypoallergenic. Further, 90 percent of people who eat only this product for several months show great improvement in symptoms and at repeat endoscopy and biopsy.

Research with the 6-Food Elimination Diet consistently reports 72 percent of people recovering from EoE. The diet eliminates fish and shellfish, dairy products, all gluten-containing grains (including wheat), nuts and peanuts, eggs, legumes, and soy at 23.8 percent. Cow's milk is the largest offender, in almost 62 percent of people, followed by wheat at 28.6 percent, eggs at 26.2 percent, and legumes and soy at 23.8 percent. Typically, when testing for allergies, skin testing for reactions is utilized. However, in this instance, there was little correlation between the skin testing and which foods actually caused EoE. The 6-Food Elimination Diet was more accurately able to pinpoint offending foods than scratch testing. Since this initial study, over 40 more papers have demonstrated the usefulness of this dietary approach.

My husband was diagnosed with EoE and took PPIs and an inhaled steroid for 3 months. When he was rescoped, there was no change at all. Then he ate the 6-Food Elimination Diet for five months. When he was scoped, he had no EoE, and for a year, he has had no recurrence of eosinophils with endoscopy. He discovered that his biggest issues were with dairy products and alcoholic beverages. His few glasses of wine and stout had to go, much to his chagrin.

The low-histamine diet has not been studied in people with EoE, yet it makes sense to me that if the 6-Food Elimination Diet doesn't get results, reducing histamine from food and taking diamine oxidase (DAO) enzymes may be useful. Again, looking at my husband's EoE, wine and beer aggravated his swallowing issues. The low-histamine diet is discussed in Chapter 14.

One study showed an atypically alkaline esophageal environment in nine out of nine children with EoE. More research on this subject is needed, but it would seem that if esophageal pH is low, you may want to try increasing your level of stomach acid to see whether this relieves the symptoms.

I have worked with several children who have EoE. One toddler began having problems immediately after an immunization, a story commonly heard from parents of autistic children. Another parent began working with an autism specialists trained in integrative medicine to heal her son's EoE. You will remember from the

DIGIN model that no matter what the diagnosis, we always use the same principles to treat digestive issues.

About half of people with EoE respond to PPIs. Some respond to use of swallowed steroids from an inhaler.

EOSINOPHILIC GASTROENTERITIS

Eosinophilic gastroenteritis (EoG) is similar to EoE, but it takes place in the stomach and small intestine rather than in the esophagus. It is quite rare. It is characterized by severe infiltration of eosinophils into the stomach, small intestine, or both. It is also called eosinophilic gastritis (when just in the stomach) and eosinophilic enteritis (when just in the small intestine). It was first discovered in 1937 by a researcher named Kaijser.

Half the children who have EoG have a history of eczema, asthma, or food allergies. Many children and adults with EoG also have more typical allergies to dust, pollen, and mold. Typical symptoms of EoG include abdominal pain, diarrhea, and pain with swallowing. Often a child will refuse to eat because it hurts. Cramping and abdominal pain may be accompanied by nausea and vomiting.

As with children with EoE, it is essential to test them for food allergies and sensitivities, especially to gluten and dairy products.

Dr. DicQie Fuller had an infant daughter, Colleen, who suffered from eosinophilic gastritis. The child was failing to thrive, and the family was told that she would likely die. In an effort to save her daughter's life, Dr. Fuller began giving her digestive and proteolytic (protein-splitting) enzyme supplements. Not only did this save Colleen's life, but she is now in mid-life and has been living a healthful life ever since.

Treating EoE and EoG
Treatments for EoE and EoG may include steroids, but they aren't often used due to the long-term side effects. At this time, medical treatments aren't that promising, and the long-term implications of having EoE or EoG are uncertain. This leads one to really use more of an integrated approach when working with these diseases. Begin with the DIGIN model.

One resource is the American Partnership for Eosinophilic Disorders: http://www.apfed.org.

Laboratory Testing for EoE and EoG
EoE or EoG is diagnosed by doing an upper endoscopy (scoping) and taking biopsies. Once diagnosed, it's also useful to explore specific food allergies and sensitivities by using the 6-Food Elimination Diet. Research finds that the diet more

effectively reflects allergies than the testing does. Still, you may find it useful to do testing to explore other underlying issues that may be contributing to the chronic immune response. Tests to consider include the following:

- Food-allergy testing/IgE
- Food-sensitivity testing/IgG and, if possible, IgM and IgA
- Urine provocation test for heavy metals
- pH test, quantitative fluid analysis, or the Heidelberg capsule test

Healing Options for EoE and EoG

Drugs currently used for EoE include steroid medications, cromolyn sodium, and leukotriene inhibitors. Initial research shows that even with medication, restriction of allergy-inducing foods is still necessary to achieve the full benefit. The other natural healing options presented herein are my own ideas, as no research has been conducted on natural therapies for EoE and EoG.

- **Try the 6-Food Elimination Diet for 3 months minimum.** Eliminate all dairy products, eggs, wheat (and other gluten-containing grains), legumes, peanuts, soy, tree nuts, fish, and shellfish. Then get rescoped to see if things have improved.
- **Try a low-histamine diet.** We have no research on a low-histamine diet and EoE, but since it's related to allergies and histamines, it makes sense to try.
- **Quercetin.** Quercetin is very effective when combined with grapeseed extract or Pycnogenol, and it diminishes, relieves, and prevents allergy symptoms and protects esophageal tissue. Adults can take 500 to 6,000 mg. A child can take 200 to 1,000 mg three to six times daily, depending on the child's size and symptom severity.
- **Probiotics.** This will balance gut ecology and immune system function. See Chapter 6 for dosages and types.
- **Consider heavy-metal toxicity.** There is some research that associates high levels of heavy metals with eosinophilic esophagitis.
- **Digestive enzymes.** Use these to enhance complete digestion of foods so that they don't become allergens. Take one capsule each time you eat.
- **DGL licorice.** This will soothe inflammation and stimulate repair. Take one to three tablets, chewables, or capsules before meals. You could also consider using the demulcent herbs marshmallow, meadowsweet, and slippery elm.
- **Folic acid.** This will protect mucous membranes from inflammation elsewhere in the gastrointestinal tract. Take 800 mcg daily.

GASTRIC HYPOFUNCTION OR HYPOCHLORHYDRIA

Hypochlorhydria (low stomach acid) has been associated with many common health problems. (See Chapters 3 and 11.) Stomach acid is used to begin the process of protein digestion. Stomach acid also provides our first defense against food poisoning, *H. pylori*, parasites, SIBO, and other infections. In addition, without adequate acid we leave ourselves open to indigestion, decreased immune resistance, mineral deficiencies, and vitamin deficiencies. A normal stomach acid level is a pH of 1.5 to 2.5. As we age, the parietal cells in the stomach lining produce less HCl. Use of acid-blocking medications increases stomach pH to 3.5 or higher.

Common symptoms of low stomach acidity include belching or burning sensations immediately after meals, bloating, a feeling that the food just sits in the stomach without digesting, and an inability to eat more than small amounts at any one sitting. Poor HCl levels have been associated with childhood asthma, chronic hepatitis, chronic hives, diabetes, eczema, gallbladder disease, lupus erythematosus, osteoporosis, rheumatoid arthritis, rosacea, underactive and overactive thyroid conditions, vitiligo, and weak adrenals.

Stomach acid is also necessary for absorption of many minerals, so mineral depletion may occur with use of these medicines. Minerals that can become depleted include iron, calcium, magnesium, zinc, and copper. Adequate HCl is necessary for the absorption of vitamin B_{12} from food. B_{12} deficiency causes weakness, fatigue, and nervous system problems. Most B-complex vitamins require normal levels of stomach acid for proper absorption. Vitamin C levels are also low in people with poor stomach acid. Acid is critical for the breakdown of protein bonds in the stomach.

Hypochlorhydria may be caused by the following: pernicious anemia, chronic *H. pylori* infection, long-term treatment with PPIs, such as Prilosec, autoimmune gastritis, and mucolipidosis type 1V; it is also common in autoimmune diseases.

Functional Laboratory Testing
- Heidelberg capsule test
- Self-test for HCl adequacy

For healing options, see Chapter 3.

FUNCTIONAL DYSPEPSIA

Functional Dyspepsia is a general term that means "bad digestion" in Latin. About 40 percent of us complain of bad digestion, which is typically self-limiting and goes away on its own. Functional dyspepsia is a catch-all phrase for "we haven't explored the underlying issues of your digestive distress". It may be due to a motility issue, digestive issue, inflammation or infection. Exploring the DIGIN model will help to figure out the root issues. If you have two or more of the following factors, it's time to see your doctor: being over age 50, loss of appetite, feeling full even though you haven't eaten much, trouble swallowing, blood in your stools or in phlegm, or abdominal masses.

GASTRITIS

In general eating smaller meals can be helpful for people with dyspepsia. The Mediterranean and FODMAP diets have also been found to be useful. Various studies have used questionnaires with people who have dyspepsia to determine foods that reduce and exacerbate symptoms. Foods that worsen dyspepsia include: alcohol, citrus foods, spicy foods, peppers, onions, sausages, bologna, vinegar, carbonated drinks, grains, salty foods, pizza, watermelon, and pasta. Foods that seem to help include rice, apples, bread, kiwi fruit, caraway seeds, dates, honey, yogurt, quinces, and walnuts.

Several studies have demonstrated benefits in dyspepsia from taking digestive enzyme supplements with meals. Acupuncture and herbal remedies can also be utilized to reduce spasms, gas, or calm the stomach, including ginger, Iberogast, peppermint and caraway oils, bitters, lemon balm, and chamomile.

Gastritis is a general name that describes any inflammation in the stomach that doesn't involve an ulcer. This could be a chronic issue or something that's acutely painful. The most common symptoms are gnawing or burning ache or pain in your stomach that gets better or worse with food, loss of appetite, bloating, belching, hiccups, indigestion, nausea, vomiting, vomiting of blood, dark stools, feeling full even if you haven't eaten much, and weight loss. It's typically found when a gastroenterologist does an endoscopy. It can be caused by alcohol, infection such as with *H. pylori*, taking NSAIDs (such as aspirin), smoking, chronic stress, bile reflux, drinking poisons or caustic substances, and autoimmune disorders.

Other causes include corticosteroids, cancer drugs, and antibiotics; excessive coffee consumption; organ failure; and severe stress or trauma. It is common in the elderly, affecting 20 percent of people between the ages of 60 and 69 and 40 percent of people over age 80. The lack of hydrochloric acid secretion in the elderly allows for bacterial growth, such as *H. pylori*; however, when treated with antibiotics, symptoms improve.

Long-term effects of gastritis include poor vitamin B_{12} status in all people. Signs of B_{12} deficiency often mimic those of senility. Many people have B_{12} deficiencies with normal serum levels. Tests for B_{12} status include methylmalonic acid and trials with B_{12} injections or sublingual B_{12}.

Gastritis is usually treated with H2 blockers or PPIs. However, there are natural solutions that don't have the long-term effects that H2 blockers and PPIs have. Looking at triggers such as stress, medications, and poor HCl production is also an important step toward prevention.

GASTRIC ULCERS AND *H. PYLORI* INFECTION

Gastric ulcers occur in the stomach and the duodenum (the first section of the small intestine), where gastric juice has burned a hole in the lining. It hurts! Gastric juice is so acidic it would burn your hand if you spilled some on it. A mucous layer protects the stomach tissue from being eaten away by pepsin (a protein-splitting enzyme) and the gastric juices. Secretions of bicarbonate (baking soda) from the stomach lining are mixed into the mucus, buffering the acid. This makes an effective barrier to keep the stomach lining from harm. Pepsin, the real villain in this story, slowly digests this mucus layer, and if the mucus isn't replaced, gastric juices come into contact with the stomach lining and ulcers occur.

About half a million Americans have ulcers. About 10 percent of us will develop ulcer disease at some point in our lives. Each year 6,000 American people die from ulcers, half from peptic ulcers and half from duodenal ulcers. In 1982, the Australian physician Barry Marshall and J. Robin Warren discovered the presence of *H. pylori* between the stomach lining and the mucous membrane. Until their discovery, ulcers were believed to be caused by stress and lifestyle alone. In 2005, Marshall and Warren won the Nobel Prize in Physiology or Medicine for this work. Also, 80 percent of ulcers are caused by *H. pylori* infections, 10 percent are caused by the use of NSAID medications, and another 10 percent are of unknown origin.

Symptoms include abdominal pain that is frequently described as burning. This pain can radiate to your back and typically occurs one to five hours after you've eaten. You may feel better if you eat, take antacids, or vomit. All of this typically is in a daily pattern that is specific to you. As if this isn't enough to alert you to see a doctor, if you have bleeding, are anemic, have unexplained weight loss, feel full even though you only ate a little bit, have increasing trouble swallowing or painful swallowing, suffer recurrent vomiting, or have a family history of GI cancer, see a doctor now. If you have sharp and sudden severe stomach pain that persists, bloody or black stools, bloody vomit, or vomit that looks like it has coffee grounds, seek immediate medical help.

On the other hand, if you are slowly burning a hole in your stomach from over-use of NSAIDs like aspirin, Motrin, Aleve, and prescription pain relievers, you may not notice a thing until you begin to see bleeding or have anemia. Continued use of these therapies has been widely shown to cause ulcers and hospitalizations. It's estimated that up to 30 percent of regular NSAID users have ulcers. NSAIDs block pain but also block healing and repair to the stomach lining by decreasing beneficial prostaglandins and cyclooxygenase. It has been estimated that 107,000 people are hospitalized each year because of NSAID complications, and at least 16,500 NSAID-related deaths occur each year among arthritis patients alone. In 2018, the Food and Drug Administration (FDA) updated warnings on NSAIDs to include increased risk of heart attack and stroke, with the risk beginning within the first weeks and increasing the longer you use them and at higher doses. This can happen even in people with no known risk for heart disease.

Ten percent of people with ulcers and gastritis do not have *H. pylori* infection, nor have they used NSAID medications. For these people, the cause of ulcers and gastritis is still a mystery. Looking at stress, diet, and lifestyle may yield important clues. Stress plays a significant role in ulcers and gastritis. While low-grade stress probably won't cause an ulcer, severe stress has been shown to cause ulcers in both animal and human studies. Psychological stress increases stomach acid and causes the mucus to become more fragile, making it easier for ulcers to form.

H. pylori

H. pylori can be diagnosed with stool, blood, and breath testing and is widely available. If you've been having severe symptoms or bleeding, your doctor may order an endoscopy.

H. pylori is also associated with gastric reflux (GERD), gastritis, stomach cancer, and stomach lymphoma. *H. pylori* induces an immune response that increases inflammation and leaky gut. Because of this, it can wreak havoc throughout the body. It has been found to play a role in atherosclerosis, heart disease, idiopathic thrombocytopenia purpura, iron-deficiency anemia, inflammation in the iris of the eye (idiopathic anterior uveitis), Parkinson's disease, autoimmune thyroid disease, GI lymphomas, ear infections, glaucoma, Sjögren's syndrome, food allergy, migraine headaches, lichen planus, prurigo nodularis, Henoch-Schonlein purpurea, psoriasis, and rosacea.

H. pylori presents a conundrum: It is present in about 50 percent of the world's population, yet only a small percentage of people get sick from it. This poses a curious question. Why do some people have *Helicobacter* infection, yet no GI upset? In fact, some scientists hypothesize that *H. pylori* actually protects us from allergies, eczema, and asthma. A recent study explored the protective effect of *H. pylori* in people from developing inflammatory bowel disease (IBD). They have found inverse relationships between the presence of *H. pylori* and the absence of these allergic conditions. It's probably due to a difference in genetics and the microbiome. A great book on this is *Missing Microbes*, by Martin Blaser, MD.

Because many people have *H. pylori* and have no symptoms, conventionally it is treated only when someone has the infection and an ulcer, gastritis, stomach cancer or precancerous lesions, mucosa-associated lymphoid tissue, or iron-deficiency anemia that doesn't respond to treatment. Conventional treatment is with triple or quadruple antibiotic therapy. Once treated, ulcers typically don't recur.

After 4 weeks, people are retested to see if the ulcer has healed and if the *H. pylori* has been eradicated. Despite treatment, 10 to 20 percent have a relapse of their ulcer within 6 months without aggravation from NSAID medications. Although this treatment has minor side effects, the overall outcome shows improved quality of living and less psychological stress after therapy.

There are many natural remedies for *H. pylori* that are being used by integrative clinicians. Many of these are supported by excellent research.

Because ulcers have been experienced throughout history, people have found effective natural therapies. Most physicians are not aware of these therapies, but nutritionally oriented physicians have been using them with promising results. Some recommend a combination of antibiotic therapy and bismuth, with DGL licorice, citrus seed extract, goldenseal, activated charcoal, and aloe vera. Glutamine, gamma oryzanol, SanoGastril, cabbage juice, comfrey, and calendula have also been shown to heal ulcers.

Other natural substances that have been shown to be effective against this bacterium include oil of oregano, turmeric, cumin, ginger, chili, borage, and licorice root. Several of these, such as turmeric, borage, and parsley, also inhibit the ability of *H. pylori* to adhere to the stomach.

Dietary recommendations for people with ulcers may be useful. Low-fiber diets may contribute significantly to ulcers. Eating probiotic-rich foods can help heal and eradicate *H. pylori* infections. Cooked broccoli sprouts or Brussels sprouts (about 3 ounces daily), cabbage juice, sauerkraut juice, cranberry juice (about 2 cups daily), green tea as you'd like, yogurt, apples, moderate amounts of red wine or red grape juice, onions, and capers all have antibacterial effects on *H. pylori*.

A recent study on the diet of people with duodenal ulcers found that people who had good vitamin A intake, followed a high-fiber diet, or ate seven or more servings of fruits and vegetables per day rather than three servings or fewer reduced risks of developing ulcers by 54 percent, 45 percent, and 33 percent, respectively. Again, this shows that a great diet can reduce your risk of all sorts of health problems.

One new therapy uses lactoferrin, which is found in colostrum and transfer factor, to eradicate *H. pylori*. Research has shown that use of triple therapy with added lactoferrin improves the success rate. Alone, it probably won't do the job. People with high levels of gastritis and *Helicobacter* also have concurrent high levels of lactoferrin in their stomach. Is the lactoferrin helping the *H. pylori* gain a foothold and helping it gain necessary iron for its metabolism? Or is the lactoferrin called in by the body's immune system to help rid us of the bacteria? At this point, no one really knows.

Research for ulcer healing has shown good results for a wide variety of natural products. You can also find relief from combination products that contain bismuth, licorice root, grapefruit seed extract, goldenseal root, aloe vera, zinc carnosine, mastic gum, quercetin, sea buckthorn, water hissop, Bolivian medicinal, traditional Chinese formulations, and other herbs. Cranberry juice, ginger juice, broccoli sprouts, Brussels sprouts, plantain (banana type), propolis, evening primrose oil and other polyunsaturated fatty acids, reishi mushrooms, green tea, turmeric or curcumin, and yogurt can also heal ulcers. One study of 1,785 people found that moderate drinking of alcohol killed *H. pylori* infection. Details on many of these follow.

Functional Laboratory Testing
- ***H. pylori* test.** This can be done through stool, breath, or blood testing. It is widely available.

Healing Options
- **Drink water.** One very simple remedy for ulcers and gastritis is to drink huge amounts of water. Drink four to six glasses of water during the pain, and it may magically disappear. A fascinating book on this subject is *Your Body's Many Cries for Water*, by Fereydoon Batmanghelidj, MD. Drink eight to ten glasses of water or more each day.
- **Try licorice.** DGL licorice helps heal the stomach's mucous lining by increasing healing prostaglandins that promote mucus secretion and cell proliferation. It also makes an environment that is inhospitable to *H. pylori* and has some weak antibiotic effects. Licorice enhances the blood flow and health of intestinal tract cells. It's considered to have the same healing effect as cimetidine (Tagamet).

It's important to use DGL licorice to avoid side effects caused by whole licorice. Take 760 to 1,520 mg chewed before each meal. Daily total dosage is 4.5 grams.

- **Use aloe vera.** Aloe vera is a folk remedy for ulcers and has been approved by the FDA for use in oral ulcers. It is soothing, reduces inflammation, and helps to heal gastric ulcers. Take 1 teaspoon of fresh gel after meals. Use gel that doesn't have skin; otherwise it can give you diarrhea. If you buy an aloe vera product, use as directed.

- **Take zinc carnosine.** Studies report 100 percent symptom relief and 80 percent healing of ulcers after taking zinc carnosine for 8 weeks. Take 75 mg two to four times daily. Stop when well.

- **Try unripe plaintain powder.** Take 5 to 10 g daily.

- **Take oil of oregano.** Try 200 mg three times daily.

- **Try gamma oryzanol.** Gamma oryzanol, a compound found in rice bran oil, is a useful therapeutic tool in gastritis, ulcers, and irritable bowel syndrome. It acts on the autonomic nervous system to normalize production of gastric juice and has also been shown to be effective in normalizing serum triglycerides and cholesterol, symptoms of menopause, and depressive disorders. Studies involving 375 hospitals in Japan indicate that gamma oryzanol was effective in reducing symptoms in 80 to 90 percent of participants, with more than half of the participants experiencing total or marked improvement. In the study, typical dosage was 100 mg three times daily for three weeks. Occasionally, the dosage was doubled, and often the therapy was used longer. Minimal side effects were experienced by 0.4 percent of these people. Take 100 mg of gamma oryzanol three times daily for a trial period of 3 to 6 weeks to determine if it relieves the problem.

- **Drink cabbage juice.** Cabbage juice is a long-standing remedy for heartburn and ulcers. Garnett Cheney MD studied people with ulcers in the late 1940's. He reported that people with ulcers resolved them within 7-10 days by drinking cabbage juice. It takes pretty horrible, so mix it with other juices to make it palatable. Drink 1 quart of cabbage juice daily for a period of two weeks.

- **Drink cranberry juice.** Cranberry juice has been well studied for helping to resolve *H. pylori*. It appears to block *H. pylori* from adhering to the stomach tissue in the same way that it does in the bladder. While it doesn't work for everyone, a Chinese study reports that 11.3 percent of people were *H. pylori* free after drinking two 9-ounce juice boxes of cranberry juice daily for 90 days. Another report states that when cranberry was used along with oregano, results improved because of the synergy. In another study, when cranberry juice was given to people along with triple therapy, results improved; 82.5 percent of people who drank 9 ounces (250 ml) of cranberry juice twice daily had normal *H. pylori* breath tests. In women results were even better: 95.2 percent had normal test results.

■ **Use mastic gum.** Several studies tout the anti-ulcer benefit of mastic gum. Take 1 gram (1,000 mg) daily in divided doses.

■ **Eat yogurt.** Eating 12 to 24 ounces of yogurt containing bifidobacteria lowered *H. pylori* in breath testing after six weeks of daily consumption.

■ **Drink a lot of green tea.** *H. pylori* was inhibited in gerbils when given green tea extract. The human dosage would be 4 to 8 cups of green tea daily using about ½ teaspoon of dried green tea per cup.

■ **Try glutamine.** Glutamine is the most popular antiulcer drug in Asia today. The digestive tract uses glutamine as a fuel source and for healing. It is effective for healing stomach ulcers, IBS, and ulcerative bowel diseases. Begin with 8 grams daily for a trial period of 4 weeks.

■ **Try grapefruit or citrus seed extract.** Citrus seed extract has widely effective antiparasitic, antiviral, and antibiotic properties. Take 75 to 250 mg three times daily.

■ **Use goldenseal.** Goldenseal is soothing to mucous membranes, enhances immune function, and has antibiotic and antifungal properties. Take 200 mg three to four times daily.

■ **Try SanoGastril.** SanoGastril is a fermented soy product that contains a specific strain of *Lactobacillus bulgaricus* (LB-15). It's a chewable tablet that buffers the acidity of the stomach. (SanoGastril is marketed in the United States by Nutri-Cology/Allergy Research Group.) A study using two tablets three times daily involved 93 people with ulcers and gastritis. After 1 month, each participant was X-rayed to see progress. At that time, 12 out of 22 people with gastric ulcer, 25 out of 58 people with duodenal ulcer, and 4 out of 12 people with gastritis were completely healed. Two tablets of SanoGastril three times daily before meals relieved heartburn completely immediately in 76 percent of 158 people. Take two tablets chewed or sucked three times daily between meals.

■ **Try catsclaw/Una de Gato.** The inner bark and stems of *Uncaria tomentosa* and *Uncaria guianensis* decrease inflammation. Take 1,000 mg capsules three to five times daily. *Caution: Do not take with Coumadin (warfarin).*

■ **Use evening primrose, borage, or flaxseed oils.** These oils increase the levels of prostaglandin E2 series, which promotes healing and repair. Take 4,000 to 8,000 mg of one of these oils or a combination oil three times a day for a trial period of four weeks.

Low dietary intake of linoleic acid, an essential fatty acid, has been associated with duodenal ulcers. Flaxseeds are excellent sources of linoleic acid. A benefit to using ground flaxseeds rather than the oil is that the mucous portion of the flaxseed buffers excess acid, which makes it ideal for inflammation in the stomach and throughout the gastrointestinal tract. Grind them fresh daily or buy products with enhanced shelf life, and store in the refrigerator. Linoleic acid is also found in pumpkin seeds, tofu, walnuts, safflower oil, sunflower seeds and oil, and sesame seeds and oil. Use 2 to 3 teaspoons in smoothies or protein drinks, or on salads and vegetables.

- **Try Turkish herbs.** Six Turkish plant medicines were studied for their effectiveness against *H. pylori* in a laboratory setting. Five were found to be highly effective, with *Cistus laurifolius* (laurel rockrose) being the most effective. The effective herbs were the flowers of *Cistus laurifolius*, cones of Cedrus libani (cedar of Lebanon), herbs and flowers of *Centaurea solstitialis* (yellow starthistle), fruits of *Momordica charantia* (bitter melon), herbaceous parts of *Sambucus ebulus* (danewort or dwarf elder), and flowering herbs of *Hypericum perforatum* (Saint-John's-wort). We may begin to see research on some or all of these plant medicines. We may also begin to see them in supplements. There have been no human studies.

- **Try melatonin.** Several studies have looked at the effect of melatonin on GERD. Melatonin is a hormone that helps us fall asleep and is a powerful antioxidant. It's also found in the hormone-producing cells in the GI wall. It works best when given along with Tagamet (cimetidine). Dosages between 3 and 6 mg before bed for 4 to 8 weeks have been found to be an effective treatment for GERD.

- **Try comfrey and calendula.** A Bulgarian study used comfrey and calendula either with antacid medications or alone in patients with peptic ulcers. Eighty-five percent of both groups felt better, but people who also used antacids felt better a few days earlier. Gastric scoping showed equal healing of ulcers in both groups. Comfrey, one of my favorite herbs, has come under fire lately. It contains small amounts of pyrrolizidine alkaloids, which have liver-damaging and possible carcinogenic effects. Although there have been no known cases of toxicity in humans from comfrey, rat testing has caused it to be removed from many products and banned in several countries. Studies were done using the specific pyrrolizidine alkaloids, but in studies with whole comfrey, no adverse reactions were found.

While the controversy continues, be cautious about using comfrey internally. Restrict its internal use to 2 weeks. Comfrey has been used medicinally for hundreds of years to promote wound and bone healing. The combination of comfrey and calendula makes sense in terms of today's triple therapy: Comfrey promotes healing and protects the gastric mucosa, while calendula has antibacterial effects. Dosage in the Bulgarian study was unclear, but comfrey leaf and calendula flower tea at 3 to 4 cups daily would be appropriate.

- **Try other natural substances.** The following have been found to be useful: Dangshen, dragon's blood (*Dracaena cochinchinensis*), ginger, Optiberry (a combination of berries), parsley, probiotics, propolis, quercetin, reishi mushrooms, seabuckthorn, swallowroot (*Decalepis hamiltonii*), turmeric, curcumin, water hyssop (*Bacopa monnieri*), and traditional Chinese medicine formulas.

GASTROPARESIS

Gastroparesis is delayed gastric emptying. It occurs when the muscles in your stomach don't open to let the food pass into the duodenum properly. It literally means "paralyzed stomach." This can be a very severe disease because your food doesn't move. Symptoms can vary but may include vomiting, nausea, feeling of fullness after eating just a bit, bloating, heartburn, lack of appetite, weight loss and malnutrition, and fluctuations in blood sugar levels. Causes vary but may include damage or unresponsiveness of the vagus nerve, diabetes, *H. pylori* infection, viral infection, autoimmune disease, nervous system disorders such as Parkinson's disease, and scleroderma. It's more common in people who have had gastric or other abdominal surgeries and in people with eating disorders, hypothyroid, scleroderma, and Parkinson's disease. Gastroparesis can result in weight loss and malnutrition, bacterial overgrowth in the stomach, or food that sits and hardens in your stomach (called a bezoar). An endoscopic exam can determine whether gastroparesis is your problem. It is diagnosed by an upper endoscopy. Ultrasound is also used to rule out gallbladder disease and pancreatitis. The SmartPill is also used to diagnose gastroparesis.

Gastroparesis is now associated with autoimmune GI dysmotility, bringing into view a new perspective on gastroparesis and dysmotility issues. They report that many people also have high anti-nuclear antibodies (ANA), which may be a tip-off. A study of 11 women with gastroparesis who were nonresponsive to other therapies reported that 50 percent responded to intravenous immune globulin therapy (IVIG), prednisolone plus mycophenolate mofetil, or mycophenolate only for 8 to 12 weeks.

The Mayo Clinic has developed a specific antibody test that looks for dipeptidyl-peptidase-like protein-6, and this is now available to physicians all over. Japanese researchers have associated antiganglionic acetylcholine receptor antibodies in about 50 percent of patients with chronic intestinal pseudo-obstruction (gastroparesis or paralytic ileus). While more research needs to be done in this area, for such a difficult condition, it is good to see new avenues of thought.

Current medical treatment typically consists of antibiotics, acetylcholinesterase inhibitors, and other drugs. Helping to increase motility may be useful. Gerard E. Mullin, MD, gastroenterologist at Johns Hopkins Hospital, recommends ginger, Iberogast, acupuncture, D-limonene, probiotics, and the traditional Japanese herbal medicine Liu Jun Zi Tang (TJ43).

When queried about which foods made them feel better or worse, people with gastroparesis listed a wide variety of foods. Bland, starchy, sweet, and salty foods were least likely to provoke issues. Restorative foods for healing, which are mainly easy-to-digest foods (discussed in Chapter 15), may be worth trying.

A lot of the medical treatments may work for a while but then stop working. Some of the integrative physicians I have met use a prescription drug called domperidone. It is used in Mexico, Canada, and many European countries for gastroparesis. Physicians like it because it works well and has few side effects. Domperidone is not legally available in the United States due to cardiac arrhythmias, cardiac arrest, and sudden death. The FDA does allow physicians to obtain domperidone for expanded access for clinical research. I could find almost *no* research on the use of natural therapies, but here are some that have worked for others and are worth trying.

Healing Options

- **Try d-limonene 1000 mg twice daily.** If you feel worse, begin taking one every other day and slowly increase. Take 30 minutes before a meal or 60 minutes after a meal with water or other beverage. Swallow the capsule whole. Do not break it open. Do not take if you are pregnant, nursing, or suspect you have an ulcer.
- **Try Iberogast.** Iberogast, formulated in Germany in 1961, comprises nine different herbs and is used for IBS, motility issues, and GI discomfort. These include German chamomile, clown's mustard, angelica, caraway, lemon balm, celandine, licorice, and peppermint. The exact mechanism isn't known but has a dual action in that it relaxes smooth muscle, helping when there is spasm, and also helps where there isn't any muscle tone. It also has anti-inflammatory and strong antioxidant properties.
- **Try ginger:** Ginger increases gastric emptying in healthy people and may help people with gastroparesis.

- **Try Liu Jun Zi Tang (TJ43):** Liu Jun Zi Tang is a traditional Kampo (Japanese) medicine. A paper reporting on a study of 22 people noted improvement in gastric emptying. Dosage: 2.5 g three times daily.

- **Try tangweikang.** A Chinese study found that the herbal combination tangweikang was effective at helping with gastric emptying and blood sugar control in people with diabetes.

- **Try magnesium.** Magnesium is used as a prokinetic in preparation for colonscopies due to its effect on increasing motility. There are no papers on this, but it seems to be worth trying. Dosage: Begin with 200 mg of magnesium citrate and increase until you get the required response. If you get diarrhea or gas, back off. Adding choline citrate will increase your body's ability to absorb magnesium.

- **Try probiotics.** We currently have no research on probiotics and gastroparesis, yet they do help with motility issues.

- **Try lipoic acid.** Richard Bernstein, MD, in his book *Dr. Bernstein's Diabetes Solution,* has an entire chapter on gastroparesis and its relationship to diabetes. Lipoic acid helps liver function and regulation of blood sugar. He recommends 600 mg of lipoic acid daily.

- **Try digestive enzymes.** While these will not change your muscle tone, Dr. Bernstein states that many of his patients find that papaya enzymes have helped with symptoms of belching and bloating and help to keep blood sugar in control.

- **Take betaine HCl with pepsin.** Dr. Bernstein also recommends betaine HCl with pepsin to help more fully digest the food into chyme. The better the food is digested, the more easily it will pass through a narrow sphincter. *Caution: This should* not *be used in people who have ulcers, gastritis, or esophagitis.*

- **Eat pureed foods.** Pureed meats, fruits, and vegetables; soups; smoothies; baby food; protein drinks; yogurt; cottage cheese; ricotta cheese; and other foods that are primarily in a liquid form are more easily digested.

- **Try biofeedback and other mind-body techniques.** I found one study where 26 people with impaired gastric emptying were given a relaxation technique, called autonomic training, along with directed imagery. The authors concluded that this technique or biofeedback therapy might be useful. We do have good research indicating that mind-body therapies, imagery, and biofeedback are useful for other GI motility issues, such as IBS, so it may also work for gastroparesis.

CHAPTER 20

The Liver: Fatty Liver Disease, Hepatitis, and Cirrhosis Q DIGIN

The liver is the most complex organ in the body. Unlike the heart, which has one major function—to beat—the liver has a multitude of functions that include regulation of blood sugar levels, making 13,000 different enzymes, humanizing food by acting as a filter, breaking down toxins, manufacturing cholesterol and bile, breaking down hormones, and more. Because of its complexity and the 10,000 pounds of substances it must filter over a lifetime, the liver can easily become overwhelmed. Often the first sign of liver disease is two elevated liver enzymes, aspartate aminotransferase (AST) and alanine aminotransferase (ALT).

Jaundice, a yellowing of your skin, is a sign that something is wrong with your liver. Common liver conditions include hepatitis, cirrhosis, hemochromatosis, and, more rarely, cancer. Current research implicates dysbiosis as the driver of cardiometabolic conditions such as fatty liver disease, obesity, and insulin resistance. Dysbiosis favors microbes that increase the number of calories that are utilized, leading to increased fat accumulation in fat cells. In turn, this leads to fatty liver.

Love your liver by helping facilitate detoxification and by supporting your microbiome health. See Chapter 17 for information on detoxification programs.

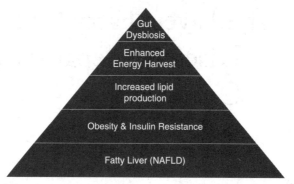

Figure 20.1 **Gut Dysbiosis leads to obesity, insulin resistance and fatty liver.**

FATTY LIVER DISEASE

Fatty liver disease is just as it sounds—your liver is accumulating fat. It's not an actual disease but can lead to cirrhosis and liver failure. It's also called nonalcoholic fatty liver disease (NAFLD) and differs from alcoholic fatty liver in one way: it's not caused by alcohol. It affects 20 percent of Americans. At this stage, it's completely reversible with changes in diet, exercise, and liver support. You probably will have *no* symptoms. If you do, you may be tired, have pain in your liver area (below your ribs to the right), or be losing weight for no reason. It's detected when your liver enzymes, ALT and AST, are elevated in a blood chemistry panel. It can also lead to, or be the result of, metabolic syndrome, which increases the risk of diabetes, obesity, and cardiovascular diseases.

A recent study conducted in San Diego found fatty liver disease in 13 percent of children who died from natural causes and were autopsied. The highest rates were in obese children: 38 percent had fatty liver. High-fructose corn syrup has been linked to fatty liver disease in several studies; however, there is some evidence that artificially sweetened soft drinks may contribute to fatty liver more than drinks sweetened with high-fructose corn syrup. Environmental toxins, junk food, and high-fat diets also contribute to fatty liver. A recent study of rats asked the question: Will pregnant moms who eat junk food predispose their children to obesity and fatty liver disease? The answer is yes. However, the study also showed that adopting a healthy diet can actually reverse fatty liver disease.

Healing Options
- **Balance your microbiome:** Implement the recommendations on balancing the microbiome given in Chapters 6 and 7.

- **Diet and lifestyle:** Changes in diet and lifestyle are the current medical recommendations for people with fatty liver. Lose weight if you are overweight. Exercise if you aren't exercising. Eat a whole-foods diet filled with fruits and vegetables. Avoid refined sugars and soft drinks. Stop drinking alcoholic beverages. Take an antioxidant supplement. Take milk thistle and lipoic acid supplements (see "Healing Options" in the "Hepatitis" section later in this chapter for dosages). Check your labs every 4 to 6 months. If your ALT and AST levels aren't responding, be more aggressive.
- **Try southern ginseng:** Gynostemma pentaphyllum is known as southern ginseng because it has similar therapeutic properties to ginseng and grows in southern China. A study that combined diet, exercise, and southern ginseng reported additional effects in weight loss, liver enzyme reduction, insulin levels, and HOMA levels. Take 500 mg three times daily.
- **Try keishi-bukuryo-gan:** There is a formula used in Japanese medicine called keishi-bukuryo-gan (KBG TJ-25). This was found to be of benefit when added to exercise, diet, and weight loss.

HEPATITIS

The eight types of hepatitis are A, B, C, D, E, autoimmune, alcoholic, and nonalcoholic steatohepatitis (NASH). Types A through E are caused by a blood-borne viral infection that causes inflammation in the liver. Autoimmune hepatitis, alcoholic hepatitis, and NASH are not caused by infection.

Hepatitis A
Hepatitis A can occur in isolated cases or spread among large groups of people. You can catch it from close personal contact with a person who has it or from food or water that has been contaminated. It is usually a self-limiting illness with flu-like symptoms. Once you've had hepatitis A, you cannot get it again. It may take several months to recover fully. A vaccine for people over the age of two is available for lifelong protection against hepatitis A.

Hepatitis B
Hepatitis B is the most common serious liver infection in the world and is more serious than hepatitis A. It can lead to cirrhosis, liver cancer, or liver failure. In most people, it is a self-limiting illness. However, 90 percent of infected babies, 30 to 50 percent of infected children, and 5 to 10 percent of infected adults will also develop

a chronic infection. A vaccine is available to help prevent hepatitis B infection. It is currently recommended by the Centers for Disease Control and Prevention (CDC) that all babies be vaccinated.

Each year, 100,000 Americans contract hepatitis B, and 5000 to 6000 Americans will die from it. It is estimated that 1.25 million Americans have chronic hepatitis B. Worldwide, it affects 400 million people, and there are 1 million deaths per year. It is passed directly through blood. Since 1992, blood collected for transfusions is carefully screened for hepatitis B (and C). Prior to that time, infection through blood transfusion was common.

You can get hepatitis B from having unprotected sex with someone who has it, by sharing needles for drug use or tattooing, or by an accidental needle poke with an infected needle. During childbirth, a mother can pass it to her child.

Hepatitis C

Hepatitis C accounts for about 15 percent of acute viral hepatitis, 60 to 70 percent of chronic hepatitis, and up to 50 percent of cirrhosis, end-stage liver disease, and liver cancer. In the United States, four million people, or 18 percent of our population, have been diagnosed with antibodies to the disease. This indicates that they currently have an infection or previously were exposed to the virus. There are 10,000 to 12,000 deaths each year because of hepatitis C. Seventy-five percent of people with acute hepatitis C will ultimately develop chronic hepatitis. Millions more of us may be infected but have not been diagnosed.

Many people with hepatitis C are asymptomatic and may not know they have the disease. In those who do have symptoms, they are generally mild and include fatigue, liver discomfort or tenderness, nausea, muscle and joint pains, and a poor appetite. Baby boomers, born between 1945 to 1965, are one of the largest groups who ought to be screened for hepatitis C.

The course of this disease varies radically. No symptoms might occur for up to 20 years and liver enzymes might not be elevated. If a liver biopsy is performed and the injury is mild, the outcome is usually good. On the other hand, if severe symptoms occur and liver enzymes are elevated, many people will ultimately develop cirrhosis and end-stage liver disease. The illness may be characterized by elevated liver enzymes with few symptoms, with an uncertain outcome. It is estimated that 20 percent of those with chronic hepatitis C will develop cirrhosis within 10 to 20 years. After that time, a small group will develop liver cancer. Hepatitis C is the most common reason for liver transplants.

Hepatitis C is passed via blood. The hepatitis C virus was only isolated in 1988, so many people were infected by blood transfusion prior to that time. Since 1992, blood has been routinely screened for hepatitis. You can get hepatitis C from having unprotected sex with someone who has it, by sharing needles for drug use or tattooing, or by an accidental needle poke with an infected needle. During childbirth, a mother could pass it to her child. In 10 percent of cases, the source of the infection is unknown.

Hepatitis C is now curable 95 percent of the time with several anti-viral medications that are on the market. If you suspect that you might have it, get screened for it and ask your doctor about treatments.

Hepatitis D

You can get hepatitis D only if you already have hepatitis B. It exists as a co-infection. You contract it the same way you contract hepatitis B and C.

Hepatitis E

Hepatitis E spreads by consuming contaminated drinking water and food. At this point in time, the only Americans who contract this form of hepatitis get it outside of the country, probably in a developing nation. For best prevention, drink bottled water when traveling, and use only ice made with bottled water. Don't eat raw shellfish, and avoid uncooked fruits and vegetables that are not peeled by you personally.

Autoimmune Hepatitis

Autoimmune hepatitis occurs when your body's immune system attacks your own liver cells, and it is probably due to a genetic defect. About 70 percent of people with this illness are women, and it's usually diagnosed between the ages of 15 and 40. It is a long-term illness and, if left untreated, can lead to cirrhosis and eventual liver failure. With treatment, about 70 percent of people with autoimmune hepatitis go into remission or experience a decrease in symptoms. It is usually treated with prednisone and azathioprine, both of which have unwanted side effects. About half of the people who are affected also have another autoimmune illness, such as Hashimoto's thyroiditis, Grave's disease, Sjögren's syndrome, ulcerative colitis, or autoimmune anemia. The most common symptoms are fatigue, enlarged liver, jaundice, itching, skin rashes, joint pain, lack of menstrual periods in women, and abdominal discomfort.

Alcoholic Hepatitis

Alcoholic hepatitis is a self-inflicted, progressive liver disease caused by the toxicity of alcohol. Unlike hepatitis A, B, C, and D, it is not an infectious disease. It is also known as alcoholic steatohepatitis, acute hepatic insufficiency of patients with chronic alcoholism, florid alcoholic cirrhosis, subacute alcoholic cirrhosis, and fatty liver with hepatic failure.

Alcoholic liver disease causes symptoms in more than two million people (1 percent of our population) but affects many more people who remain completely asymptomatic. It is the fourth leading cause of death in urban adult men ages 24 to 65. It is estimated that up to 35 percent of heavy drinkers have alcoholic hepatitis. This is often undetected until the disease has progressed. Women and nonwhite males are more susceptible to alcoholic liver damage with smaller amounts of alcoholic consumption. On average, it is estimated that men develop cirrhosis taking in about two ounces daily of ethanol, and women with less than one ounce daily. This is an illness that can kill you. Overall, the one-year survival rate after hospitalization for alcoholic hepatitis is about 40 percent.

Symptoms, when present, can include abdominal pain, fever, jaundice, and liver failure. It can progress to cirrhosis or liver cancer.

The long-term outcome depends on whether the person stops drinking alcohol and whether the illness has progressed to cirrhosis. If you have this and keep drinking alcohol, you will develop cirrhosis. If you stop drinking, it gradually resolves over a period of weeks to months. People may experience a worsening of liver function during the first weeks of abstinence. Because of alcohol excess, many people with alcoholic hepatitis are malnourished and deficient in antioxidant nutrients. They drink instead of eating. Use of acetaminophen (Tylenol) while drinking alcoholic beverages is well documented to accelerate liver disease. No one should drink booze and take acetaminophen (Tylenol).

N-acetyl cysteine (NAC), catechin (from green tea), and milk thistle (silymarin) have been shown to be helpful in recovery.

Nonalcoholic Steatohepatitis (NASH)

NASH is another noninfectious type of hepatitis. It also is called pseudoalcoholic hepatitis, diabetic hepatitis, fatty-liver hepatitis, and alcohol-like hepatitis. It causes few problems in most people who have it but can lead to cirrhosis. Children especially may experience vague discomfort located at the liver. It often goes unrecognized but is common in those with elevated liver enzymes who have no other diagnosis. In a recent study of children with NASH, nearly all were obese.

NASH was first discovered in 1980. Until recently, it was believed to be primarily a disease that affected obese, diabetic women. However, recent studies have shown that healthy, lean men, women, and children can all be affected. Inflammation of the liver, mitochondrial damage, and free radical pathology are apparent in this disease. Liver enzymes are elevated, and there is an increased need for antioxidant nutrients. Iron, on the other hand, is a pro-oxidant. It has been shown that high iron levels accelerate progression of NASH.

Ultimately, NASH is diagnosed with a liver biopsy. It is believed that a rich diet and lack of exercise can cause this illness. It can also be caused by drugs such as amiodarone, perhexiline maleate, glucocorticoids, synthetic estrogens, and tamoxifen. Surgeries, such as jejunal bypass, gastroplasty (stomach stapling), biliopancreatic diversion, or extensive small bowel resectioning can also trigger NASH. I even had one client who developed NASH from aggressive herbal treatment prescribed by a doctor. This resolved with clean food and some simple recommendations.

If you are trying to lose weight, be sure to do so gradually. Quick weight loss can aggravate the disease.

Diagnosis and Treatment of Hepatitis

Many people with hepatitis have no obvious symptoms, but when they do, the most common ones are fatigue, mild fever, headache, muscle aches, tiredness, loss of appetite, nausea, vomiting, and diarrhea. As the illness progresses, sufferers become jaundiced, which is evident by the yellow color of the skin and whites of the eyes. They may experience stomach pain and have dark-colored urine with pale-colored bowel movements.

Diagnosis of hepatitis is done with a routine blood test for liver enzymes. Further testing needs to be done to determine which type of hepatitis is present. A liver biopsy may be performed.

If you have been diagnosed with hepatitis C, there are now antiviral drugs that cure nearly everyone. Ask your physician to prescribe these for you. If you have other types of hepatitis, consider the recommendations given here. It is remarkable how many substances will help to lower a viral load.

It is well documented that people with hepatitis have an increased need for antioxidants. While much more research could be done in this area, taking antioxidants offers a simple and effective way to help protect liver function. It is advisable to take several antioxidant nutrients either in combination or separately. Antioxidants include vitamins C and E, selenium, N-acetyl cysteine, S-adenosylmethionine (SAMe), lipoic acid, and flavonoids; many herbs have antioxidant properties as well. In foods, they are found in fruits and vegetables, preferably fresh and organically grown.

Bert Berkson, MD, is an expert on lipoic acid. He reports that a combination of lipoic acid, selenium, and milk thistle rapidly dropped viral levels and brought viral and lab values down in three of his patients with hepatitis C who had serious complications due to the infection. All three were able to avoid liver transplants as a result of this inexpensive antioxidant therapy. Dosages were 300 mg of lipoic acid twice daily, 300 mg of milk thistle three times daily, and 200 mcg of selenomethionine once daily. In a 1976 German study, 42 patients with hepatitis were given intravenous (IV) lipoic acid. The treatment showed promise for many of the patients and, because of the low toxicity and lack of side effects, was recommended for long-term treatment.

Rest, sleep, and healthful eating help with an easy recovery. It's also critically important not to drink any alcohol because alcohol is a direct liver toxin.

If you are planning to travel outside of North America, check to see if you are going to a country with known hepatitis problems. You may want to get vaccinated against hepatitis A and B before you go.

There are a huge number of nutrients, antioxidants, herbs, flavonoids, and phytonutrients that may be beneficial in helping reduce symptoms and the long-term effects of hepatitis and cirrhosis. Supplements and herbal products that have been found to be beneficial in people with liver disease include: B-complex vitamins, phyllanthus, shiitake mushrooms, astragalus, fenugreek, schizandra, andrographis, phosphatidylcholine, thymus extract, chlorophyll, and many more natural compounds. I could have spent weeks researching this one topic because there are so many agents that help lower viral loads and the symptoms of hepatitis.

Functional Laboratory Testing

Routine medical testing is adequate for diagnosis of hepatitis. People who are infected may also want additional information. Tests to consider include the following:

- Vitamin and mineral status
- Antioxidant status
- Glutathione levels
- Small intestinal bacterial overgrowth testing

Healing Options

Hepatitis is a serious illness. For best results, these healing options are meant to be used in combination. You don't need to use them all, but pick several at least.

- **Avoid alcoholic beverages.** Alcohol is damaging to the liver. Don't drink if you have any type of hepatitis.
- **Eat lots of fruits and vegetables.** They contain antioxidant nutrients, vitamins, and minerals that help support your immune system. Eat at least five servings daily, preferably a lot more. Fresh juicing of organic vegetables is a great way to quickly multiply your nutrients and antioxidants.
- **Take a multivitamin with minerals.** Cover your bases. A good multivitamin will have base amounts of antioxidants, vitamins, and minerals. Look for one

with at least 400 IU of vitamin E, 200 mcg of selenium, and 250 mg or more of vitamin C.

- **Balance the microbiome with food and probiotics.** See previous chapters for more information.
- **Take vitamin C.** Studies have shown vitamin C levels to be very low in people with hepatitis. Vitamin C is well known for its antiviral and antioxidant effects. Much research was also done in the 1970s and early 1980s on vitamin C's ability to naturally stimulate interferon production. Interferon is the drug treatment of choice for people with chronic hepatitis (hepatitis C). Interferon is isolated at great expense, it is only 30 percent effective, and the side effects make many people decide not to even try it. Linus Pauling theorized that vitamin C could be used to increase natural production of interferon. Other researchers also reported that this was so.

    Robert Cathcart, MD, a long-standing advocate of complementary medicine, uses high doses of IV vitamin C for hepatitis. He found that with doses of 40 to 100 grams, he was able to greatly improve symptoms in two to four days and clear jaundice within six days. Other people have found similar effects. Taking as little as 2 grams prevented hepatitis B in hospitalized patients. However, there is little published research specifically on vitamin C and hepatitis.

    At a minimum, take 2,000 mg of vitamin C daily. Preferably, use dosages up to bowel tolerance and recalibrate your dosage every week. Determine your personalized dosage with a vitamin C flush. (See Chapter 17.)
- **Try milk thistle or *Silybum marianum* (silymarin).** Milk thistle has been used for liver protection for centuries and has few side effects. We have excellent animal data on milk thistle and hepatitis but less in people. Silymarin, the most studied active component in milk thistle, has anti-inflammatory effects, protects the liver from fibrosis, scavenges for free radicals, upregulates bile flow, and has many more actions. When used along with antiviral drugs, silymarin has a beneficial effect. At this time, it is not recommended to use milk thistle alone for the treatment of hepatitis. It does not appear to be more effective than placebo for lowering liver enzyme levels. Look for a product that has been standardized for silymarin content. A company that has done that will clearly label it on the bottle. Take 420 mg daily.
- **Take zinc.** People with hepatitis are commonly zinc deficient. Zinc helps with healing of tissues and is important for prevention of scarring. Take 50 to 75 mg daily.
- **Try whey protein or transfer factor.** There are numerous studies on the use of transfer factor in people with hepatitis. They have been very positive. Transfer factor is isolated from cow colostrum and is loaded with protective antibodies

that help us fight infection. A current study also demonstrates that a whey protein product called Immunocal was effective in patients with hepatitis B, but not hepatitis C. Take 12 to 30 grams of whey protein daily and 300 mg transfer factor, once or twice daily.

- **Try NAC.** Several research studies have found that glutathione levels are inversely related to the viral loads for hepatitis B and C. German researchers found that when NAC was added to hepatitis cultures, viral load decreased 50-fold. Take 1,000 to 2,000 mcg twice daily.

- **Try lipoic acid.** Lipoic acid, also called thioctic acid, is a strong antioxidant and has been shown to protect the liver in mushroom and chemical poisoning. In studies with chemically induced hepatitis, lipoic acid has been shown to be effective in treatment. Take 200 to 300 mg twice daily.

- **Try SAMe.** In one study, 220 patients with liver disease were given 1,600 mg of SAMe daily. Twenty-six percent of the participants had hepatitis. The study found the use of SAMe resulted in a reduction of symptoms of itching and fatigue and an improved sense of well-being. Laboratory testing confirmed these benefits with improvement of conjugated bilirubin and alkaline phosphatase, two laboratory markers that are elevated in people with hepatitis.

- **Take vitamin E.** People with hepatitis have lower levels of vitamin E. A 2001 pilot study published in *Antiviral Research* investigated people with hepatitis B. In the study, 32 patients were given either 300 IU of vitamin E twice daily for three months or no treatment. They were followed for one year. In the vitamin E group, 47 percent (seven patients) had normalized ALT, a liver enzyme. Only one of the controls normalized ALT. Hepatitis B DNA was normalized in 53 percent of the vitamin E group and in only 18 percent of the control group. A normalization of both ALT and DNA was seen in 47 percent of the vitamin E group and none of the control group.

In another study, people with hepatitis B were given 600 IU of vitamin E daily for nine months. All symptoms of hepatitis disappeared in 5 of the 12 people tested.

In yet another study, looking this time at people with hepatitis C, there was some additional improvement when people were given 544 IU of vitamin E with interferon therapy. And in a different study, in which people with hepatitis C were given 400 IU of vitamin E twice daily for 12 weeks, there was improvement in 11 out of 23 patients (48 percent). ALT levels were decreased by 45 percent, and AST, a liver enzyme, decreased 37 percent after a six-month follow-up. Vitamin E is nontoxic and worth trying in all types of hepatitis. Take 600 to 1,000 IU of vitamin E daily. Look for d-alpha-tocopherol and mixed tocopherols, rather than dl-alphatocopherol.

- **Try *Picrorhiza kurroa*.** Picrorhiza, an herb commonly used in Ayurvedic medicine, has been less well studied than milk thistle, but studies indicate that it is equally effective with nearly identical effects. It has anti-inflammatory and liver-protective properties. Indian researchers also used *Picrorhiza* in acute hepatitis A and it proved to be helpful in a speedy recovery. Take 400 to 1,500 mg in capsules.
- **Try licorice.** Licorice has been shown to reduce elevated liver enzymes in people with hepatitis. It appears to be the glycyrrhizin that tempers NF-kappaB and inflammatory cytokines. It also naturally raises the body's interferon levels. In Japan, it is often used intravenously for hepatitis B and C. Glycyrrhizin can elevate blood pressure levels, so use with caution.
- **Try sho-saiko-to.** Sho-saiko-to is a Chinese remedy that contains bupleurum and other traditional Chinese herbs. Several trials were done in people with hepatitis B infection and one small trial in people with hepatitis C. Sho-saiko-to helps reduce symptoms and normalize blood liver enzymes in people with active viral hepatitis. It has also been found to help reduce the incidence of liver cancer in people with hepatitis. Take 2.5 grams three times daily. *It should not be used in combination with interferon therapy.*
- **Drink Rooibos tea (*Aspalathus linearis*).** Rooibos tea is also called red tea. It is a relatively new food product and offers a delicious, caffeine-free alternative to people who drink tea. Research was done in rats, and I was delighted to see that, at least in this initial report, it showed a regression of liver damage and cirrhosis and a lowering of liver enzymes (ALT and AST). The researchers consider it to be a useful plant for patients with liver disease. Other studies show it to have antioxidant effects. It appears to have the same properties as green tea. I recommend that you drink it as often as you like.
- **Try quercetin with amla.** Another flavonoid with antioxidant effects is quercetin. Although studies need to be done in people, animal research shows that treatment with quercetin dehydrate reduced oxidative damage from hepatitis twofold. Another mouse study found liver-protective effects of quercetin when combined with amla. *Bougainvillea spectabilis* has been used in Chinese folk medicine for treatment of hepatitis. The active component of *Bougainvillea* is quercetin. Take 1,000 to 3,000 mg of quercetin daily, plus 900 to 2,700 mg of amla daily.

CIRRHOSIS

Cirrhosis is an advanced disease of the liver. Scar tissue replaces normal tissue and blocks the flow of blood and nutrients. It kills about 26,000 Americans each year and is the 12th leading cause of death. The most common causes of cirrhosis are alcoholism and hepatitis. Some people have diseases that may lead to cirrhosis, such as alpha-1 antitrypsin deficiency, hemochromatosis, Wilson's disease, galactosemia, and glycogen storage diseases. NASH can also lead to cirrhosis. NASH is a condition where fat accumulates in the liver and eventually causes scarring. It is usually associated with diabetes, protein malnutrition, obesity, heart disease, and treatment with steroid medications. Blocked bile ducts can also cause cirrhosis, called *biliary cirrhosis*. Because the liver is our body's main filtering system for drugs and toxins, bad reactions to them may also lead to cirrhosis. Overdosing with vitamin A supplements is another cause of cirrhosis. Vitamin A toxicity in the liver is accentuated in an alcoholic.

About one-third of people with cirrhosis have no symptoms during the initial stages of the disease. Loss of liver function may be picked up on routine blood testing. As the scarring progresses, liver function begins to fail. People with cirrhosis may experience some of the following symptoms: exhaustion and fatigue, loss of appetite, nausea, light-colored stools, weakness, weight loss, abdominal pain, or spiderlike blood vessels that break out on the skin. Cirrhosis may also lead to water retention, bruising and bleeding, jaundice, itching, gallstones, increased sensitivity to medication and environmental contaminants, increased insulin resistance, diabetes, liver cancer, osteoporosis, impotence, and infection in other organs.

The scarring caused by cirrhosis cannot be reversed, but treatment can help stop or slow the disease progression. The liver is remarkably able to recuperate when we eliminate the factors that hurt it. Many find that with a nutritious diet, rest, and supplements, they can begin to feel healthy again. It is critical that you stop drinking all alcoholic beverages if you are diagnosed with cirrhosis. Alcohol is known to cause cirrhosis, liver cancer, and liver failure and generates a large need for antioxidant nutrients, such as vitamin E, selenium, vitamin C, and N-acetyl cysteine. Alcoholics are notoriously deficient in B-complex vitamins.

If possible, stop using hazardous chemicals. If you do need to use them, protect your skin, be in a well-ventilated area, and wear a breathing apparatus. If your work involves the use of paint, solvents, cleaning products, or other chemicals, it's probably time to look for a different job. Use greener cleaning supplies, shampoos, and other toiletries. Long ago, I worked with a man who had cirrhosis that was due to his job in an auto body shop, where he spray-painted cars.

Research indicates that many people with cirrhosis have increased intestinal permeability, which can lead to infection and problems elsewhere in the body. Nutrients such as glutamine, quercetin, and probiotics can help heal a leaky gut.

Methionine, an amino acid, from our food is metabolized in the liver into SAMe. People with cirrhosis have problems metabolizing methionine. SAMe increases glutathione levels, a vital antioxidant for detoxification. SAMe is an important methyl donor and is used as a supplement for people with elevated homocysteine levels, heart disease, joint diseases, and depression.

Functional Laboratory Testing

- Functional liver testing
- Intestinal permeability testing
- Vitamin and mineral analysis

Healing Options

- **Avoid alcoholic beverages.** Alcohol is damaging to the liver. Don't drink at all if you have hepatitis or cirrhosis. If you are an alcoholic, you might find Alcoholics Anonymous or a residential program to be of benefit. Support helps ease the way.
- **Eat lots of fruits and vegetables.** They contain antioxidant nutrients, vitamins, and minerals that help support your immune system. Eat at least five servings daily, preferably a lot more. Fresh juicing of organic vegetables is a great way to quickly multiply your nutrients and antioxidants.
- **Stay nourished and get enough protein:** Your body needs nutrients to heal and reduce inflammation. The current recommendation is that people with cirrhosis get 1 gram of protein daily for each kilogram of body weight. So, for a 150-pound person, that would be about 68 grams of protein daily. Using a protein powder and adding branched amino acids may be useful.
- **Take a multivitamin with minerals.** Cover your bases. A good multivitamin will have base amounts of antioxidants, vitamins, and minerals. Look for one with at least 400 IU of vitamin E, 200 mcg of selenium, at least 250 mg of vitamin C, and at least 15 mg of zinc.
- **Take an antioxidant supplement.** In addition to a good multivitamin with minerals, it would be wise to take additional antioxidants. These can be found in a combination supplement and may include mixed carotenoids, selenium, vitamin E, vitamin C, N-acetyl cysteine, lipoic acid, and more. Or you could use what are known as powdered greens or reds. These products typically contain dehydrated green vegetables and grasses or red and orange fruits and vegetables. It's a quick way to get a ton of antioxidants and vegetables in one swoop.
- **Try lipoic acid.** Lipoic acid is a strong antioxidant and has been shown to protect the liver in mushroom and chemical poisoning. In studies with chemically induced hepatitis, lipoic acid has been shown to be effective in treatment. Take 200 to 300 mg twice daily.

- **Try SAMe.** In one study, 220 patients with liver disease were given 1,600 mg of SAMe daily. A total of 68 percent had cirrhosis, 6 percent had biliary cirrhosis, and 26 percent had hepatitis. A reduction of symptoms of itching and fatigue were noted, along with an improved sense of well-being.

- **Try sho-saiko-to.** Sho-saiko-to, also called TJ-9, is a Chinese remedy that contains bupleurum and six other herbs. It is being extensively used in Japan for people with hepatitis and cirrhosis and to prevent the development of liver cancer. Take 2.5 grams three times daily. *It should not be used in combination with interferon therapy.*

- **Try milk thistle or *S. marianum* (silymarin).** Milk thistle has long been used for all liver disease. It appears to retard progression of cirrhosis, primarily through its antioxidant effects. Animal research has been consistent in its results; human research has been less so. Still, there is little or no risk and the possibility of great benefit. Take 420 mg daily. Look for a product that has been standardized for silymarin content. A company that has done that will clearly label it on the bottle.

- **Take zinc.** People with cirrhosis often have a zinc deficiency. Get your red blood cell zinc level checked. If it's low, take 50 to 75 mg of zinc daily.

- **Drink Rooibos tea (*A. linearis*).** Rooibos tea is also called red tea and is a relatively new food product. It offers a delicious caffeine-free alternative for tea drinkers. Research was done in rats, and I was delighted to see that, at least in this initial report, it showed a regression of liver damage and cirrhosis and a lowering of liver enzymes (ALT and AST). The researchers consider it to be a useful plant for patients with liver disease. It contains small amounts of vitamin C, iron, magnesium, phosphorus, sodium, chloride, and potassium. Other studies show it to have antioxidant effects. For dosage, I recommend that you drink as much as you like.

- **Take probiotics:** Probiotics are of benefit in people with cirrhosis and may even be of benefit in improving liver function in people who are stable.

- **Take L-carnitine:** Check serum carnitine levels to see if carnitine supplementation is needed, or just try using it empirically. Many people with cirrhosis have low carnitine levels. Supplementation with carnitine can be helpful in lowering ammonia levels and reducing muscle cramps. Dosage: 3 grams daily.

CHAPTER 21

The Pancreas: Pancreatic Insufficiency, Pancreatitis, and Diabetes ⌕ D I G I N

The pancreas has two main functions in the body. The first is digestive (exocrine function): to produce digestive enzymes to break down fat, carbohydrate, and protein; and bicarbonate to neutralize stomach acid once the food moves from the stomach to the duodenum. The second function of the pancreas (endocrine function) is production of insulin and glucagon to regulate blood sugar levels. Insulin tells your body to store glucose as glycogen; glucagon tells your body to raise blood glucose levels, turning glycogen back into glucose.

The main health problems with the pancreas are insufficiency of enzymes, acute or chronic pancreatitis, pancreatic cancer, diabetes, and cystic fibrosis. In type 1 diabetes, the pancreas is no longer able to produce insulin. Many people with type 2 diabetes have insulin resistance, which can overwhelm the pancreas so that it stops producing enough insulin. Some of the medications used in type 2 diabetes can also affect the beta cells so that they stop producing insulin.

If you have pancreatitis, you will have elevated serum lipase and amylase levels. To assess pancreatic insufficiency, stool testing for pancreatic elastase or chymotrypsin is used. You will often have levels of pancreatic elastase that are less than 400 mcg/g, which indicates pancreatic insufficiency. If pancreatic elastase levels are less than 200, pancreatic insufficiency may be a lifelong issue. For chymotrypsin, the lowest normal value is 100 or 72 mcg, depending on the study. Low chymotrypsin levels were found in people with celiac disease, psoriasis, and gastric surgery. Pancreatic elastase is not affected when you take digestive enzymes; chymotrypsin is.

PANCREATIC INSUFFICIENCY

If your pancreas cannot secrete enough enzymes, you have pancreatic insufficiency. While in conventional medical terms, pancreatic insufficiency is rare, those of us working in integrative health see it all the time. How would you diagnose it?

- Abdominal discomfort
- Bleeding tendency (vitamin K deficiency)
- Bloating
- Inability to gain weight
- Failure to thrive in children
- Fatigue for no obvious reason
- Food sensitivities
- Gas
- Hypoglycemia
- Malabsorption
- Steatorrhea—pale, tan colored stools
- Stools that float (fat maldigestion)
- Undigested food in your stools

Pancreatic insufficiency is common in people who have celiac disease, psoriasis, cirrhosis, pancreatitis, and cystic fibrosis. Other triggers are parasites, bacterial overgrowth, dermatitis herpetiformis, inflammatory bowel disease (IBD), Zollinger-Ellison syndrome, and AIDS. Stress (mental and physical), getting older, nutritional deficiencies, poor diet, eating only cooked foods, exposure to radiation or toxins, hereditary weaknesses, drugs, and infections also contribute to pancreatic insufficiency.

Functional Laboratory Testing
- Stool pancreatic elastase test
- Stool chymotrypsin test
- 72-hour fecal fat test. This is done by a gastroenterologist
- Food allergies—IgE test; food sensitivities—IgG or IgG4 test

Healing Options
- **Improve your eating habits.** Eat in a relaxed manner. Chew your food thoroughly. Limit beverage intake with meals. Drinking liquids at meals dilutes the gastric juices in the stomach and pancreatic juice in the small intestines.

- **Take pancreatic enzyme supplements.** Clinical experience shows that pancreatic enzymes work well as a digestive aid. Glandular-based supplements, like pancreatic enzyme preparations, are directed to specific tissues, helping to initiate repair. Pancreatic enzymes also help restore the balance of gastrointestinal (GI) flora. In studies done on monkeys, it was shown that pancreatic enzymes were able to kill *Clostridium*, bacteroides, *Pseudomonaceae, Enterobacter, Escherichia coli*, and *Klebsiella*. Continued use of pancreatic enzymes can help with repair and maintenance of pancreatic tissue.

    The United States Pharmacopoeia (USP) regulates the strength of pancreatic enzymes. Take one to two tablets or capsules at the beginning of meals.
- **Try vegetable enzymes.** For people who would rather have a vegetarian alternative to pancreatic enzymes, vegetable enzymes are a suitable option. These enzymes are derived from a fungus called *Aspergillus oryzae*. Take one to two capsules at the beginning of meals.

PANCREATITIS

Pancreatitis is an inflammation of the pancreas. There are two types of pancreatitis, acute and chronic. Acute pancreatitis is typically caused by gallbladder disease or alcohol abuse. The typical symptoms are abdominal pain, nausea, vomiting, and loss of appetite. Serum amylase and lipase levels are elevated. In acute pancreatitis, it's important to keep electrolytes in balance. People are hospitalized and given intravenous (IV) solutions or medical foods until the inflammation has calmed down.

Chronic pancreatitis is an ongoing inflammation of the pancreas. In 70 percent of people, it's alcohol induced, while 7 percent of people with pancreatitis have genetic alterations in either the cystic fibrosis gene (CFTR), the serine protease inhibitor gene (SPINK 1/PSTI), or the cationic trypsinogen gene (PRSSI). If it's inherited, it often begins in childhood or adolescence with acute pancreatitis, which eventually becomes chronic. Other causes include tropical pancreatitis (due to unknown nutritional issues), hyperparathyroidism with high calcium levels, extremely high levels of triglycerides, and obstruction of the pancreatic duct.

The main symptom of chronic pancreatitis is a dull pain around the stomach with pain that radiates to the middle of your back. The pain is intermittent and gets worse if you eat. People with pancreatitis gradually lose weight. If the pancreas isn't producing enough lipase, stools will get lighter, float, and have a bad odor. You may need to urinate often and have symptoms of vitamin A, D, E, and K deficiencies. Sometimes people get jaundiced.

It's important to consider the entire DIGIN model in people who have chronic pancreatitis. It's also important to check micronutrient levels; people with pancreatitis may be low in many minerals and vitamins, including magnesium, calcium, zinc, and iron. One paper reported that nearly half of people with pancreatitis had hypochlorhydria, so testing for that could be useful.

Healing Options

- **Stop drinking alcohol.** Easier said than done, but essential. If necessary, join Alcoholics Anonymous or enter treatment.
- **Use a restorative healing diet.** See Chapter 15 for details.
- **Use medical foods.** In some cases, eating predigested foods can provide calories and needed nutrients.
- **Take pancreatic enzymes.** There are many prescription and over-the-counter pancreas enzymes. According to Maurice E. Shils, et al., in *Modern Nutrition in Health and Disease, 10th Edition*, from 4,500 to 20,000 USP will be needed with a minimum of 28,000 IU of lipase. Take one tablet with the first bite of your meal and continue sprinkling your tablets throughout the meal.
- **Take vitamins.** You are likely to be deficient in many nutrients, especially vitamin B_{12} and the fat-soluble vitamins A, D, E, and K. Take an excellent multiple vitamin and have your vitamin and mineral levels assessed.
- **Increase antioxidants to reduce inflammation.** Eat more fruits and vegetables. Make fresh vegetable and green juices. Use wheat grass juice. Use powdered greens or powdered reds, which typically contain dehydrated green vegetables and grasses or red and orange fruits and vegetables, to add antioxidants. Take antioxidant supplements.
- **Try Chinese medicine and acupuncture.** Several studies looked at the combined effect of Chinese herbs with Western treatment for pancreatitis. Patients who received traditional Chinese medicines had better outcomes. Miltiorrhiza, known as red sage, Chinese sage, tan shen, or dan shen, was given to rats and people with pancreatitis, with protective effects. There are lots of other studies coming out of China on pancreatitis and herbs. I recommend finding a doctor of oriental medicine to help you with this.

DIABETES

Diabetes is a worldwide epidemic that's increasing fast. In 1985, 30 million people worldwide had diabetes. Today, one billion people have diabetes, and a third of the children born each day are expected to have diabetes later in life. In the United

States, according to the American Diabetes Association, 30.3 million Americans (9.4 percent) have diabetes. Diabetes is found in 25.2 percent of people over the age of 65. Diabetes rates are highest in Native American populations, where 45 percent of children and 17 percent of the overall population have it. Blacks, Hispanics, and Asians are also more likely to develop diabetes than whites. Most people with diabetes have never been diagnosed. If you've never had your blood sugar levels looked at, do so.

Diabetes Basics

You may recall that glucose is the main energy source for most of our cells; when blood glucose levels rise, the pancreas normally secretes the hormone insulin, which acts as a transporter, allowing glucose and amino acids to leave the bloodstream and be taken into the cell. This process, however, can go awry. Diabetes occurs when the body.

- Doesn't produce insulin,
- Makes insufficient amounts of insulin, or
- Is resistant to insulin.

Diabetes is a common chronic illness that runs in families, so children with parents or grandparents who have diabetes are more likely to develop diabetes than other children are.

Symptoms of Diabetes

- Blurred vision
- Darkened and velvety areas of skin, most typically in the armpits and neck folds
- Fatigue
- Frequent infections
- Frequent urination
- Increased appetite
- Increased thirst
- Irritability (in children mainly)
- Skin tags
- Slow healing of sores
- Weight loss

Monitoring Diabetes

If you have diabetes, a hemoglobin A1c (HmgA1c; also called glycosylated hemoglobin) test is a simple way to monitor your blood sugar levels. It gives a three-month average of the sugar levels on the outside of red blood cells. Imagine a gum drop. Recall that it has sugar crystals on the outside of it. Imagine that your red blood cells look like gum drops. The more sugar crystals they have on the outside, the more damaging those crystals are inside a person's blood vessels, heart, eyes, and kidneys and the greater risk of long-term health issues relating to the diabetes. Healthy levels of HmgA1c are less than 7 percent of total hemoglobin. Keeping levels as low as possible helps prevent damage throughout the body.

Uncontrolled diabetes of either type can lead to serious complications later in life. High blood glucose level is the most significant risk factor for developing heart and vascular disease, and diabetes is the leading cause of kidney failure and adult blindness. Careful blood sugar control is essential for preventing these and other complications, including nerve problems and gum disease.

Type 1 Diabetes

Type 1 diabetes is considered to be an autoimmune disorder. It is typically diagnosed in children and young adults. Statistics show that 5 to 10 percent of people with diabetes have type 1 diabetes. Type 1 diabetes, which used to be called juvenile diabetes, is more specifically termed insulin-dependent diabetes mellitus (IDDM). Diagnosed in about 13,000 children in the United States each year, its onset is usually sudden and can occur at any time during childhood. People with type 1 diabetes require injections to replace the insulin that their bodies can no longer make. Children with type 1 diabetes are usually thin, and they may complain of thirst. Type 1 diabetes is often triggered by an infection, typically a virus. The body's immune system mounts an attack on the infection and also mistakenly attacks and destroys the insulin-secreting beta cells in the pancreas. Allergy to milk has also been implicated as a possible trigger for diabetes.

New Ideas About Underlying Causes of Type 1 Diabetes. Accumulating research findings suggest that the gut immune system plays an important role in type 1 diabetes. Like all autoimmune diseases, there is a growing consensus in research indicating that people with type 1 diabetes have increased intestinal permeability (leaky gut) and dairy allergy, gluten intolerance, or celiac disease. Alessio Fasano, MD, medical director at the Center for Celiac Research at University of Maryland School of Medicine, and his research group believe that intestinal permeability is a necessary ingredient for the development of autoimmune conditions, along with genetic and environmental factors. Outi Vaarala and her group report that a disordered gut microbiota contributes to the development of type 1 diabetes. High levels of zonulin have been found in people with type 1 diabetes. Zonulin is a protein that contributes to leaky gut by opening up the tight junctions between cells. Zonulin levels can increase on exposure to specific foods and bacteria. Animal studies show that if zonulin is blocked, destruction of the pancreatic beta cells can be prevented.

There is a small but important crossover in people with type 1 diabetes and celiac disease. Kaur, in a 2018 paper published in *Digestive Disease*, reports that 8 percent of people with type 1 diabetes have celiac disease, and that this "is a gross underestimation" in people with silent celiac disease. A study of 141 children with type 1 diabetes, for example, found elevated antigliadin antibodies in more than 8 percent and found celiac disease in almost 3 percent, which is 10 times the average incidence. Another study of 331 children with type 1 diabetes from 1987 through 2004 reported 6.6 percent of the children had celiac disease as well (determined by elevated tTg levels and confirmed with biopsy). Interestingly, the incidence of celiac in these children rose from 3.3 percent in 1994 to 10.6 percent in 2004. One has to ask the question: What specifically has changed in this decade?

Children with type 1 diabetes have higher incidences of allergic conditions: rhinitis, asthma, and eczema. Getting screened for allergies and avoidance could help calm the immune system. A considerable amount of research has shown a link between infant allergy to cow's milk and development of type 1 diabetes. Initially, it appeared that the link was strong; yet the association weakened as more research was conducted. Still, testing for milk-protein allergy and lactose intolerance can be useful. In a similar vein, an epidemiological study in 40 countries found that the incidence of type 1 diabetes in children was highest in the countries with the highest consumption of dairy and other animal foods. In children who develop both celiac disease and type 1 diabetes, celiac disease often precedes or develops at the same time as the diabetes. (See sections on celiac disease and autoimmune disease in Chapters 23 and 26, respectively, for a more complete analysis of the gut-autoimmune connection.)

Children eating a mainly vegetarian diet had a lowered incidence of type 2 diabetes. This needs to be explored more fully to determine what components of a vegetarian diet helped to protect these children. What can be supposed is that vegetarian diets have a higher level of polyphenols and fiber, which both have protective properties.

Food Sensitivity and Diabetes. Looking for food sensitivities and allergies may help stabilize blood sugar levels and reduce the need for medications in people with type 1 diabetes. A study done by Russell M. Jaffe, MD, PhD, and colleagues looked at the role of diet and food intolerance in 26 adults with type 1 diabetes. The control group ate their regular diabetic diet and followed their usual lifestyle program. The test group ate a dairy-free diet, removed any additional foods that showed antibody reactions, and were given specific nutritional supplements. After six months, the test group showed significantly greater improvement in blood glucose levels and hemoglobin A1c than the control group. Clinical nutritionist Jayashree Mani reports that by working with an allergen-free and alkalizing diet, she was able to lower blood glucose levels in a type 1 diabetic teenage boy from 350 to 125 mmol/l, while also reducing his insulin needs by more than a third.

In my practice, I've counseled people to use glucose monitoring 30 to 60 minutes after a meal to determine specific foods and/or meals that spike or drop their glucose levels. It helps people to discover food reactions to optimize what they eat.

Type 2 Diabetes
Type 2 diabetes, which used to be called adult diabetes, is more specifically termed non-insulin-dependent diabetes mellitus (NIDDM). Type 2 diabetes occurs mainly in adults over the age of 45 and constitutes 90 to 95 percent of all diabetes cases. Type 2 diabetes was virtually unknown in children 30 years ago, but it is on the rise. In some Native American communities, it occurs in 45 percent of children. In children, it is first diagnosed between the ages of 10 and 19 years, and the hormonal changes around puberty seem to be an important trigger. Between 45 percent and 80 percent of children with type 2 diabetes have a parent with diabetes. Children with type 2 diabetes are commonly overweight but typically have no other symptoms until they are diagnosed.

Type 2 Diabetes Is Largely Preventable. Type 2 diabetes at first appears to be a disorder of overly elevated blood glucose (blood sugar) levels. Yet for most people with type 2 diabetes, disordered glucose levels are just the end of a long road that led to diabetes in the first place. Type 2 diabetes is often the result of lifestyle choices. In other words, we "earn" it. It's often termed "a feast in the middle of a famine" because your blood has excessive amounts of glucose (the feast) while your cells starve for the sugar they desperately need to produce energy. If left unchecked, high insulin levels affect our kidneys, eyes, and heart and are linked to fatty liver, nerve damage, brain compromise, gastroparesis or dumping syndrome, maldigestion and malabsorption, sexual dysfunction, and problems with the genitourinary system, such as polycystic ovary disease.

Eating a low-nutrient, highly refined diet; eating a diet low in antioxidants and polyphenols and fiber; obesity; lack of exercise; and lack of sleep all help us build to a point where our metabolism begins showing signs of metabolic syndrome: weight gain around the middle (apple shape or beer belly), low serum high-density lipoprotein (HDL) cholesterol levels with high low-density lipoprotein (LDL) cholesterol levels, high insulin levels, rising blood pressure, and/or rising triglycerides. In metabolic syndrome, also called Syndrome X, we don't have the right cellular conditions to properly use glucose. Our pancreas responds by making more insulin to get the glucose into the cells. This is called insulin resistance, which leads to more weight gain and even more insulin resistance, in a vicious circle. Eventually we cannot overcome this by just producing more insulin, and our blood sugar levels skyrocket. This condition is diabetes. Often we have decades of warning signs before we are diagnosed with diabetes. We can stop metabolic syndrome by changing our lives, and in most cases we can prevent diabetes.

Eating a low-glycemic diet, getting plenty of exercise, and having the right nutrients can turn type 2 diabetes and metabolic syndrome around.

Gestational Diabetes

A third type of diabetes is called gestational diabetes. It occurs only during pregnancy and typically resolves once the baby is born. This affects about 4 percent of all pregnant women. It's important that these women be closely monitored during pregnancy for the safety of the mom and baby. Babies born of women who developed gestational diabetes are more likely to develop type 2 diabetes later in life.

Other Types of Diabetes

There are three other types of diabetes that have been more recently codified.

- Latent autoimmune diabetes of the adult (LADA) happens in people who are not obese but have antibodies to insulin. They typically have signs of metabolic syndrome, so if monitored they can prevent diabetes decades earlier.
- People with type 1.5 diabetes have anti-insulin antibodies and are typically obese and insulin resistant.
- Some people who have Alzheimer's disease have insulin dysregulation in their brain; this is called type 3 diabetes. Type 3 diabetes occurs when people have insulin resistance in the brain. Insulin is probably the most inflammatory molecule in our bodies. When insulin levels increase in the brain, we have accelerated oxidative stress, nerve damage, cell damage, and early death. This can cause memory loss as well.

Functional Laboratory Testing

- Certainly do all of the regular medical testing for diabetes, including fasting glucose and hemoglobin A1c levels.

- Blood sugar levels: Buy a glucose monitor and monitor your blood sugars daily or more often. There are excellent apps that connect your glucose monitor now.
- One- and two-hour postprandial insulin testing: This is done 1 to 2 hours after a high-carbohydrate meal or with a glucose drink.
- Anti-insulin antibodies test.
- Salivary cortisol: Cortisol levels are often high in diabetes.
- Vitamin and mineral assessments, especially B-complex vitamins, red blood cell (RBC) zinc, magnesium, and antioxidant status.
- Food sensitivity testing.
- Celiac testing.

Healing Options for All Types of Diabetes

If you are taking medication for your diabetes, it is critical to use it *consistently and exactly as prescribed*. If you need an insulin pump, you'll need specific instructions on its use from your physician or diabetes educator. There are also apps that hook up to your cell phone to monitor glucose levels continuously. They measure glucose levels through the skin, so they do not require drops of blood. These are often replacing the use of insulin pumps.

Historically, people worldwide have used various natural remedies to control blood sugar levels: glucomannan fiber, young barley shoots, prickly pear cactus juice, fenugreek—the list is long. As we integrate this sort of information, many more options may become available. You can find many of the herbs and nutrients in the following list in products that combine them to help with glucose regulation.

- **Buy a glucose monitor or use a glucose-monitoring app with your phone.** Monitoring your glucose levels is essential. By monitoring glucose after meals, you can to determine which foods and meals keep your glucose levels in an optimal range, and which foods and meals spike it. These will be specific to you. I had a client with Type I diabetes. Every time she ate just a bit of papaya or white rice, her blood sugars went soaring. Her body reacted to even tiny amounts of these specific foods. A glucometer is an easy way to determine your best diet. Keeping your glucose levels normalized and having a hemoglobin A1c level below 7 will help to prevent much of the damage caused by high insulin levels.
- **If you are overweight, normalize your weight.** Obesity puts an enormous burden on the body. Losing weight can go a long way toward normalizing insulin and glucose levels.
- **Exercise regularly.** Regular exercise helps to lower blood glucose levels, reduce medication needs, and balance mood and behavior. It is essential that you find some type of exercise you enjoy and can do nearly daily. In type 2, exercise can often make oral medications unnecessary.

- **Get psychological support.** Seek support to help manage the times when you just can't cope. Managing a chronic disease can be difficult. Having a sick family member puts a strain on everyone in the family; you all may need individual and/or family counseling from time to time.
- **Decrease inflammation.** Eat a diet rich in fruits, vegetables, legumes, nuts, and seeds. These contain anti-inflammatory antioxidants and polyphenols. Monitor first morning pH to ensure that you are getting as much as your body needs. You cannot put out a forest fire with a bucket.
- **Find the diet that works best for you.** Most people with diabetes will find that a low-glycemic diet works best. Vegetarian diets, which are richer in fiber, antioxidants, and minerals than meat-based diets are, can help reduce the incidence of type 2 in children and adults. Yet Loren Cordain, PhD, professor at Colorado State University and researcher and author on Paleolithic diets reports that a Paleolithic diet devoid of grains reverses diabetes. James Anderson, MD, from the University of Kentucky, has demonstrated extraordinary benefits from diets that are high in fiber, high in legumes, and rich in complex carbohydrates. If you monitor your glucose levels carefully, you will discover the best type of diet for you.
- **Implement a high-fiber diet.** Use fiber to regulate blood glucose levels. Research shows that eating a high-fiber diet slows the release of glucose into the bloodstream over time. Peas and beans, fruits, vegetables, and whole grains, and especially high-fiber cereals containing 9 or more grams of fiber per serving, can be extremely useful.
- **Add insulin- and glucose-modulating foods to your diet.** Cinnamon, oat bran, fibers, ginger, rosemary, green tea, cranberries, blueberries, lemon balm, fenugreek, holy basil, and bitter melon are all beneficial. So add some cinnamon to that oat bran!
- **Discover your food sensitivities.** Figure out if you have celiac disease, gluten intolerance, or other food sensitivities. I have seen people whose glucose levels spiked with a single bite of carrot or papaya. Monitoring your glucose levels carefully can help you figure this out. Arthur F. Coca also developed the pulse test. Often your resting pulse will rise more than 16 beats per minute 30 minutes after a meal in response to a food that bothers you.
- **Take a multivitamin and mineral supplement.** Take these supplements to counteract inadequacies in basic nutrients.
- **Take an antioxidant supplement.** Use antioxidants to reduce inflammation and help prevent damage throughout the body. An antioxidant supplement will most probably contain carotenoids, vitamin E, selenium, and glutathione or n-acetyl cysteine, and may also contain lipoic acid and additional nutrients. Find a good antioxidant supplement and use as directed. In addition, take lipoic acid, 100 to 600 mg daily.

- **Try magnesium.** Take this to counteract probable deficiency and insulin resistance. Along with supplements, eat magnesium-rich foods such as green leafy vegetables (like kale, broccoli, spinach, chard, and collards) and whole grains. Magnesium glycinate, malate, succinate, orotate, ascorbate, and fumarate are best absorbed. Start with 100 mg daily; increase the dose by 100 to 200 mg until you get diarrhea; then reduce it 100 to 200 mg until your bowels are normal. *Note:* If the necessary magnesium dosage is higher than 1,000 mg daily, 1 or 2 teaspoons of choline citrate daily can help with absorption and allow the dosage to be reduced.
- **Try chromium.** This nutrient will help reduce insulin resistance, improve blood sugar regulation, decrease visceral fat, and increase lean body mass. Take 800 to 1,000 mcg daily, whether from nutritional yeast or a chromium supplement. *Note:* Increase dosage slowly, especially if you are taking medication or insulin, because blood sugar levels can drop suddenly.
- **Take vanadium.** Vanadium helps to move glucose into cells without raising insulin levels. Vanadium ascorbate, citrate, fumarate, malate, glutarate, and succinate are much better utilized than vanadyl sulfate. Take 250 mcg daily.
- **Take gymnema sylvestre.** Try this to improve your body's ability to use insulin effectively and stimulate insulin production. In type 1 diabetics, it lowered insulin needs and hemoglobin A1c levels. Take 400 to 800 mg daily in divided doses. Look for a product that has been standardized to 25 percent gymnemic acids.
- **Take carnitine.** Low blood levels of carnitine, a nutrient needed for burning fat and proper functioning of heart muscle, have been found in children and teens with type 1 diabetes. Take 500 to 3,000 mg daily. Dosage can also be determined through testing.

Healing Options That Are Specific for People with Type 1 Diabetes and Autoimmune Diabetes

The treatment goal for children with type 1 diabetes is to minimize the amount of insulin needed and prevent long-term complications by prolonging pancreatic islet beta cell functioning for as long as possible, maintaining good glucose control, and maximizing helpful lifestyle changes. It is unlikely that you will need to use every suggested healing option.

- **Consider autoimmunity.** Autoimmune antibodies against the thyroid, parietal cells, adrenal glands, and endomysium have been found in adults with type 1 diabetes. People with one autoimmune disease are more likely than other people to develop another. Checking for autoantibodies could prevent damage to other organs and glands. If they are high, you'll know to be more aggressive about allergy reduction in your environment and foods.

- **Take digestive enzymes.** Research shows that people with type 1 diabetes often lack pancreatic enzymes. Use of digestive enzymes can enhance digestive function. Take one to two capsules with each meal or snack. The dose depends on the type of enzyme product and the size of the meal.
- **Use nicotinamide.** Nicotinamide has been shown to reduce progression of the disease in newly diagnosed children. It can put some children into remission, improve glucose control, and help preserve some of the beta cell function. Children should take 25 mg/kg body weight daily (1 kg = 2.2 pounds).
- **Take folic acid.** Folic acid can protect against vascular damage. Take 800 mcg daily.
- **Take thiamine.** Thiamine can reduce numbness and tingling, protect beta cells, and help normalize megaloblastic anemia. The dosage varies, but typically, it is between 50 and 200 mg daily.

Healing Options Specific for People with Type 2 Diabetes

The treatment goal in type 2 diabetes is to maximize lifestyle changes and minimize medication use.

- **Use a glucose-control supplement.** These supplements help regulate blood glucose levels with a combination of vitamins, minerals, and herbs. They commonly contain B-complex vitamins, chromium, vanadium, bitter melon, and gymnema; they may also contain biotin, vitamins E and C, magnesium, CoQ10, lipoic acid, and/or carnitine. Ask at your local health food store for recommendations. Use as recommended on the bottle.
- **Try holy basil.** Holy basil is used to help regulate blood glucose levels. When I lived in Hawaii, my diabetic clients swore that eating three leaves of holy basil daily helped normalize their blood glucose without medication. Hairy basil seed has been used for the same purpose. Nontoxic and tasty—you can even make pesto out of it.
- **Eat bitter melon.** Bitter melon is a food that helps regulate blood glucose levels. This is a common food in the Philippines. It's pretty bitter and is an acquired taste. It can also be used as a tea (1 to 2 cups daily). If you purchase this in supplement form, use as directed.

CHAPTER 22

The Gallbladder: Gallstones and Cholecystectomy ⌕ D I G I N

The gallbladder, a pear-shaped organ that lies just below the liver, stores and concentrates bile that is manufactured in the liver. When we eat a meal that contains fat, the liver and gallbladder are stimulated to release bile. Each day, the liver secretes about a quart of bile, which is absorbed into the body from the ileum and colon and returned to the liver to be used again. Between meals, the gallbladder concentrates bile. Bile emulsifies fats, cholesterol, and fat-soluble vitamins by breaking them into tiny globules. These create a greater surface area for the fat-splitting enzymes (lipase) to act on for digestion. As a result, people who have poor gallbladder function will likely be deficient in fatty acids and fat-soluble vitamins (A, D, E, and K). The detoxification properties of bile are of great interest to me. Bile removes heavy metals, drugs, chemicals, cholesterol, metabolic waste, and excess hormones from the body.

The most common digestive problem associated with the gallbladder is gallstones. One in five Americans over the age of 65 has gallstones, and most people who have gallstones are never bothered by them. Medical treatment for gallstones consists of an injection of a drug that dissolves the stones, oral medication to dissolve stones, lithotripsy that breaks stones with sound waves, or surgical removal of the gallbladder. Half a million cholecystectomies (i.e., gallbladder removal surgeries) are performed each year. Most help to solve the problem. Risk factors for gallbladder removal include hypothyroidism, diabetes, losing weight rapidly, being very obese, having liver cirrhosis, and using total parenteral nutrition. After cholecystectomy about 10-15 percent of people complain of persisting symptoms which typically resolve within six months. There are rare cases in which symptoms of gallbladder disease persist.

Women are two to four times more likely to be affected by gallstones than men. An inflammation of the gallbladder can lead to pain and discomfort. Symptoms can take the form of abdominal discomfort, vomiting, bloating, nausea, belching, or food intolerances. When you have more than one stone, you may experience a sharp pain or a spasm under the ribs on the right side. Occasionally, the pain will be felt under your right shoulder blade. These pains are typically strongest after eating a high-fat meal. If you experience pains like these, see your doctor or, if they are severe, go to the emergency room.

Diet plays an important role in prevention of gallbladder disease. Low-fat, low-meat, and vegetarian diets are recommended, as is a low-sugar, high-fiber intake. In fact, a recent study of more than 1,100 people found that none of the 48 vegetarians in the group had any gallstones at all. There was an increase in gallstones in people who were heavy coffee drinkers. Dennis Burkitt, a British physician who lived and worked in Africa for 20 years, performed only two surgeries for gallbladder removal among Africans eating an indigenous diet. So, eating a high-fiber whole foods diet may be of benefit.

If you are overweight, losing weight will reduce your risk of developing gall-stones. Be careful, though; several studies have shown that fasting and extremely low-fat, low-calorie diets increase your risk of developing gallstones. Fasting for more than 14 hours raises the risk of problems due to gallstones. So easy does it while dieting. And always eat breakfast.

Exercise is also important for the prevention of gallstones. In one study, men who watched fewer than 6 hours of television per week had a gallstone rate lower than that of men who watched more than 40 hours. The researchers concluded that 34 percent of the cases of symptomatic gallstone disease in men could be prevented by increasing exercise to 30 minutes of endurance-type training five times per week.

Physicians familiar with natural therapies have seen favorable results treating gallstones without use of drugs or surgery by having their patients detoxify the liver and strengthen liver function. Metabolic cleansing or other detoxification programs are a critical first step in treatment. Food sensitivities also play an important role in the development of gallstones—most patients with gallbladder disease have them, and they must be identified.

Functional Laboratory Testing

- Liver function profile
- Home test for bowel transit time
- Test for hydrochloric acid (HCl) adequacy
- Food sensitivity testing
- Acid-alkaline home testing

Healing Options

- **Make dietary changes.** Low-fat diets help prevent gallstones and also reduce pain and inflammation associated with gallstones. Saturated fats found in dairy products, meats, coconut oil, palm oil, hydrogenated oils, and vegetable shortening stimulate concentration of bile. While a low-fat diet is optimal, essential fatty acids are vital to gallbladder function and overall health. Make sure you get 1 to 2 tablespoons of uncooked expeller-pressed oils or extra-virgin olive oil each day—the easiest way is in homemade salad dressing. Also, vegetarian diets have been found to be helpful in reducing the incidence of gallbladder disease.

  Several studies have indicated that people who consume a lot of sweets are more likely to develop gallstones. On the other hand, people who eat a high-fiber diet are less likely to develop gallstones.

  Decrease coffee intake and increase water consumption. Coffee may trigger gallbladder attacks in susceptible people. Use of either regular or decaffeinated coffee raises levels of cholecystokinin, a hormone that stimulates the release of bile from the gallbladder and digestive enzymes from the pancreas, and causes gallbladder contractions. Stop drinking coffee and see what effect this produces. Some people get horrible headaches or flu-like symptoms when they withdraw from caffeine. If you do, wean yourself gradually. And don't forget to drink six to eight glasses of water every day.

- **Reduce bowel transit time.** People with gallstones have significantly slower transit times than healthy people. Eat more high-fiber foods, drink more fluids, get more exercise, and make sure that your magnesium status is good.

- **Investigate food sensitivities.** In 1968, James Breneman, a pioneer in the area of food allergies, reported that food sensitivities play a role in gallbladder disease. He put 69 patients on an elimination diet consisting of beef, rye, soy, rice, cherry, peach, apricot, beet, and spinach. After three to five days, all people were free of symptoms. With a slow reintroduction of foods they were sensitive to, symptoms returned. The most common food offenders were pork (64 percent), onions (52 percent), and eggs (3 percent). Interestingly, beef and soy are often trigger foods for food sensitivity reactions.

- **Rule out deficient levels of HCl.** A study published in *The Lancet* found that about half of the people with gallstones had insufficient levels of HCl. A Heidelberg capsule test or SmartPill test can determine if you have sufficient levels of HCl. You can also do a home test. (See Chapter 11 for more information.)

- **Try milk thistle (silymarin).** Extracts of the herb milk thistle have been used historically since the 15th century for ailments of the liver and gallbladder. It helps normalize liver function; detoxify the liver, which it does gently and thoroughly; and improve the solubility of bile. Silymarin promotes the flow of bile and helps tone the spleen, gallbladder, and liver. Take three to six 175-mg capsules daily of standardized 80 percent milk thistle extract with water before meals.

- **Try lipotropic supplements.** Lipotropic supplements contain substances that help normalize liver and gallbladder functions. They may contain dandelion root, milk thistle, lecithin or phosphatidylcholine, methionine, choline, inositol, vitamin C, black radish, beet greens, artichoke leaves (*Cynara scolymus*), turmeric, boldo (*Peumus boldo*), fringe tree (*Chionanthus virginicus*), greater celandine, and ox bile. Lipotropics may also contain magnesium and B-complex vitamins (B_6, B_{12}, and folate) to enhance their function. Use lipotropic supplements as directed on the label, and take 1,000 mg each of methionine and choline daily.

- **Try lecithin or phosphatidylcholine.** Phosphatidylcholine, and lecithin have been shown to make cholesterol more soluble, which reduces formation of gallstones. Studies have shown that as little as 100 mg of lecithin three times daily will increase lecithin concentration in bile. I recommend 500 mg daily.

- **Take vitamin C.** Vitamin C has been shown to prevent formation of gallstones. Vitamin C is required for the enzymatic conversion of cholesterol to bile salts. People with high risk for developing gallstones have low ascorbic acid levels. Take 1 to 3 grams daily of vitamin C. I prefer mineral ascorbates as the best form.

- **Try black radish.** Lately, I've been seeing black radishes at the grocery store. Black radish (*Raphanus sativus niger*) has long been used as a folk remedy to stimulate bile production and aid in the digestion of fats. Radishes of all types seem to be of benefit. A recent study of rats showed that inflammation and other abnormal parameters observed in those that were fed a fat-rich diet were reversed with treatment with black radish. Radishes are also high in bioflavonoids and other immune-protective substances. You can eat radishes for the same benefit. Daikon radish, an Asian variety, is a mild-tasting radish for those of us who aren't radish lovers. Or you can take black radish in capsule or tablet form.

- **Try bile salts.** These are useful for people who have already had their gallbladders removed. Take one to two tablets or capsules with fatty meals.

- **Try lipase-loaded digestive enzymes.** Taking digestive enzymes that contain extra fat digestion enzymes, lipase, can be extremely useful in preventing the need for surgery, or after you've had a cholecystectomy. Take one with fat-containing meals and snacks.

- **Do a liver or gallbladder flush.** Anecdotes about people showing up at their doctor's office with a jar full of stones after a gallbladder flush are abundant, but there is little documentation to validate whether what they passed are really gallstones or just congealed olive oil. Nonetheless, many people testify to the benefits of the gallbladder flush. Do this procedure at home only under the supervision of a clinician.

From Monday through Saturday, drink as much natural apple juice as possible. Continue to eat normally and take your usual medications or supplements. On Saturday, eat a normal lunch at noon. Three hours later (at 3:00 PM), dissolve 1 tablespoon of Epsom salts (magnesium sulfate) in 1/4 cup of warm water and drink it. This is a laxative and helps peristalsis move the stones through your digestive system. It doesn't taste great, so you may want to follow it with some orange or grapefruit juice. Two hours later (at 5:00 PM), repeat the Epsom salts and orange or grapefruit juice. For dinner, eat citrus fruits or drink citrus juices. At bedtime, drink 1½ cups of warm extra-virgin olive oil blended with 1½ cups of lemon juice. Go to bed immediately and lie on your right side with your knees pulled up close to your chest for half an hour. On Sunday morning, take 1 tablespoon of Epsom salts in 1½ cup of warm water an hour before breakfast. If you have gallstones, you will find dark green to light green stones in your bowel movement on Sunday morning. They are irregular in shape and size, varying from small, like kiwi seeds, to large, like cherry pits. If you have chronic gallbladder problems, you may want to repeat this therapy in two weeks. The flush can be repeated every three to six months if you continue to form stones.

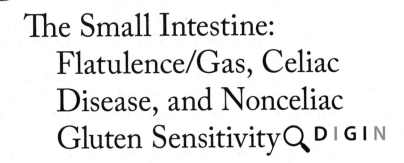

The Small Intestine: Flatulence/Gas, Celiac Disease, and Nonceliac Gluten Sensitivity

Gas and bloating are the most common symptoms of small intestinal problems. Other problems that occur in the small intestines are parasites, celiac disease, food sensitivities, and increased intestinal permeability (leaky gut). All of the DIGIN approaches can be used to work with these issues.

FLATULENCE OR INTESTINAL GAS

Everyone has gas. It's normal. In fact, we "pass gas" an average of 10 to 15 times a day. Yet, when our digestive system is working well, we may not pass much gas at all. Most of our gas comes from swallowed air. Chewing gum, drinking carbonated beverages, and eating whipped foods such as egg whites and whipped cream all contribute to swallowed air. The gas we pass is mainly nitrogen (up to 90 percent), carbon dioxide, and oxygen, all of which are odorless. Gas and bloating are also a product of the fermentation of small pieces of undigested foods by the bacteria in our intestines. Fermentation produces stinky gases like methane and hydrogen sulfide, which have the odor of rotten eggs. Other substances, like butyric acid, cadaverine, and putrescine, are present in tiny amounts, but they are noted for the mighty fragrance they give to gas.

Some of us experience excessive amounts of gas, which can be not only embarrassing but also an uncomfortable sign that something is out of balance. Millions of people have bloating and discomfort associated with gas. If you've ever made wine, you'll recall putting a balloon on the top during the fermentation process that allowed for expansion of the gases produced. Our bellies act like a balloon, expanding to contain the gas produced by fermentation.

Foods from the cabbage family, dried and sulfured fruits, and beans all contain sulfur, which gives gas a rotten-egg odor; however, sulfur also has critical uses throughout our bodies. Cucumbers, celery, apples, carrots, onions, and garlic are all commonly known to cause gas. People with lactose intolerance often experience gas when they eat dairy products. Eating a high-fiber diet is healthful but can cause gas until your intestinal flora adjusts. You may have insufficient levels of hydrochloric acid (HCl), intestinal flora, pancreatic enzymes, or a dysbiosis that is causing your problems. Food sensitivities, especially to wheat and grains, can also cause excessive gas.

You will probably find the answers to your gas issues in the DIGIN model. If they're not solved by these suggestions, look deeper. I remember one man whose flatulence was causing difficulties at work. His coworkers complained. He went through stool testing and discovered he had parasites. Once treated, his gas normalized.

Functional Laboratory Testing
- Small intestinal bacterial overgrowth (SIBO) test
- Organic acid testing
- Comprehensive digestive stool analysis with parasitology
- IgE and IgG allergy testing
- Lactose breath test
- Self-test for lactose intolerance by eliminating all dairy from your diet

Healing Options
- **Test for dysbiosis.** An imbalance of bacteria, yeast, or parasites often causes fermentation of sugars, fruits, and starches that we feel as gas and bloating. A comprehensive digestive stool analysis, organic acid test, or small intestinal bacterial overgrowth (SIBO) test can determine whether you have dysbiosis or other dysbiotic imbalance.
- **Chew your food well and eat slowly.** These simple activities can have far-reaching effects on healthy digestive processes and gas reduction.
- **Increase fiber gradually.** Most of us need to dramatically increase the amount of dietary fiber we eat, but raising these levels too quickly can cause a lot of gas and discomfort. Our flora goes wild with sudden increases in dietary fiber, and the fermentation causes gas. Increasing your fiber intake more slowly will solve this problem. High-fiber foods include whole grains, beans, and many fruits and vegetables.

- **Consider possible lactose intolerance.** The inability to digest lactose, the sugar in milk, is a frequent cause of gas. Eliminate all dairy products for at least two weeks and see if there is improvement. Make sure to eliminate all hidden dairy products found in foods. Products such as Lactaid and Digestive Advantage LI really help for the times you do eat dairy products.

- **Supplement with probiotics.** Use of a supplemental probiotic bacteria can make a tremendous difference in your ability to digest foods. Beneficial flora can help reestablish the normal microbial balance in your intestinal tract. Take one to two capsules or powdered probiotic supplement as directed on the label. Products differ in dosage. Mix a powdered supplement with a cool or cold beverage; hot drinks kill the flora.

- **Try digestive enzymes.** Many people find that supplementation at meals with digestive enzymes, either vegetable, bromelain, papaya, or pancreatic enzymes, really helps prevent gas. Take one to two digestive enzymes with meals.

- **De-gas your beans.** Beans are an excellent source of vegetarian protein, containing both soluble and insoluble fibers, as well as sitosterols, which help normalize cholesterol levels. However, beans are notorious for their gas-producing effects. They contain substances that are difficult for us to digest. For instance, beans, grains, and seeds hold their nutrients with phytic acid. Soaking or sprouting releases the nutrients so that we can absorb more of them. First, soak the beans for 4 to 12 hours, then drain off the water, replace with new water, and simmer for several hours until they are soft. Some people find that putting a pinch or two of baking soda in the water helps reduce gas. Others add kombu, a Japanese sea vegetable, or ginger. Beano is a product that contains the enzymes necessary for digestion of beans. Place a drop or two on your food; it helps reduce flatulence for most people. Beano is sold widely in drugstores and health food stores.

  Also recall that we produce digestive enzymes for foods we commonly eat. If you rarely eat beans, start by eating a tablespoon or two each day. Your body may begin to produce the enzymes necessary for their digestion.

- **Explore food sensitivities.** Although lactose intolerance is the most common food sensitivity, people can be sensitive to nearly any other food. The most likely culprits are sugars and grains. Careful charting of your foods and flatulence levels can help you detect which foods are giving you the most trouble. Food sensitivities don't usually exist by themselves. If you have a number of food sensitivities, check for dysbiosis.

- **Avoid alcohol sugars.** Sorbitol, maltitol, isomalt, and xylitol are indigestible alcohol sugars found in most sugarless candy and gum. They are used by diabetics and dieters because these sugars are sweet but don't affect blood sugar levels.

Large amounts of sorbitol and xylitol cause gas, but even small amounts can cause a problem for those who are sensitive.

■ **Take chlorophyll.** Chlorophyll liquid or tablets can help prevent gas. Take 1 tablet two to three times daily with meals.

■ **Use ginger, fennel, and anise.** Most of us have at least one of these spices in our kitchen, and they are valuable tools for reducing gas. Put a few slices of fresh ginger or ½ teaspoon of dried ginger in a cup of boiling water and steep until cool enough to drink. It will soon begin to dispel your gas from both ends, and you'll be much more comfortable. Fennel and anise can be used in tea or you can simply chew on the seeds to relieve gas. In Indian restaurants, you find small bowls of these seeds. They also cleanse the palate with their sweet pungency.

■ **Use herbs and drink herbal teas.** Traditionally, herbs and spices were added to foods to aid digestion. Nearly all our common kitchen herbs and spices have a beneficial effect, including basil, oregano, marjoram, parsley, thyme, celery seed, peppermint, spearmint, fennel, bayberries, caraway seed, cardamom seed, catnip, cloves, coriander, lemon balm, and sarsaparilla. You can find many digestive herbal tea blends in health food stores.

■ **Try activated charcoal tablets.** Charcoal absorbs toxins and gases and can be found in nearly any pharmacy or health food store. Your stools will turn black—that's the charcoal leaving your body. It has been rated "safe and effective" by the Food and Drug Administration (FDA) for acute poisoning. It's inexpensive and very helpful. Take one to four tablets as needed, with a meal or immediately if you are having gas problems.

CELIAC DISEASE AND NONCELIAC GLUTEN INTOLERANCE

Celiac Disease

Celiac disease, also called gluten-sensitive enteropathy, is a genetic autoimmune disease that affects about 3 million people in the United States. When people with celiac eat gluten-containing grains, there is inflammation, and ultimately the villi erode and the absorptive capacity of the small intestine gets diminished. It is often discovered in childhood, but it can go on for decades before being recognized. If the disease is left unchecked, people often have other diseases as a result of the undiagnosed celiac. The typical signs of celiac are indigestion, abdominal pain and bloating, diarrhea, inability to gain weight, and anemia. Celiac disease is like a chameleon: only 1 out of every 8 to 15 people present this way; most people with celiac don't have

SIGNS AND CONDITIONS ASSOCIATED WITH CELIAC DISEASE

There is an increased incidence of the following conditions in people with celiac disease. Obviously, many of these symptoms and conditions exist in people who do not have celiac disease or gluten intolerance. For example, celiac disease is found in a small percentage of people with type 1 diabetes or schizophrenia. For those few people, knowing that they have celiac is life-changing.

- Abdominal cramps
- Addison's disease
- Allergies/hay fever
- Anemia
- Asthma
- Ataxia
- Autism
- Bloating
- Bowel movements that won't flush
- Bruising easily
- Calcium deficiency
- Carpal tunnel syndrome
- Cerebral vasculitis
- Dairy intolerance
- Dementia
- Depression
- Dermatitis herpetiformis
- Dizziness
- Down's syndrome
- Ear infections
- Epilepsy
- Failure to thrive
- Fatigue/general weakness
- Feeling unwell or tired without other symptoms
- Fibromyalgia
- Fluid retention
- Gas
- Gastroesophageal reflux disease (GERD)
- GI hemorrhage
- Gray or tan-colored stools
- Hives
- Infertility
- Inflammatory bowel disease
- Interstitial cystitis
- Intestinal cancer
- Irritable bowel syndrome
- Juvenile idiopathic arthritis
- Kidney disease (increased risk)
- Liver disease
- Magnesium deficiency
- Migraine headache
- Miscarriages
- Multiple sclerosis
- Muscle wasting
- Muscle weakness
- Myopathy
- Neurological issues
- Nosebleeds
- Obesity
- Oily stools
- Osteoporosis/ osteopenia
- Palor (paleness)
- Panic attacks
- Peripheral neuropathy
- Psoriasis
- Red urine (hematuria)
- Rheumatoid arthritis
- Schizophrenia
- Sjögren's disease
- Small intestinal bacterial overgrowth
- Stomach rumbling
- Stunted growth
- Thyroid disease
- Turner syndrome
- Type 1 diabetes
- Uncoordinated/ clumsy
- Vitamin deficiencies
- Weight loss
- Williams syndrome

Sources: www.celiac.com; www.celiaccentral.com; Alessio Fasano, "Celiac Disease Insights: Clues to Solving Autoimmunity," *Scientific American* (Aug. 2009); Institute of Functional Medicine, GI Module 2010.

any gastrointestinal (GI) symptoms at all. Only half of people present with diarrhea at diagnosis. Other common presentations are depression, bone loss, dental erosion, arthritis/joint pain, mouth sores, muscle cramps, skin rashes, irritability, stomach discomfort, and neurological problems.

In 72 people who had been diagnosed with celiac disease, 28 percent had migraines, 20 percent had carpal tunnel syndrome, 35 percent reported psychiatric issues or depression, and 35 percent had sensory loss. A friend of mine loses his hearing for a few days if he accidentally eats a tiny bit of gluten. In teens with celiac disease, often depression or disruptive behaviors precede the diagnosis of celiac.

In children the most common symptoms are abdominal pain, bloating, diarrhea, constipation, weight loss, failure to thrive, and vomiting. Malabsorption of nutrients can cause far-reaching health problems. Often by the time of diagnosis, people have other health issues, such osteoporosis, infertility, neurological issues, or other autoimmune conditions, that are a result of this. Dr. Marios Hadjivassiliou and colleagues have estimated that 57 percent of people with neurological dysfunction of unknown cause have gluten sensitivity. Thyroid disorders have been found in 30 to 43 percent of people with celiac disease. There is an eightfold incidence of cirrhosis in people with celiac. The World Health Organization believes that a policy of mass screening for celiac disease is warranted because it is common and because avoiding gluten-containing grains is an effective treatment.

The recognition of celiac disease and gluten intolerance is rising, although it still takes someone with celiac disease an average of 6 to 10 years and at least five doctors to be diagnosed. It affects about 1 in 100 people, and the incidence is rising, partly due to better detection and partly for unknown environmental reasons. Some speculations and research about causes include early-life infections, gastroenteritis as an adult, dysbiosis, increased consumption of wheat globally, change in the type of wheat eaten since the 1970s, increase in wheat gluten or tissue transglutaminase enzymes added to baked goods, increased overall environmental and personal stress, increased incidence of leaky gut, and the widespread use of glyphosate as a herbicide.

Ninety-five percent of people with celiac are thought to be undiagnosed. Nearly all people who have celiac disease have the genetic predisposition by having either the HLA-DQ2 or HLA-DQ8 genes. Thirty-five percent of us have these genes, yet only one percent of us develop celiac disease. As with all of the genetic diseases, three conditions need to be met for it to be expressed: having the right genes, having the right environment to trigger the disease, and having a leaky gut. Changes in the microbiome can predispose us to celiac. This is why some people develop celiac in early childhood and other people are diagnosed well into adulthood. If you have a relative with celiac or other autoimmune diseases (such as type 1 diabetes, rheumatoid arthritis, or lupus), your risk is 8 to 15 times higher than the general population.

Gluten is a protein component of wheat and several other grains. It's what makes bread and pastries elastic and "gluey." Gluten is a complex, unusual molecule rich in proline and glutamine; digesting it thoroughly is something we humans find difficult to do. Part of the molecule is impervious to our digestion. In healthy people, the molecule stays inside the gut lumen and is passed as waste in stool. In people with leaky gut, the molecule passes through the gut, where it plays havoc. In people with celiac, this molecule provokes immediate and ultimately chronic inflammation and malabsorption. In 2010, at the Defeat Autism Now conference, Dr. Alessio Fasano, who is one of the foremost celiac researchers in the world, showed a video of two mice, one of which had been exposed to gluten and one that had not been exposed to gluten. In the mouse that was exposed, there was a buildup of intraepithelial lymphocytes (IELs) at the inside of the gut lumen. IELs are white blood cells that immediately release cytokines to get rid of molecules that don't belong there. Dr. Fasano states that this happens in *all* of us when we eat gluten-containing grains. If we have a leaky gut, then it becomes an issue because every time we eat gluten-containing grains, there is more immune involvement.

If you've been diagnosed with celiac disease, it is essential that you avoid gluten 100 percent of the time. This isn't a condition where you can sneak a bit of gluten once in a while, you can't. If you do, your risk for developing additional auto-immune diseases increases. I knew a woman who was diagnosed with lupus and subsequently with celiac disease. She kept eating gluten and within a year she had been diagnosed with Crohn's disease. If you have celiac disease, take it seriously. Working with an expert and finding out the hidden sources of gluten will minimize your risk of developing problems and additional autoimmune diseases. The lucky part about celiac is that if you completely stop eating gluten-containing grains, the body heals. You will see big changes almost immediately, and over 3 to 12 months, the small intestine will heal. For some people, discovering additional food sensitivities and actively healing the gut are also needed. So, if eliminating gluten doesn't make you feel amazingly better, use the DIGIN model to find additional issues. Think of it this way: If you are sitting on two tacks and you take one away, you might not feel 50 percent better. Avoiding all gluten is easier than it used to be, but still it can be daunting. How deeply you have fallen into the celiac rabbit hole will determine how long it will take for you to be renourished and how well some of the coexisting conditions will heal.

About half of all people with celiac disease are also lactose intolerant at the time of their diagnosis. Lactase, the enzyme required to split lactose, is manufactured at the tips of the villi. Because these villi are damaged in people with untreated celiac disease, their bodies can't manufacture the lactase. Once people have gone onto a gluten-free diet and the intestinal lining is repaired, some will be able to tolerate dairy products.

Researchers are working hard to find additional approaches for people with celiac, but right now the *only* safe treatment for celiac is to avoid gluten 100 percent. There is some promise with the use of digestive enzymes to break down gluten. Others are trying to inhibit tissue transglutaminase (tTG) so that it doesn't modify undigested gluten particles, causing them to bind to the HLA-DQ2 and DQ8 proteins. Dr. Fasano is currently studying a drug, Larazotide, that blocks zonulin (which opens the tight junctions in the intestine, increasing leaky gut). Still others are working on possible vaccines. It's too soon to know for sure what will be discovered, but keep your eyes open.

Nonceliac Gluten Sensitivity (NCGS) and Nonceliac Wheat Sensitivity (NCWS)

Many people do not have celiac disease, but they have sensitivity to gluten or wheat. Although first described in 1978 by Ellis Linaker, the idea didn't get traction until 2012, in a number of publications that began teasing out the difference between nonceliac gluten sensitivity (NCGS) and nonceliac wheat sensitivity (NCWS), determining them to be discrete from celiac disease. Research is emerging and our understandings are evolving, but there is still much that is unknown.

NCGS and NCWS have symptoms that overlap with celiac disease, both digestive and systemic. Common symptoms of NCGS include abdominal pain, diarrhea, gas, bloating, irritable bowel syndrome (IBS), fatigue, eczema, headaches, depression, anemia, numbness, joint and bone pain, muscle cramps, osteoporosis, and glossitis of the tongue. The mechanisms are varied and those believed to be the issue include reactions to gluten, fructans or possibly other fermentable oligo-, di-, monosaccharides and polyols (FODMAPs), histamine, wheat agglutinin, amylase-trypsin inhibitors, lipopolysaccharides, or true wheat allergies.

Due to the many causal issues and the lack of precise testing, estimates of NCGS range from 0.6 percent to 10.5 percent of the population and 20 percent in people who have IBS. Another confounder is the fact that many people choose a gluten-free lifestyle, either because they feel better on it or because they think it's healthier for them. In people who feel better off without gluten, they have a small but real chance of having undiagnosed celiac disease (2 to 7 percent). Therefore, follow-up testing to determine whether celiac is present in that particular person is important.

Gluten intolerance may or may not be permanent. If you can discover underlying causes in the DIGIN model, you may be able to heal your gut and tolerate gluten again. The very best method of testing yourself for gluten sensitivity is to avoid all gluten for three months.

Testing for Celiac Disease and Gluten Intolerance

Gastroenterologists feel that the most accurate diagnosis of celiac disease is done through jejunal biopsy. I have worked with many people who have negative biopsies yet still get sick on even small bits of gluten. The most specific and accurate blood test for celiac is antibodies to tissue transglutaminase (tTG). If positive, you have celiac disease. There are false negatives, however; tTG testing is negative 31 percent of the time in people with celiac disease. If it's not full-blown, it's not discovered.

Testing for Celiac Disease

Testing to Diagnose Gluten-Related Disorders

Celiac Disease

- Tissue transglutaminase IgA and IgG
- Total IgA (if low, then it negates other IgA tests)
- Antideaminated gliadin IgA and IgG
- Anti-endomysial antibodies IgA
- Biopsy of the duodenum
- In people who have dermatitis herpetiformis, biopsies of skin lesions
- Genetic testing: Because so many people have the HLA-DQ2 and HLA-DQ8 genes, this is not a good screening test for celiac disease except for:
  - People who have been gluten free for 3 or more months
  - Relatives of people with celiac disease

NCGS

- There is no test that will diagnose everyone with NCGS. Some that are useful include:
- Gluten-free diet trial
- Fructan-free diet trial if gluten-free trial fails
- IgG antigluten antibodies
- Alpha gliadin antibodies IgA and IgG
- Tissue transglutaminase IgA and IgG
- Activation of IELs
- Novel Laboratory testing:
  - Cyrex Labs has been testing for a variety of wheat and gluten proteins.
  - Wheat Zoomer from Vibrant America Labs
  - IgG food sensitivity panels indicate gluten issues 50% of the time.
  - Alcat and MRT/Leap testing
  - Elisa Act testing
- See more extensive lists in Chapter 11.

Wheat Allergy

- IgE testing for wheat allergy
- Antigliadin antibodies
- May also be non-IgE mediated, so a negative test does not rule out wheat allergy.
- When exposed to wheat, people experience GI symptoms, lung and breathing issues, and skin reactions, including itching, eczema, and hives.

Genetic testing is useful but limited, since 35 percent of us have the right genetics to develop celiac disease. IgG and IgA antibodies to gluten and gliadin can help to determine whether you have gluten intolerance yet these tests are only positive in about 50 percent of people with gluten issues.

Eating a gluten-free diet will quickly tell you if gluten-containing grains are an issue. If you embark on one, do it 100 percent. Otherwise, you may not get the definitive results you seek. If you feel better, consult with your physician to rule out celiac disease.

People with celiac disease have malabsorption, so typically they have nutritional deficiencies. It's useful to test for these and/or take a good multivitamin with minerals.

Laboratory Testing

The following tests can help determine if there are additional factors in celiac disease. If NCGS is suspected and IBS or other issues are present, remember to go back to the DIGIN model.

- Vitamin and mineral testing
- Organic acid testing
- Comprehensive digestive stool analysis with parasitology
- Intestinal permeability testing
- Lactose breath test
- Food sensitivity testing

Healing Celiac and Gluten Intolerance

- **Avoid all gluten-containing grains and any products that contain them, even in small amounts.** Gluten is found in many grains, including wheat (couscous, semolina, orzo, bulgur, graham, and farina), rye, barley, millet, spelt, kamut, and triticale. Oats don't contain gluten but are often contaminated with gluten from farming practices, transportation, or manufacturing. In addition to obvious sources of gluten, many products have hidden sources. Salad dressings, some hot dogs, ice cream, bouillon cubes, chocolate, and foods containing hydrolyzed vegetable protein may contain gluten.

Gluten-free grains and grain substitutes include:

Almond meal flour	Potato flour
Amaranth flour	Potato starch
Amaranth grain	Roasted kasha (buckwheat)
Brown rice flour	Quinoa flour
Buckwheat	Quinoa grain
Coconut flour	Sorghum
Cornmeal	Sorghum flour
Cornstarch	Tapioca
Guar gum	Tapioca flour
Millet	Teff
Millet flour	White rice flour
Pecan meal	Xanthan gum

Although giving up gluten will be difficult at first, it has become easier over the past few years with the growing number of products, restaurants, and bakeries offering gluten-free options. You'll be able to find delicious breads, pastas, cookies, crackers, and more.

■ **Try digestive enzymes.** Either pancreatic or vegetable enzymes can be used to enhance digestive function. Take one to two with each meal. Specific amylase enzymes can be of particular benefit.

■ **Supplement with probiotics.** Probiotic flora enhances digestive function. Either eat cultured and fermented foods or take probiotic supplements.

■ **Try gut-healing nutrients.** Glutamine, N-acetyl-D-glucosamine, and gamma oryzanol are all healing to the intestinal lining. While no specific testing has been done on therapeutic use of these nutrients in people with celiac disease, clinical experience with celiac indicates their usefulness.

■ **Take a multivitamin with minerals.** Zinc, selenium, folic acid, iron, and vitamins A, B_6, D, E, and K have all been shown to be deficient in people with celiac disease. Get a good-quality multivitamin with minerals. Look for a supplement that is hypoallergenic and contains no grains or dairy.

Resources: Celiac Foundation: www.celiac.com, National Foundation for Celiac Awareness: Alessio Fasano, *Gluten Freedom.*

The Colon or Large Intestine: Constipation, Diarrhea, Diverticular Disease, Irritable Bowel Syndrome, Inflammatory Bowel Disease, and Hemorrhoids Q DIGIN

Common problems in the large intestine, also called the colon, include constipation, diarrhea, diverticular disease, irritable bowel syndrome (IBS), inflammatory bowel disease (IBD), ulcerative colitis, Crohn's disease, hemorrhoids, polyps, and colon cancer. Proper functioning of the colon requires a high-fiber diet. The colon is where most of the microbiome in your body lies, including tens of trillions of beneficial bifidobacteria and other flora that ferment dietary fiber that, in turn, produce short-chain fatty acids (SCFAs), butyric acid, valerate acid, propionic acid, and acetic acid. These SCFAs are the primary fuel of the colonic cells and are needed to maintain and build new colonic cells. Without adequate fiber and prebiotics, we starve the colonic cells and weaken the integrity of the colon. Butyric acid has been shown to stop the growth of colon cancer cells in vitro and is used clinically to heal inflamed bowel tissue.

The colon's main functions are the many functions of the microbiome, as discussed in previous chapters, and to recycle nutrients and water back into our bodies and eliminate waste products. Adequate hydration is essential for good colon health. Water is our best choice, followed by fresh vegetable juices, diluted fruit juices, herbal teas, coconut water, and fruits and vegetables.

CONSTIPATION

Constipation affects up to 28 percent of North Americans. Physicians write more than a million prescriptions for constipation relief annually, and in the United States, we spend $1.26 billion a year on laxatives. Constipation is defined differently by different people, and it is often subjective: I feel constipated if I have only one bowel movement a day. The Rome IV criteria for constipation includes two or more of the following signs for at least three months, with symptoms that began at least 6 months ago: straining for at least 25 percent of bowel movements; lumpy or hard stools at least 25 percent of the time; sensation of incomplete evacuation in at least 25 percent of bowel movements; sensation of obstruction at least 25 percent of the time; manual maneuvers to facilitate evacuation at least 25 percent of the time; fewer than three bowel movements a week. An additional symptom is hard stools unless you use laxatives. There is a lot of overlap between constipation and constipation-type IBS. Long-standing constipation could also be a sign of small intestinal bacterial overgrowth (SIBO). Constipation affects women twice as often as men and is more common in people over age 65.

A total of 50 percent of people have bowel movements daily; many people do not have a bowel movement every day; most people are irregular and may not have the same number of bowel movements every day or at the same time of day. In integrative circles, it is considered normal to have one to three soft bowel movements each day. Optimal bowel transit time is 12 to 24 hours, so if you are having only three bowel movements each week, you have a transit time of 56 hours, which is way too long. This makes sense in light of current theories about fecal transit time. If you haven't done the transit time self-test, now would be a good time. (See the section on bowel transit time in Chapter 2.)

Bowel movements should be painless. If you experience pain, see your physician. You may have a structural abnormality, fissure, hemorrhoid, or more serious problem. Pain during bowel movements can cause a muscle spasm in the sphincter, which can delay a stool. Magnesium helps relieve and prevent muscle spasms.

Causes of Constipation
Although aging is commonly listed as a cause of constipation, it is due more to the results of lifestyle. Elderly people often eat low-fiber foods, rely on packaged and prepared foods, take medications that interfere with normal bowel function, and have decreased mobility. Medications that constipate include opiate medications, antidepressants such as Elavil and Tofranil, anticonvulsants, iron supplements, calcium channel blockers like Cardizem and Procardia, and antacids that contain aluminum, such as Amphojel and Basaljel.

Many other factors can be the underlying cause of constipation. Dysbiosis and lack of gut microbiome balance are often overlooked causes of constipation. Recent research has confirmed that people who are chronically constipated often have positive methane breath testing, which indicates SIBO. In fact, the more severe the constipation, the more likely that SIBO is present. Magnesium deficiency slows peristalsis, causing constipation. Hormones play a role. Women often notice that their bowel habits change at various times in their menstrual cycles. Pregnancy is a common, but temporary, cause of constipation. Constipation can also be caused by an underactive thyroid. Some diseases can affect the body's ability to have bowel movements. Parkinson's disease, scleroderma, lupus, strokes, diabetes, kidney disease, low or high thyroid function, and certain neurological or muscular diseases, such as multiple sclerosis or spinal cord injuries, can cause constipation. Colon cancer can also cause it. Neurological problems, such as injuries to the spinal column, tumors that sit on nerves, nerve disorders of the bowel, and certain brain disorders are other causes.

Dennis Burkitt, MD, father of the fiber hypothesis, studied the bowel habits of Africans living in small towns and large cities. He was the first person to theorize that it was the lack of fiber in the diets of Western cultures that was the root cause of many diseases. He found that people who ate indigenous, local foods had an average of a pound of feces each day, with 12-hour transit times. On the other hand, Burkitt found that those who lived in cities on Western diets excreted only five and a half ounces of stool each day, with average transit times of 48 to 72 hours. People on native diets had extremely low incidences of diseases common to Western civilization, such as appendicitis, diabetes, diverticulitis, gallstones, coronary heart disease, hiatal hernia, varicose veins, hemorrhoids, colon cancer, and obesity. When these people moved into cities and ate a Westernized diet, they too developed these diseases. Dr. Burkitt attributed much of this disease to poor dietary fiber intake in a modernized diet.

Overuse of laxatives is common and compounds the problem. Chronic use of laxatives, even herbal laxatives, causes the bowels to become lazy, and the muscles become dependent on laxatives to constrict. Some laxatives can cause damage to the nerve cells in the wall of the colon. If you have used laxatives, you need to retrain your body to have bowel movements on its own. Try sitting on the toilet each morning for 20 minutes and relax. Over time your body will remember how to relax and function normally.

Solving the Problem

For most people, eating more of a whole-foods diet, exercising, and drinking plenty of fluids normalizes bowel function.

Pay attention to your body's needs. When your body gives you the signals that it's time to defecate, stop what you are doing and go to the bathroom as soon as practical. When you ignore your body's urges, the rectum gets used to being stretched and fails to respond normally. Feces back up into the colon, causing discomfort. If you dislike having a bowel movement at work, school, or in a public restroom, readjust your attitude and get used to the idea. Everybody's doing it.

Healing Options

- **Look for infection.** Bacterial, fungal, and parasitic infections can cause constipation. SIBO is evident in many people with chronic constipation.

- **Double your fiber intake.** Most of us eat only half the amount of dietary fiber that is recommended. Legumes, such as kidney, navy, pinto, and lima beans, have a large amount of dietary fiber. Make whole grains the rule and processed grains the exception. The addition of high-fiber cereals at breakfast can make a big difference. Brussels sprouts, asparagus, cabbage, cauliflower, corn, peas, kale, parsnips, flaxseeds, and potatoes contain high amounts of fiber. Ground hempseed meal, chia seeds, or ground or soaked flaxseeds also work well to soften stools and normalize bowel movements. Make these changes slowly. A quick change to a high-fiber diet can cause gas and bloating. As your body gets used to this new way of eating, it will adapt. Remember that the requirements for most of us are to double our daily fiber intake.

- **Hydrate.** Be sure to drink six to eight glasses of water, juices, or herbal teas and eat at least five servings of fruits and vegetables each day.

- **Exercise if you don't already do so.** Exercise helps relieve constipation by massaging the intestines. Many of my clients have found that regular exercise keeps their bowels regular.

- **Try psyllium seed husks.** Stop using laxatives and enemas and start using psyllium seeds. They add bulk and water to stool, which allows for easy passage. A recent study compared the use of psyllium seeds, a fiber supplement, with the use of docusate sodium, a common stool softener. The psyllium was more effective at relieving constipation than the stool softener. So use psyllium and eat more fiber. Though not a laxative, psyllium seeds do regulate bowel function, are beneficial for both diarrhea and constipation, and do not cause harmful dependencies. Build up gradually to 1 teaspoon of psyllium with each meal to avoid gas and cramping from sudden introduction of fiber.

- **Try wheat bran, flaxseeds, hempseeds, or corn bran.** These can all be used in the same way as psyllium seeds. They add bulk and moisture to stool, which allow it to pass more easily. Build up to 1 to 2 tablespoons daily.

- **Improve bowel habits.** Ignoring your body's natural urge to defecate can cause constipation. Take time each morning to have a bowel movement. If you go when nature calls, it takes just a minute or two.

- **Improve bowel flora.** Poor bowel flora causes the digestive system to move sluggishly. Eat cultured and fermented foods and/or take a probiotic supplement two to three times daily. If you are able to digest yogurt, it has a normalizing effect on the bowels and can be helpful for either constipation or diarrhea.

- **Add magnesium.** Magnesium helps keep peristalsis—rhythmic muscle relaxation and contraction—working by proper relaxation of muscles. Americans have widespread magnesium deficiency that contributes to constipation. According to recent studies, 75 percent of magnesium is lost during food processing, and 40 percent of Americans fail to meet the recommended daily allowance (RDA) levels for daily magnesium intake. Take at least 400 mg daily. I've had clients who initially needed 2,000 mg of magnesium. Eventually, their deficiency shrinks, and they need less. If you need large amounts of magnesium, you may want to use 1 teaspoon daily of choline citrate to increase absorption. Too much magnesium can cause diarrhea.
- **Take digestive enzymes.** Many people report that they have more regular and easier bowel movements when they take digestive enzyme supplements.
- **Address lactose intolerance**. People with lactose intolerance sometimes become constipated from dairy products.
- **Assess stress.** See Chapter 16 for stress-management ideas.
- **Evaluate medications.** Many medications can cause constipation: pain relievers, antacids that contain aluminum, antispasmodic drugs, antidepressants, tranquilizers, iron supplements, anticonvulsants, diuretics, anesthetics, anticholinergics, blood pressure medication, bismuth salts, and laxatives. If you noticed that constipation occurred suddenly after you began to take a new medication, discuss it with your doctor.
- **Investigate food sensitivities, dysbiosis, and leaky gut syndrome**. People with chronic constipation who do not respond to diet, fiber, liquids, and exercise should have digestive testing to see if dysbiosis, food allergies, or parasites are the underlying problem.
- **Take vitamin C.** Vitamin C can help soften stool. The amount varies depending on individual needs. Use a vitamin C flush to determine your daily needs. (See Chapter 17.)
- **Try biofeedback.** Biofeedback has been used successfully to treat constipation in people who have problems relaxing the pelvic floor muscles.

DIARRHEA

Diarrhea is a symptom, not a disease. Your body is telling you: "Get this out of me and fast!" If you have chronic diarrhea, it's important to find the underlying cause. Chronic diarrhea can be the result of drugs, diverticular disease, foods or beverages that disagree with your system, infections (bacterial, fungal, viral, or parasitic), inflammatory bowel disease, IBS, malabsorption, lactose intolerance, laxative use and abuse, contaminated water supply, or even cancer. People with gallbladder problems often experience diarrhea after a fatty meal. With careful questioning and laboratory testing, your physician will be able to find the cause. Once you have a diagnosis, you can decide how to approach the problem.

Diarrhea occurs when you have a bowel transit time that is too fast. Feces don't sit in the colon long enough for water to be absorbed back into your body, so the stool comes out runny. (It's truly amazing how much water is usually absorbed through the colon—two gallons every day.) If you have chronic diarrhea, you aren't getting the maximum benefit from foods because you aren't absorbing all the nutrients. Loss of fluids and electrolyte minerals can make us disoriented and weak. In infants, small children, and the elderly, dehydration can be dangerous and can happen suddenly. It's important to replace lost fluids to prevent dehydration. Drink eight to ten glasses of water, fruit and vegetable juices, or broths each day. Infants can be given a Fleet enema, which is easily purchased at drugstores. Follow the directions on the package.

Most diarrhea is self-limiting. It is the body's way of getting rid of something disagreeable—food, microbes, or toxins. So for acute diarrhea, just let it flow and keep drinking plenty of water and fluids. If you have severe abdominal or rectal pain, fever of at least 102°F, blood in your stool, signs of dehydration—dry mouth, anxiety, restlessness, excessive thirst, little or no urination, severe weakness, dizziness, or light-headedness—or your diarrhea lasts more than three days, call your doctor. Be more cautious with small children, people who are already ill, and the elderly.

You usually aren't very hungry when you have acute diarrhea. Many foods "feed" the bugs, and you instinctively stop eating. The diet recommended for people with diarrhea is called the BRAT diet, which stands for bananas, rice, applesauce, and toast. These foods are bland and binding. You can make a pretty tasty rice pudding with apples, rice, eggs, and cinnamon. Soda crackers, chicken, and eggs can also be eaten.

With chronic diarrhea, think about food sensitivities, celiac disease, or low-grade underlying bacterial, fungal, or parasitic infection.

Many other substances can cause diarrhea, including an excess of vitamin C or magnesium. For instance, antacids that contain magnesium salts can cause diarrhea. Sorbitol, mannitol, and xylitol are sugars found in dietetic candies and sweets that can cause diarrhea, even in small amounts. Some people have the same reaction to fructose or lactose. Too much of a good thing can also cause diarrhea. I once worked with a man whose diarrhea was caused by drinking a half-gallon of fresh vegetable juice each day. When he drank less, the diarrhea stopped.

Functional Laboratory Testing

Prolonged diarrhea is a symptom that warrants thorough investigation. These are a few of the tests that may give you information about what's causing your problem.

- Comprehensive digestive stool analysis with parasitology
- Hydrogen breath test for SIBO
- Lactose breath test
- Food allergy and sensitivity testing—IgG and IgE

Healing Options

Healing options depend on the cause of the diarrhea. See the appropriate sections for complete healing options. Do testing to discover if there is a correctable underlying cause.

- **Use *Saccharomyces boulardii.*** This friendly yeast probiotic has been used successfully to prevent and treat diarrhea caused by antibiotics, traveler's diarrhea, and diarrhea associated with AIDS. It boosts levels of secretory IgA, which is a protective part of the immune system. It is safe for all ages. Take two to six capsules daily.
- **Supplement with probiotics.** These beneficial bacteria help normalize bowel function. They ferment fiber, which produces SCFAs to fuel the colonic tissue. You can also take probiotic supplements to help prevent traveler's diarrhea. Take two to six capsules daily.
- **Wash your hands frequently.** The simple act of washing your hands with soap can help reduce the incidence of ongoing diarrhea. In a study done with mothers of children with prolonged diarrhea, the mothers were simply asked to wash their own hands with soap and water before preparing food and eating and to wash their children's hands before eating and as soon as possible after a bowel movement. There was an 89 percent reduction in diarrhea in the handwashing moms' group in comparison with the control group.
- **Investigate food allergies and sensitivities.** Diarrhea is a common symptom of food sensitivities and allergies. Lactose intolerance is a common source of diarrhea. Avoid milk and dairy foods for two or three weeks to see if the diarrhea stops. Try an elimination diet, and get tested for food sensitivities.
- **Take goldenseal.** This herb is highly effective for treatment of acute diarrhea caused by microbial infection. Be sure to use goldenseal in recommended dosages, as it may also cause diarrhea if used in excessive amounts.

- **Eat yogurt.** This can help stop diarrhea. Yogurt contains active bacteria, *Lactobacillus thermophilus* and *Lactobacillus bulgaricus*, which help prevent and stop diarrhea. There have been several studies showing yogurt's effectiveness.
- **Use olive oil.** One study showed that oleic acid, the main fatty acid in olive oil, slowed down transit time in people with chronic diarrhea. Because it's so non-toxic, it's worth a try. Oleic acid is also found in olives, almonds, and avocados.
- **Increase fiber.** Adding psyllium, flax, hemp, or other fiber as a daily supplement can help solidify stools. Begin with 1 to 2 teaspoons in at least 8 ounces of water.
- **Avoid alcohol sugars.** Sorbitol, mannitol, maltitol, isomalt, and xylitol are indigestible sugars found in sugar-free candy, gums, and snack bars. They can easily cause diarrhea, gas, and bloating.
- **Take zinc.** Much research has been done on zinc and diarrhea in children. It shortens the duration of acute diarrhea by boosting the body's immune system. Children can take 20 mg daily and adults can take 50 mg daily for up to two weeks.

DIVERTICULAR DISEASE

Diverticula are pea-sized pouches that have blown out of the intestinal wall, primarily in the colon. There hasn't been much research on the underlying cause of these diverticula. It's commonly believed that a low-fiber diet, constipation, and getting older predispose us. Soft, bulky stools easily pass through the colon and respond to peristaltic waves; hard, dehydrated stools are more difficult to push along, and the bowel wall has to work harder. As a result, the muscles in the colon thicken to help this abnormal situation, which results in greatly increased pressures within the bowel. Over time, this prolonged pressure can push out portions of the bowel wall, causing diverticular pouches. It's like pushing on a balloon.

Although diverticulitis was unknown until 1917, currently about half of all people over the age of 60 have diverticular disease, and about 10 percent of the population will have it by the age of 40. It occurs more commonly in women than in men and with increasing frequency with age. In three-fourths of us, diverticula will never cause any problem or issue. When these diverticular pockets don't bother us, we call it diverticulosis.

When the diverticula become infected, it's called diverticulitis. Infection of the diverticular pockets can be a very serious illness. The suffix "-itis" means "inflammation." You will experience pain, most commonly around the left side of the lower abdomen (except in Asians, who present most often on the right side) and often a fever with or without nausea, vomiting, chills, cramping, and constipation. It is usually at this point that a physician will order tests to discover diverticulitis and diverticulosis. These infections are treated with antibiotics, such as Rifaximin, mesalazine, probiotics, and a soft-fiber diet or liquid. In most cases, taking antibiotics will clear up the diverticulitis. New research reports that there is no benefit to using antibiotics in people who have uncomplicated diverticulitis; and that antibiotics should be used only for people who have complicated diverticulitis. In uncomplicated cases, people had similar recovery to people who took antibiotics. If you've already had diverticulitis, taking 5-aminosalicylic acid and probiotics may prevent a recurrence. Talk with your doctor about treatment. If your diverticulitis doesn't respond, you may be in the small minority of people who require surgery. The possible complications of diverticulitis are bleeding, bowel obstruction, fistulas, abscesses, perforation, and peritonitis.

Diverticular pouches don't go away; however, once the inflammation goes away, a high-fiber diet will prevent most future attacks. Repeated episodes of diverticulitis may require surgery. Diverticular disease, a disease of Western civilization, rarely occurs in people who consume a high-fiber diet. There is no evidence to support the notion that people with diverticular disease need to avoid nuts, seeds, or corn once inflammation has resolved.

To prevent diverticulitis or to limit recurrence or complications, consider the following suggestions: Make sure you are eating enough fiber. Low vitamin D levels can worsen diverticulitis. One small study by Korowitz in 2014, reports benefits in taking supplemental sodium butyrate at 300 mg/day. Have your levels checked and supplement with vitamin D_3 if they are low. If you are obese, find a program to help you to lose weight. Use of aspirin and nonsteroidal anti-inflammatory drugs twice or more a week has been associated with more complications in diverticulitis.

Healing Options

- **Consume a high-fiber diet.** A high-fiber diet is of first and foremost importance for preventing the development and recurrence of diverticular disease. If you are recovering from a flare-up of diverticulitis, begin with a soft-fiber diet. Cook vegetables until fairly soft, eat cooked fruits, use easy-to-digest grains like oatmeal, and make vegetable soups with tofu. Foods with seeds (such as strawberries, poppy seeds, sesame seeds, pumpkin seeds) can catch in your diverticula and cause irritation. Until healed, avoid seed foods.

  Once you are feeling well, establish a high-fiber diet as a normal part of your life. Focus on fruits, vegetables, whole grains, and legumes. Meat, poultry, fish, and dairy products contain zero fiber and need to be eaten in moderation. Psyllium seeds are a good fiber supplement choice because they are nonirritating. Studies have shown that people eating a high-fiber, low-fat diet lower their risks of diverticular disease significantly. (Men who eat a high-red-meat, low-fiber diet have even higher incidences.) It may take you some time to get accustomed to a high-fiber, low-fat diet, but it will be worth the effort. The benefits reach further than your digestive tract, lowering your risk factors for cancer, heart disease, and diabetes. Be certain to drink plenty of water and other healthy beverages.

- **Try butyrate supplements**. Butyrate is the main energy source for the colon. One small study done in 2014 using a microencapsulated sodium butyrate dose of 300 mg daily demonstrated reductions in episodes of flare-up, hospitalization, and surgery in the tested group compared to the control group. Butyrate is available as a nutritional supplement.

- **Supplement with probiotics**. Friendly flora can help fight the infection while it's active and protect you from future infection. We still need a lot more research on the use of probiotics and diverticulitis, and yet they are being used commonly.

- **Take gamma oryzanol**. While studies of gamma oryzanol, a compound in rice bran oil, were not directly involved with diverticulitis, gamma oryzanol is known to have a healing effect on the colon. (See the discussion of gastric ulcers and gastritis in Chapter 19.) Take 100 mg three times daily for three to six weeks.

- **Take protective omega-3 fatty acids.** I can find no research on this in relation to diverticular disease, but fish oils and protective omega-6 oils such as evening primrose oil and borage oil increase the levels of prostaglandin E2 series, which promote healing and repair. Take 1,000 to 2,000 mg three times a day.

- **Take aloe vera.** Aloe vera, which contains vitamins, minerals, and amino acids, has been used by many cultures to heal the digestive tract. Its anti-inflammatory properties are soothing to the mucous membranes, and it has been shown to reduce pain. Again, I cannot find any published research in connection to diverticulitis, but use of aloe makes sense. Aloe reduces bleeding time, which is important with ruptured diverticula. Dosages vary from product to product, so read the label.

- **Take slippery elm bark.** Slippery elm bark has demulcent properties and is gentle, soothing, and nourishing to mucous membranes. Drink as a tea, chew on the bark, or take in capsules. To make a tea, simmer 1 teaspoon of slippery elm bark in 2 cups of water for 20 minutes and strain. Sweeten if you want and drink freely; it can be used in large amounts without harm. Or take two to four capsules three times daily.

IRRITABLE BOWEL SYNDROME (IBS)

IBS affects 10 to 15 percent of all American adults and is the most common gastrointestinal (GI) complaint. Of those affected, 75 percent never seek a physician's help—they just learn to live with it. Over the years, IBS has had a variety of names: spastic colon, spastic bowel, mucous colitis, colitis, and functional bowel disease. It accounts for 10 percent of all doctor's visits and 50 percent of referrals to gastroenterologists. The quality of life for someone who has IBS is affected, and people miss between 8 and 22 days of work each year due to it. Because of the symptoms of the disease, many people cannot leave their homes before noon each day, go to parties, date, travel, excel in jobs, or engage in other activities. It affects women three times as often as men. It runs across all socioeconomic groups.

Associated symptoms are abdominal pain and spasms, bloating, gas, and abnormal bowel movements. Bowel movements usually relieve the discomfort. Diarrhea alternating with constipation is the most common pattern, although some people are diagnosed with IBS for chronic constipation. People with IBS may also experience fibromyalgia, low back pain, poor sleep, headache, restless leg syndrome, migraines, chronic fatigue, irritable bladder, and other symptoms. (See "Constipation" earlier in this chapter; the lines between IBS-type constipation and chronic constipation are blurry.)

Anemia, weight loss, rectal bleeding, and fever are *not* symptoms of IBS. Bowel changes accompanied by these symptoms need to be checked out by a physician to discover the cause.

The Rome III criteria break IBS into different types: IBS-C for constipation, IBS-D for diarrhea dominant, or mixed. However, naming something gets us no closer to finding the root cause(s).

IBS has often been treated as a psychosomatic illness or just a lack of dietary fiber. Yet the quality of life for someone with IBS is equal to that of someone undergoing chemotherapy for cancer or living with rheumatoid arthritis.

IBS sufferers often have reason to feel stressed, nervous, and depressed about their condition. Stressful situations can trigger IBS symptoms. IBS can significantly restrict one's lifestyle.

Underlying Causes of IBS

There is no single cause for IBS. IBS is a symptom of an underlying issue, and a catch-all name for a constellation of symptoms that can have many different causes.

The first place to begin is to look for small intestinal bacterial overgrowth (SIBO). If IBS is accompanied by either fibromyalgia, ME/CFS, or restless leg syndrome, the diagnosis of SIBO is pretty assured. Review papers demonstrate that 60 percent of people who have IBS-like symptoms actually have SIBO. If so, then your IBS can be treated, and you can feel better. (See Chapter 7 for more information.)

IBS can also be caused by other infections, food sensitivities, celiac disease, leaky gut, imbalances in serotonin, lactose or other sugar intolerance, infection, mind–body interaction, malabsorption of nutrients, fructan intolerance, magnesium deficiency, low-fiber diet, undiagnosed celiac disease, undiagnosed inflammatory bowel disease, undiagnosed diverticulitis, hormonal imbalances, endometriosis, AIDS, environmental sensitivities, and more.

In about 25 percent of people, IBS is initially triggered by infection, such as food poisoning, characterized by symptoms of vomiting, fever, and bloody diarrhea. Often the symptoms come on suddenly and while traveling. The infection causes inflammation in the mucosal tissues, which stimulates T-cell-mediated and smooth muscle changes. When this inflammatory response continues over time, the bowels learn to be overreactive or underreactive to stimuli. People with postinfection IBS are more likely to have diarrhea-type, as well as high serotonin levels. There is usually a good response in postinfectious IBS with use of probiotic supplements. Use of COX2 inhibitors helps to normalize bowel motility. Natural COX2 inhibitors include turmeric, boswellia, and Kaprex (a product by Metagenics).

Parasites and candida overgrowth are overlooked causes of IBS. One study showed that 18 percent of the study participants had treatable parasitic infections, while another found giardia in 9 percent and parasites in 15 percent of the study population. Even benign pinworms can cause severe colonic cramping at a certain stage of their life cycle. Ask your doctor to order a comprehensive digestive stool analysis with parasitology to determine if parasites or candida are making you sick. (See Chapter 7, on dysbiosis, for more information.)

Women may experience a flare-up in their symptoms around their menstrual period. The most common symptom associated with IBS and menstruation is pain.

Other people have an insulin rise after meals, causing an increase in serotonin, which can cause diarrhea.

Food and IBS

Dietary recommendations need to be tailored to your personal reactions. It is commonly advised to avoid alcohol and monitor sugar intake, coffee, beans, and cabbage family foods (broccoli, Brussels sprouts, cauliflower) because they can be difficult to digest. You need avoid those foods only if they bother you. I find that an elimination diet gives better results than simply eliminating these specific foods.

Food sensitivities are found in one-half to two-thirds of people with IBS and are more prevalent in those who have allergies or come from allergic families. The most common foods that trigger IBS are wheat, corn, dairy products, coffee, tea, citrus fruits, and chocolate. In a study in which people were put on an elimination diet for a year, bloating and distension were relieved by 88 percent, colic pain was reduced by 90 percent, diarrhea was reduced 85 percent, and constipation improved in 54 percent. Also, 79 percent of people who had other symptoms, such as hay fever, asthma, eczema, and hives, saw these symptoms improve.

Undiagnosed lactose intolerance is often the cause of IBS. In a recent study of 242 people, it was found that 43 percent had total remission of IBS when they excluded dairy products from their diet, and another 41 percent had partial improvement. Taking the lactose hydrogen breath test is a valuable way to discover who would benefit from a lactose-free diet. (See Chapter 11 for more information.) You can also discover this by avoiding all dairy foods and any products that contain dairy foods for at least two weeks to see how you feel. If you have only moderate improvement, other foods may also be playing a role in your symptoms.

Lactose is not the only sugar to cause problems. Our cells use single-sugar molecules (monosaccharides), but many foods contain two-molecule sugars (disaccharides) that must be split. New research suggests that many people are unable to split mannitol, sucrose, sorbitol, fructose, and other disaccharides, and a high percentage of IBS sufferers are intolerant of one or more of these sugars. The result is diarrhea, gas, and bloating. Fructose malabsorption has been found in 22 to 46 percent of people with IBS. These people find that fruit, especially citrus fruit, aggravates their symptoms. For these people the Specific Carbohydrate Diet, Atkins Diet, or a Paleolithic-type diet works best. It's also important to rule out dysbiosis.

Research on the fermentable oligosaccharides, disaccharides, monosaccharides, and polyols (FODMAP) diet has demonstrated relief of symptoms in people with IBS. The FODMAP diet restricts lactose and fructose, which can cause IBS in many people. The diet is also a low-prebiotic diet, which can help to starve dysbiotic microbes and fungi.

Breath tests can diagnose fructose, disaccharide, and lactose intolerance. You can do a self-test by avoiding all fruit and sugar for at least 10 days. Be sure to read labels carefully and avoid any product that contains glucose, sucrose, malt, maltose, corn syrup, fructose, brown sugar, honey, maple syrup, molasses, and lactose. You'll find that sugar is everywhere, but if disaccharides are the cause of your IBS, it is worth the time and trouble. If sugars and fruits make you feel worse, do the self-test and a blood or stool test for candida infection or bacterial infection.

Antibiotics are well-known causes of temporary diarrhea and gastrointestinal (GI) problems. Steroid medications can also affect the balance of flora. The good flora are eliminated, especially in people who are on repeated doses of antibiotics, which allows other microbes to dominate the intestinal tract. Acidophilus, bifidobacteria, and *Saccharomyces boulardii* supplements can help restore intestinal balance.

Mind-body techniques can help with IBS. There are good studies on yoga, biofeedback, counseling, and more.

Functional Laboratory Testing

- Comprehensive digestive stool analysis with parasitology
- Lactose breath test
- Hydrogen breath test for methane levels
- Food allergy and sensitivity testing
- Intestinal permeability screening
- Organic acid testing

Healing Options

- **Look for infection.** Since most people with IBS have SIBO, this is a terrific place to begin your quest. It's possible that someone with IBS has a fungal infection, *Clostridium difficile,* or another type of bacterial infection, or *Blastocystis hominis* or other parasitic infection. (See treatment recommendations in Chapter 9 and testing in Chapter 11.)
- **Go back to Chapter 14.** Choose one of the dietary approaches from that chapter. The Elimination Diet, FODMAP Diet, or Paleo Diet may provide quick relief often can provide quick information and relief from IBS.
- **Increase fiber intake.** High-fiber diets are recommended for people with IBS. You can use high-fiber cereals to boost fiber content, but recent research indicates that wheat bran made the problem worse in 55 percent of cases, whereas it improved symptoms in only 10 percent of patients. This is not surprising because a significant number of people with IBS have a hypersensitivity to wheat products. If you want to add a fiber supplement, use psyllium seeds, flaxseed, or hemp seed. In a study in which psyllium was given to people with IBS, it improved several parameters by increasing the number of bowel movements per week, enlarging stool weight, and speeding up transit times. No negative side effects were reported.
- **Evaluate possible lactose, fructose, and sucrose intolerance.** Many people consume more sugar than their microbiome can properly handle. Most of us are

lactose intolerant. Some people with IBS are fructose intolerant. Either eliminate sugar, or dairy, or both from your diet or do breath testing.

- **Add probiotics.** In numerous studies, probiotic supplements have been shown to help regulate IBS. Products with multiple strains of microbes would be best. Make sure they at least include lactobacilli and bifidobacteria. Studies on the *Escherichia coli* strain Nissle have also shown much promise.
- **Explore behavioral therapies.** Biofeedback, self-hypnosis, and other relaxation techniques are widely used to help people with IBS. Stress often triggers bowel symptoms, and learning stress-modification techniques can alter our reactions. If we don't react with alarm to a situation, our body doesn't sense it as stressful.

After you've tried dietary approaches, consider these additional options:

- **Add glutamine.** Glutamine, the most abundant amino acid in the body, is used by the digestive tract as a fuel source and for healing IBS. Take 4 to 8 grams daily for a trial period of four weeks.
- **Take eicosapentaenoic acid (EPA)/docosahexaenoic acid (DHA) fish oil.** Fish oils inhibit the formation of inflammatory prostaglandins and leukotrienes. They may be effective in reducing the pain and inflammation associated with IBS. Take 1,000 to 2,000 mg daily in fish oil capsules, or 300 mg daily of Neuromins.
- **Take peppermint oil.** Peppermint oil is a muscle relaxant that is widely used in England for IBS. More recently, there was a published case study on using peppermint oil for a patient with SIBO. That makes sense, since these two diagnoses are interwoven. To get the oil into the intestines intact, use enteric-coated peppermint oil. (The coating prevents it from dissolving in the stomach.) Take one to two capsules daily between meals. During a spasm, you can rub a drop or two of the oil inside your anus with a finger. Caution: it stings!
- **Try herbs.** Chamomile, melissa (balm), rosemary, and valerian all have antispasmodic properties. They help relieve and expel gas, strengthen and tone the stomach, and soothe pain. Valerian, hops, skullcap, and passionflower are all calming herbs and can be found in a combination product. Antidepressant medication is often used by physicians for IBS; these gentle, effective calmatives may give you similar results. Use these herbs in capsules, tinctures, and teas.
- **Eat ginger.** Ginger, either fresh or powdered, helps relieve gas pains. It can be added to foods or used in tea. Within 20 to 30 minutes, you'll be belching and/or passing gas, which will relieve the discomfort. To make a tea, take two or three slices of fresh ginger or ½ teaspoon dried ginger in 1 cup of boiled water.

Combine it with other herbs, such as peppermint or chamomile, to enhance the effect.

- **Try melatonin.** Studies have demonstrated benefits in some people with IBS. Melatonin helps regulate gut motility. People reported improvements in abdominal pain. Melatonin also has anti-inflammatoy properties as well as hormonal properties. In some people, it can cause daytime drowsiness, nightmares, and disturbed sleep. Take 3 mg at bedtime.
- **Take calcium-magnesium citrate.** Anecdotally, many people have found that calcium-magnesium supplements prevent or alleviate the muscle spasms associated with IBS. Take 500 to 1,000 mg calcium, and 300 to 750 mg magnesium. Be aware that too much magnesium will cause diarrhea.

INFLAMMATORY BOWEL DISEASE: CROHN'S DISEASE, ULCERATIVE COLITIS, MICROSCOPIC COLITIS, AND ISCHEMIC COLITIS

IBD includes four distinct illnesses: ulcerative colitis, Crohn's disease, microscopic colitis (lymphoid and collagenous), and ischemic colitis. Each of these autoimmune diseases has slightly different characteristics, although the treatment for all of them is aimed at reducing inflammation and rebalancing the microbiome. IBD affects one million to two million Americans; ulcerative colitis rates are about 2 people per 1,000; and Crohn's disease rates are about 1.7 per 1,000. Rates have risen since 1940 and are rising in other parts of the world where Western diets are becoming the norm. Most cases are diagnosed before age 40. Environmental issues associated with increased risk include infections, being bottle-fed as an infant, antibiotics, use of nonsteroidal anti-inflammatory drugs (NSAIDs), eating a Western-style diet, and stress. Antibiotic usage during childhood is associated with increased risk of developing Crohn's disease. The more rounds of antibiotics taken, the higher the risk. IBD tends to run in families and is more prevalent among people of Jewish descent. There is a higher incidence of IBD in women who take oral contraceptives. Women with a history of IBD or with a family history of IBD may want to choose a different form of birth control.

IBD shares many of the symptoms of IBS, but they are very different problems. IBD involves inflammation of the digestive tract, which can occur anywhere from the mouth to the rectum. Malnutrition and malabsorption are common in people with active IBD. Symptoms include abdominal pain, bloody diarrhea, and cramping. If you are having these symptoms, go see your physician. These symptoms may also be accompanied by fever, rectal bleeding, abdominal tenderness, abscesses, constipation, weight loss, awakening during the night with diarrhea, and a failure to thrive in children. Symptoms come and go and can go into remission for months or years. About half of the people with IBD have only mild symptoms. People with IBD often develop complications, which include inflammation of the eyes or skin, arthritis, liver disease, kidney stones, and colon cancer.

IBD is considered an autoimmune disease (your body begins attacking itself). The causes are many and have produced much debate. Current theories suggest that Crohn's and ulcerative colitis have a genetic component, which is triggered to a greater or lesser extent by either infection, a hypersensitivity to antigens in the gut wall, an inflammation of the blood vessels that causes ischemia (a lack of blood supply to the tissues), or food sensitivities. In 2017, 201 genes had been associated with IBD and this is probably the tip of the iceberg. The best known associations are in Crohn's disease with the CARD15 and NOD2 genes, which modulate innate immunity. The NOD gene is found in only 10 to 15 percent of people with Crohn's. Other genes (LAMB1 and HNF4a16) seem to have to do with increased intestinal permeability and regulate autophagy, inflammation and other aspects of metabolism. Genes are expressed and have different effects in Asian, Caucasian, and African populations than in others, adding to the complexity.

TYPES OF INFLAMMATORY BOWEL DISEASE

Ulcerative Colitis

Ulcerative colitis is a continuous inflammation of the mucosal lining of the colon and/or rectum. In the descending colon it is sometimes called left-sided disease, and in the rectum it is called distal disease, ulcerative proctitis, or proctosigmoiditis. If sores are present, they are shallow, and when in the rectum, it's generally milder and easier to treat. The most common symptoms are abdominal pain, diarrhea, and blood in stool, making it maroon colored. Often people note mucus or pus in their stool.

Of people with ulcerative colitis, 20 to 25 percent eventually require surgery because of massive bleeding, chronic illness, perforation of the colon, or risk of colon cancer. About 5 percent of people with ulcerative colitis ultimately develop colon cancer.

The current medications for ulcerative colitis have focused on decreasing inflammation and TNF-alpha. Drs. O. Brain and S. P. Travis at Oxford Radcliff Hospital suggest that this may be wrong. They postulate that defects in barrier function (leaky gut) and innate mucosal immunity (such as a poor ability to kill bacteria) may be the primary causes. These issues then lead to inflammation. If they are correct, then building immunity and healing a leaky gut play a leading role.

Crohn's Disease

The most common symptoms of Crohn's disease include abdominal pain, diarrhea, weight loss, and malnutrition. Crohn's disease can occur anywhere along the digestive tract, from mouth to rectum, but is most common in the colon and ileum near the ileocecal valve. It is sometimes called right-sided disease. Frequent symptoms are fevers that last 24 to 48 hours, canker sores in the mouth, clubbed fingernails, and a thickening of the GI lining, which may cause constrictions and blockage. Inflammation develops in a skip pattern, a little here and a little there, and goes more deeply into the tissues than with ulcerative colitis. In later stages, it can form abscesses and fistulas, little canals that lead to other organs or form tiny caves. If they become serious, surgery may be recommended. If you require surgery for Crohn's disease, it is important to know which part of the intestines were removed and which nutrients may have inadequate uptake. (See Figure 2.1 in Chapter 2 for an absorption chart.)

Some people with Crohn's disease have flare-ups in a seasonal cycle, which suggests an allergy component to the illness. While studies have shown that allergy is a factor in a small number of people, a survey of members of the National Foundation of Ileitis and Colitis showed that 70 percent of people with IBD listed other symptoms that were probably allergy related. This led one researcher to say that "inflammatory bowel disease is just another possible facet of allergy." Mold sensitivity and allergies to candida and other types of fungus have also been proven to provoke IBD symptoms.

Microscopic Colitis

Microscopic colitis is a newer diagnosis. It is characterized by diarrhea, cramps, and abdominal pain. The diarrhea may be continuous or can come and go. There can also be fatigue, fever, or joint pain. When a colonoscopy is done, all looks normal, yet when cells are biopsied under a microscope, inflammation is seen. Microscopic colitis is often misdiagnosed because a biopsy is needed to make a definitive diagnosis. Microscopic colitis doesn't appear to morph into Crohn's disease, ulcerative colitis, or cancer. There is some genetic component; it often runs in families.

There are two types of microscopic colitis: collagenous colitis and lymphocytic colitis. In collagenous colitis, there is a thickening of the collagen layer in the colon and an increase in inflammatory cytokines. There may also be an increase in lymphocytes, a type of white blood cell. Lymphocytic colitis is characterized by increased numbers of intraepithelial lymphocytes (IELs), which are specific types of white blood cells. This results in watery, nonbloody diarrhea. About half of people have a sudden onset and know exactly when it began. A common trigger is dysentery, giardia, or other intestinal infection.

There are several theories about the origins of microscopic colitis. Some believe it is an autoimmune disease; others suggest that it is caused by a virus, bacteria, or bacterial toxin; and another theory is that it is aggravated or triggered by use of NSAIDs. Probably it's a combination of these that triggers the illness. Like Crohn's disease and ulcerative colitis, microscopic colitis can come and go with flare-ups and healing.

Both types are most often seen in middle-aged women, but they can be found in men, women, and children of all ages. Some cases resolve on their own without any treatment. Fiber and fluids are recommended. Sometimes people might be given a medication to stop the diarrhea. *Saccharomyces boulardii* is a probiotic that is useful for diarrhea from all causes. If the flare-up is severe, anti-inflammatory drugs, steroids, or antibiotics may be used.

Ischemic Colitis

Ischemic colitis typically occurs in people over the age of 60 and is associated with cardiovascular disease. It occurs when blood flow from arteries to a part of your colon is reduced. Most often this is due to atherosclerosis, a buildup of fatty deposits in your arteries. This results in inflammation that can cause temporary or permanent damage to your colon. It can occur anywhere but most often happens on the left side of the colon. When this occurs on the right side of the colon, it can be more serious because the same arteries also feed the small intestine. The most common presentation includes abdominal pain, rectal bleeding, and often urgent bowel movements, nausea, diarrhea, or vomiting. This usually presents as a flare-up and then subsides. Treatment is typically rest, lots of fluids, and possibly intravenous (IV) antibiotics. Once treated, this condition typically doesn't recur.

Ischemic colitis can also be caused by or related to other conditions, including vasculitis (inflamed blood vessels), diabetes, blood clotting, radiation treatment to the abdomen, infections (such as *C. difficile*, shigella, and *E. coli*), and dehydration. In rare cases, medications can precipitate ischemic colitis, including the use of birth control pills, estrogen replacement, NSAIDs, migraine medications (triptan and ergot types), antipsychotic drugs, pseudoephedrine, alosetron (Lotronex for IBS), and cocaine.

Mental Health and IBD

IBD is not caused by emotional illness or psychiatric disorder, though the condition may cause emotional problems because of its chronic nature, painful episodes, and lifestyle limitations. Prolonged treatment with steroid medications can cause side effects of depression, mania or euphoria, and bone loss.

FACTORS IN INFLAMMATORY BOWEL DISEASE

In all types of IBD, looking for underlying causes or triggers is important. Using the DIGIN model can be extremely useful. People with active IBD have increased intestinal permeability. Once the inflammation is under control, the permeability normalizes. Zinc, probiotics, and butyrate have all been helpful in healing leaky gut in IBD patients.

Probiotics in IBD

Where this takes us on a practical level is to look at what we can do to have a healthy gut bacterial environment. Numerous studies have shown that use of probiotic supplements is beneficial for people with IBD. They have been shown to help maintain remission of flare-ups in Crohn's disease, ulcerative colitis, and pouchitis. Probiotic bacteria, like *L. acidophilus*, bifidobacteria, and the Nissle strain of *E. coli* 1978, VSL#3, and *Lactobacillus* GG have been shown to have benefits. Commensal bacteria stimulate our immune response, increase beneficial antibodies such as sIgA, IgM, and IgG, balance pH, and enhance tight junction integrity. Probiotic therapy with *E. coli* strain Nissle has been shown to be effective in treatment for ulcerative colitis and was found to be equivalent to the drug mesalamine for short-term maintenance of the disease and after use of steroid treatment for remission. VSL#3 is a high-dose, multistrain formula that has been used for pouchitis and to bring flare-ups under control.

More research needs to be done on IBD and probiotics. Different combinations will work for different people and to greater or lesser effect.

Although there is not much research on the yeast connection to IBD, clinicians have often found antifungal therapies to be useful. Friendly flora have been found to be dramatically out of balance in people with IBD, so use of probiotic supplements is highly recommended. Use of the comprehensive digestive stool analysis with parasitology screening and intestinal permeability tests will uncover many of these problems.

Dysbiosis and IBD

Research indicates that dysbiosis plays a significant role in IBD. Given that the gut microbiome is the center of our immune system, this makes sense. Studies have reported increased levels of gram negative anaerobic bacteria, such as *Bacteroides* species, and lower levels of bifidobacteria species in Crohn's disease, ulcerative colitis, and pouchitis (infection of the diverticula). *E. coli* has also been implicated in Crohn's disease. In a study with 137 patients, SIBO has also been reported in 45 percent of people with Crohn's disease and in 17.8 percent of people with ulcerative colitis. In Crohn's disease, fungal overgrowth has also been implicated. Bacterial infections occur in one-quarter of all recurrence of IBD.

People with IBD typically have lower levels of microbial diversity in their microbiome, higher levels of Firmicutes, lower levels of short-chain fatty acid (SCFA) producing bacteria, and increases in pathogenic bacteria, mucus-degrading bacteria, and sulfate-reducing bacteria. This leads to decreases in SCFA, which produces energy in the colon, altered T-cell function, and loss of biofilm integrity, leading to increased risk of dysbiosis, inflammation, and increased leaky gut.

Some of the current medications used to reduce inflammation and prevent flare-ups in IBD also have mechanisms that modulate the microbiome, including mesalazine, and anti-tumor necrosis factor (TNF)-α antibody therapy. A lot more research is needed on the use of probiotics, prebiotics, treating known infection, and breaking up the biofilms with probiotics, enzymes, and fiber in these conditions. People with IBD are more likely to have periodontal disease. Make sure that you are taking good care of your gums. (See Chapter 18 for more information and Chapter 28 for more on cardiovascular disease.)

Probiotics in IBD

While more research is needed, probiotics have proved helpful in IBD, with the best research on *E. coli* Nissle 1917 strain, VSL#3, and *L. rhamnosus* GG (Culturelle). Commensal bacteria stimulate our immune response; increase beneficial antibodies such as sIgA, IgM, and IgG; balance pH; and enhance tight junction integrity. Probiotic therapy with *E. coli* strain Nissle has been shown to be effective in treatment for ulcerative colitis and was found to be equivalent to the drug mesalamine for short-term maintenance of the disease and after use of steroid treatment for remission. VSL#3 is a formula with eight probiotic species that has been used for pouchitis.

Much more research needs to be done on IBD and probiotics. Different combinations will work for different people and to greater or lesser effect. You'll have to experiment with different brands and see which are most helpful. Remember to begin with a small dosage and increase slowly. You are changing your gut ecology, and you want to do it gradually. You can think of them as a medicine that you'll probably need to take daily for life.

Although there is not much research on the yeast connection to IBD, clinicians have often found antifungal therapies to be useful. Friendly flora have been found to be dramatically out of balance in people with IBD, so the use of probiotic supplements is highly recommended. Use of the comprehensive digestive stool analysis with parasitology screening and intestinal permeability tests will uncover many of these problems.

Treatment

Medical treatment for IBD consists of anti-inflammatory drugs (e.g., sulfasalazine [Azulfadine], mesalamine [Asacol], olsalazine, balsalazide), steroids (e.g., prednisone), immune suppressors (e.g., azathioprine, cyclosporine, methotrexate), and sometimes antibiotics and biological medications such as azathioprine (Imuran), infliximab (Remicade), certolizumab pegol (Cimzia), adalimumab (Humira), golimumab (Simponi), and others that suppress TNF-alpha. While these medications can often relieve symptoms of IBD, they carry their own risks. Some specific drug side effects include bone loss and low cortisol levels due to use of steroid medications, and folic acid deficiency from use of sulfasalazine. Imuran has been associated with a small rise in the incidence of lymphoma.

Medications are often necessary, but use of complementary therapies can reduce the need for them, so that when you really need medication during a flare-up, it works effectively. For example, repeated use of prednisone can lead to its failure as an available therapy.

The good news is that effective natural therapies address the underlying factors of the disease, reduce the need for prescription medications, and heal the bowel. Among the hundreds of patients with IBD that Drs. Jonathan Wright and Alan Gaby, two nutritionally oriented MDs, have seen, most have improved, many dramatically. The key to success appears to be getting people into remission as fast as possible. To do this effectively, a combination of medication and supplements may be necessary. Once a flare-up has died down, natural therapies are highly successful in preventing a recurrence. It's also really important to take care of yourself when you are well and to practice stress-management techniques to help reduce the number and severity of flare-ups.

One of the most promising new therapies is the use of phosphatidylcholine. People with ulcerative colitis have been found to have low levels of phosphatidylcholine in their colonic mucus. Phospholipids are essential for the mucous barrier to protect us. When these levels are low, we are likely to have leakiness. Some people are able to stop steroid medications when taking sustained-release phosphatidylcholine at levels of 2 to 4 grams daily. There have been three studies on this therapy, all from the same research group, one of which holds a patent on this particular form of phosphatidylcholine. This gives a possible bias. Also, I wonder whether regular phosphatidylcholine might work as well.

Diet and Nutritional Deficiencies Associated with IBD

Elimination diets are being utilized for people with inflammatory bowel disease with the goal of reducing inflammation and normalizing gut microbiota. Food sensitivities play a significant role in a subset of people with IBD. Studies have shown reduction in symptoms and inflammation in people who adhere to a hypoallergenic diet because it reduces inflammation and improves balance of the microbiome. People with bowel disease are especially sensitive to most grains. Truly, nearly any food can cause problems. In various studies, citrus, pineapple, dairy, coffee, tomatoes, cheese, bananas, sugar, additives, preservatives, spices, beverages other than water, and bread have all been implicated. One study found that 13 percent of children with IBD were allergic to cow's milk during infancy.

Many IBD patients report significant improvement with use of an elimination diet over a three-week period. After this, they gradually add foods back into their diet to determine which ones provoke bloating, pain, diarrhea, bleeding, or other symptoms. Get tested for both IgE and IgG antibodies to determine your food sensitivities. Testing of IgA and IgM antibodies is also useful.

In IBD, it's important to customize plans, look for micronutrient insufficiencies, and rebalance DIGIN. Micronutrient needs that have been shown to be greater in people with IBD include vitamin D, zinc, beta-carotene, vitamins B_1, B_6, B_{12}, K, folic acid, selenium, manganese, and iron. Food additives have been shown to increase IBD inflammation. These include carrageenan, maltodextrin, sodium caprate, polysorbate 80, and carboxymethyl cellulose.

Diet is a great starting place for maintenance and prevention of flare-ups. For specifics, refer to Chapter 14.

Parenteral and enteral feeding has been used in medical settings and hospitals for decades and includes intravenous feeding (paraenteral) and enteral diets such as the elemental diet (discussed with SIBO), semi-elemental diet, and polymeric diet. None tastes good, yet all give the digestive system a rest and starve out the microbiome, reducing inflammation. In children, parenteral feeding works as well as steroids in bringing Crohn's disease into remission; however, it does not seem to work as well in adults.

In several small studies, the Specific Carbohydrate Diet (SCD) has shown great promise in children with Crohn's disease and in adults with either Crohn's disease or ulcerative colitisin several small studies. A larger, multicentered study in Crohn's disease compared the SCD with the Mediterranean diet. In 50 adults with Crohn's and ulcerative colitis, the SCD improved diversity, decreased symptoms, and improved quality of life. There is currently an on-going study comparing the Mediterranean diet and the SCD in people with Crohn's disease in 34 centers.

There is some research demonstrating the effectiveness of the fermentable oligosaccharides, dissacharides, monosaccharides, and polyols (FODMAP) diet. In a small, but promising, study, 33 percent of people with ulcerative colitis and 57 percent of people with Crohn's disease saw improvement while on this diet.

Other diets have also been utilized, including a semi-vegetarian plan, the paleolithic diet, Maker's diet, vegan diets, and others. These have little or no data, but all are lower carbohydrate diets that are whole foods based.

The idea behind all of these diets is to use them as a therapeutic protocol for 2 to 4 months and then begin reintroducing foods to see what is tolerated.

A low-sulfur diet may be of benefit in Crohn's disease. Studies have shown an increase in sulfur-eating bacteria in people with bowel disease compared with other people. In a 1998 study by Dr. William Roediger, four people were advised to avoid high-sulfur foods, including eggs, cheese, whole milk, ice cream, mayonnaise, soy milk, mineral water, sulfited drinks (including wine), nuts, and cruciferous vegetables (broccoli, cabbage, cauliflower, Brussels sprouts, and so forth), and to reduce red meats. They were advised to get protein from fish and chicken. Dr. Roediger found significant changes—participants had no relapses or attacks while on the diet, and there were no adverse effects from the diet itself. The expected relapse rate had been 22.6 percent. Of the four people in the study, one was able to stop taking steroid medication and had been attack free for 18 months, compared to the four attacks experienced in the 18 months before the dietary changes. The other three showed microscopic improvement of inflammation. The average number of daily bowel movements in all four was reduced from six to one and one-half. Since then, no additional papers have been published on low-sulfur diets in IBD. Yet, we do have more research on dysbiotic microbes that thrive on sulfur.

Diets that are low in fiber and high in animal fat and sugar have been implicated in the development of IBD. Cigarettes and fast foods have also been implicated in IBD. Eating fried potatoes has been implicated in increased IBD as well. It's believed that the glycoalkaloids (alpha-solanine and alpha-chaconine), which become concentrated when potatoes are fried, increase gut permeability.

Because of bleeding and continued irritation, malabsorption of nutrients is often found in people with IBD. These same nutrients are often vital for repair, so the cycle worsens. Low serum levels of zinc, an important nutrient for wound repair, are often found in people with IBD. Folic acid helps repair tissue and prevents diarrhea.

Prolonged bleeding can cause deficiencies of copper, zinc, iron, folic acid, and vitamin B_{12}.

Studies have shown an increased need for antioxidant nutrients such as vitamins A, B_3 (niacin), C, E, and K, selenium, calcium, phosphorus, copper, iron, zinc, glutathione, and superoxide dismutase (SOD). Many also have anemia, which is related to iron, B_{12}, copper, and/or folic acid deficiencies.

Several studies have shown bone loss in people with Crohn's disease and ulcerative colitis. While incidence of loss in some studies is correlated with use of steroid medications, in others it appears to be independent. It is advisable to do at least a baseline bone density study to see if you are at risk. Also check vitamin D levels and try to keep them in the higher end of the normal range. If risk of bone loss is determined, increasing all bone nutrients would be advised. A study on low-impact exercise in people with Crohn's disease found that bone density was significantly increased. So get out there and exercise regularly.

Nicotine and IBD

One unusual twist in the story is that nicotine appears to be protective for ulcerative colitis, while it makes Crohn's disease worse. Although normally I wouldn't recommend nicotine patches, the severity of the disease could warrant a try. Nicotine is certainly less toxic than the usual drugs that are used. The studies show positive results, using 15 to 25 mg patches over periods of four to six weeks along with mesalamine. Many people stayed in remission for up to three months after stopping the patch. One study gave people who were in relapse either nicotine or prednisone with mesalamine for five weeks. The relapse rate was much better in the nicotine group—only 20 percent in comparison to a 60 percent relapse rate for those on prednisone. In the long term, nicotine patches appear to help with flare-ups and maintenance when used with mesalamine.

Less Conventional and Highly Effective Approaches to IBD

There are many additional approaches for IBD, including several studies on the use of beneficial worms (helminths), such as rat tapeworm and *Trichuris suis* ova (TSO) whipworms, to modulate the immune system and halt flare-ups in IBD. (See Chapter 8 for more information on this.) One promising approach involves photopheresis, a process that exposes blood to light and many herbal therapies. Natural COX2 inhibitors, such as curcumin, green tea, and boswellia, also show promise.

Fecal microbial transplant (FMT), while 90 percent effective in people with recurring *C. difficile*, has been shown to be less effective in IBD. Research is growing in this area, but FMT seems to provide a significant benefit in some people with ulcerative colitis and Crohn's disease. Between 23 and 32 percent of people with ulcerative colitis in controlled studies, as well as 50 percent of people with Crohn's disease in uncontrolled studies, obtained remission with FMT. While researchers are still working to figure out who will best be helped, FMT has a very low downside, so it is worth trying.

Functional Laboratory Testing

- Comprehensive digestive stool analysis with parasitology
- Lactose breath test
- Food and environmental sensitivity testing
- Calprotectin or lactoferrin (great for diagnosis and monitoring treatment)
- Intestinal permeability screening
- Antioxidant analysis
- Bone density testing and vitamin D levels
- Immunogenetics testing
- Nutritional analysis of blood
- Testing trimethylamine N-oxide (TMAO) levels

Healing Options

- **Make dietary changes.** Begin by eliminating simple sugars, alcohol, and fast foods (one study showed that flare-ups occurred almost four times as frequently in people with ulcerative colitis when fast foods were eaten twice a week). Grains and dairy products often aggravate the condition.
- **Use one of the therapeutic dietary approaches mentioned previously and in Chapter 14.** These are short-term diet plans that reduce inflammation and get your microbiome back into better balance.
- **Maintain a normal weight.** While dietary changes can be useful, don't limit your food so severely that you lose weight and muscle mass. Especially in people with Crohn's disease, malnutrition is common. Find a diet that works for you and helps you maintain your weight and health. Don't limit wheat, dairy, other grains, nuts, or seeds unless you are pretty sure that they are causing problems.
- **Correct anemia if present. Correct other vitamin and mineral deficiencies if present. Correct vitamin D levels if they are low. Take a multivitamin with minerals and antioxidant nutrients.** Because of general malabsorption and poor dietary habits in people with Crohn's disease and ulcerative colitis, it is wise to closely measure yourself for nutritional status with testing. Also add a good-quality multivitamin with minerals to your daily routine. Deficiencies of many nutrients have been found in people with IBD: calcium/magnesium; folic acid; iron; selenium; vitamins A, B_1, B_2, B_6, C, D, and E; and zinc. Because oxidative

damage plays a significant role in IBD, the supplement should contain adequate amounts of antioxidant nutrients: at least 10,000 IU of beta-carotene or other carotenoids, 400 IU of vitamin E, 250 mg of vitamin C, 200 mcg of selenium, 5 mg of zinc, plus other nutrients. It may also contain CoQ10, glutathione, N-acetyl cysteine (NAC), Pycnogenol, SOD, and other antioxidants. It is best to buy a supplement that is free of foods, herbs, colorings, and common allergens.

- **Explore possible lactose intolerance.** Hydrogen breath testing or elimination of all dairy products and foods containing dairy from your diet for at least two weeks can help determine whether lactose intolerance is contributing to your problem. Definitely eliminate dairy during a flare-up of your illness.
- **Consider food sensitivities.** Food sensitivities play a significant role in ulcerative colitis and Crohn's disease, occurring approximately half the time. Try an elimination diet, SCD, or gut and psychology syndrome (GAPS) diet. The most common offenders are dairy products, grains, and yeast, followed in frequency by egg, potato, rye, coffee, apples, mushrooms, oats, and chocolate.
- **Try the Specific Carbohydrate Diet (SCD).** Many people have found relief from using the Specific Carbohydrate Diet outlined in Elaine Gottschall's book *Breaking the Vicious Cycle.* Unfortunately we don't yet have any clinical research on the SCD. This diet can be beneficial because it eliminates most foods that cause sensitivities—grains and dairy products. Similar to the candida diet (see Chapter 7), it helps restore intestinal balance. While going on the diet alone may be effective, it is most effective after laboratory testing has determined your unique biochemistry.
- **Take glutamine.** Glutamine is the first nutrient I recommend for bowel and intestinal health. It is the most abundant amino acid in our bodies. The digestive tract uses glutamine as the primary nutrient for the intestinal cells, and it is effective for healing stomach ulcers, irritable bowel syndrome, and ulcerative bowel diseases.

Douglas Wilmore, MD, has done a lot of clinical research giving high doses of glutamine to people who have short bowel syndrome. This occurs when only a short portion of the colon remains after surgery. These people develop chronic diarrhea and often cannot tolerate any real food. With a high-fiber, high-glutamine diet, and short-term use of growth hormones, Dr. Wilmore was able to normalize bowel function. Glutamine is also great for building muscle mass. Begin with 8 to 20 grams daily for a trial period of four weeks. In clinical settings, up to 40 grams daily have been used.

A study of Nigerian rabbits reported that when honey was added to glutamine supplementation after bowel resectioning, rabbits who got honey had better healing. The researchers report that this might also have benefits in people who have had bowel-resectioning surgery.

- **Try bromelain.** Bromelain, a protein-splitting enzyme derived from the green stems of pineapple, was studied and shown to reduce the incidence and severity of ulcerative colitis with no negative effects even in large doses. Dosages were not listed in this study. Typical doses of bromelain range from 1,000 mg to 3,000 mg daily.

- **Try tormentil.** Tormentil (Potentilla tormentilla), an herb and member of the rose family, is being studied for its effectiveness in treating ulcerative colitis. According to Grieve's *A Modern Herbal*, it nourishes and supports the bowels and stops diarrhea. It's been reported to have high antioxidant properties and polyphenols. While in early clinical testing, one study with 16 people reported improvements in those treated with 2,400 mg daily. Although the study was done on ulcerative colitis, the benefits could certainly extend to other inflammatory bowel conditions.

- **Take sustained-release phosphatidylcholine.** Recent research on the use of sustained-release phosphatidylcholine in people with ulcerative colitis looks quite promising. Effective doses appear to be 2 to 4 grams daily.

- **Try wheatgrass juice.** People with ulcerative colitis have had great results reducing flare-ups of the disease by drinking wheatgrass juice. In 2002 Israeli researchers finally put it to the test. Twenty-three people with active distal ulcerative colitis were given either 3½ ounces (100 cc) of wheatgrass juice daily or a green placebo daily for one month. People who received the wheatgrass juice had less severe flare-ups of the disease and less blood loss. Wheatgrass juice is high in glutathione. Low glutathione levels have been found in people with inflammatory bowel disease. There was also improvement in sigmoidoscopy. This is certainly a nontoxic and easy remedy to try.

- **Increase glutathione naturally.** Inflammatory bowel disease is one of increased free radicals. One of the most important reducers of inflammation due to toxicity is glutathione. Two of the simplest ways to increase your glutathione levels are to use a good quality whey protein powder daily and take NAC. Dosages of NAC range from 500 to 2,000 mg daily.

- **Increase consumption of omega-3 fatty acids.** Salmon, mackerel, herring, tuna, sardines, and halibut are all excellent sources of EPA/DHA oils. Eating these fish several times a week can supply your body with these essential fats. Seaweeds also provide generous amounts of omega-3 oils, but carrageenan, an extract from seaweed, may increase the inflammation in the colon. While carrageenan is used in animals to produce IBD, in humans the research is not yet clear. To be on the safe side, avoid red and brown seaweeds.

You can also take capsules of EPA/DHA oils daily. In a recent study, it was found that the use of Max/EPA decreased disease activity by 58 percent over a period of eight months. No patient worsened, and eight out of eleven were able to reduce or discontinue use of medication. The dosage was 15 capsules of Max/EPA, which contains 2.7 grams of EPA and 1.8 grams of DHA, per day. Many other studies also show the benefit of fish oils with dosages between 3.5 and 5.5 grams daily.

- **Take probiotics and prebiotic fibers.** *E. coli* strain Nissle 1917 was found in three studies to be equal to the use of 5-ASA medication. VSL#3 has also been studied to keep people in remission and prevent pouchitis. There is much that is unknown, yet probiotics and prebiotics play an important role in modulation of inflammation and immune response. The dose ought to be in proportion to the level of inflammation. (See Chapter 6 for more on probiotics.)

- **Consider beneficial helminth therapy.** Use of benign whipworm eggs can modulate your immune system to calm down and prevent flare-ups. There is a growing body of research on this in IBD. (See Chapter 8 for more information.)

- **Consider fecal transplant therapy.** Fecal transplants help many people who have IBD. Currently, though, there are few centers utilizing this therapy except in research.

- **Take gamma oryzanol.** Gamma oryzanol, a compound found in rice bran oil, is a useful therapeutic tool for gastritis, ulcers, and irritable bowel syndrome. Try taking 100 mg three times daily for a period of three to six weeks. (See Chapter 19 for more on gamma oryzanol.)

- **Take boswellia.** Boswellia has been used in Ayurvedic medicine as an anti-inflammatory for ulcerative colitis. Only one study has been done so far, but in comparison with sulfasalazine, it was equivalent. Take 350 mg three times daily.

- **Try butyrate enemas.** Butyrate is the preferred fuel of the colonic cells. It is produced when fiber in the colon is fermented by intestinal flora, predominantly bifidobacteria. A few studies have shown that butyrate enemas, taken twice daily, helped heal active distal ulcerative colitis.

- **Explore herbal remedies.** Demulcent herbs—marshmallow, slippery elm, acacia, chickweed, comfrey, mullein, and plantain—are beneficial and soothing to the intestinal membranes and help stimulate mucus production. All are gentle enough to be used at will; try them in capsule or tea form. Other herbs used by people with bowel disease include wild indigo, purple cornflower, echinacea, American cranesbill, goldenseal, cabbage powder, wild yam, bayberry, agrimony, neem, aloe vera, chamomile, feverfew, ginger, ginkgo biloba, Saint-John's-wort, milk thistle, valerian, peppermint, hawthorn, and Lapacho.

- **Drink aloe vera juice.** Aloe vera juice has been used as a traditional remedy for digestive disorders of all types. A randomized, double-blind, placebo-controlled trial was done using oral aloe vera gel in people with active colitis. A total of 44 people were given 3 ounces daily of either aloe vera gel or a placebo for four weeks. People who received the aloe vera had a significant reduction of all disease symptoms in comparison with people who received the placebo.
- **Try bovine cartilage**. Bovine cartilage is shown to have anti-inflammatory and wound-healing properties. Its benefit has been documented in many illnesses, including ulcerative colitis, hemorrhoids and fissures, rheumatoid arthritis, and osteoarthritis.

HEMORRHOIDS

About half of Americans over the age of 50 have hemorrhoids. They are not life-threatening or dangerous, but they can be painful and might bleed. They occur when blood vessels in and around the anus get swollen and stretch under pressure, similar to varicose veins in the legs. They are found either inside the anus (internal hemorrhoids) or under the skin around the anus (external hemorrhoids). Internal hemorrhoids may become so swollen that they push through the anus. When they become irritated, inflamed, and painful, they are called protruding hemorrhoids.

Straining during bowel movements is a common cause of hemorrhoids. The most common symptom is bright red blood with a bowel movement. Hemorrhoids are also common but temporary during pregnancy. Hormonal changes cause the blood vessels to expand. During childbirth, extreme pressure is put on the anus. Hemorrhoids also occur in people with chronic constipation or diarrhea. Sitting for long periods, heavy lifting, and genetics are other influential factors. In most cases, hemorrhoids go away in a few days. If you have bleeding that lasts longer, have your doctor examine you to rule out a more serious problem.

Fiber and Hemorrhoids

A high-fiber diet with plenty of fluids—water, fruit juices, and herbal teas—helps prevent hemorrhoids because fiber and fluids soften stool so they pass through easily. No straining with bowel movements means less pressure on the blood vessels near your anus. So, increase your intake of fruits, whole grains, legumes, and vegetables, especially those containing the most fiber: asparagus, Brussels sprouts, cabbage, carrots, cauliflower, corn, peas, kale, and parsnips. Eating a high-fiber breakfast cereal significantly increases your fiber intake.

Could It Be Pinworms?

Hemorrhoids generally don't itch. If your anus itches mainly at night, you might have pinworms. The best time to check for them is at night while you itch. Place a piece of tape around your finger, sticky side out. Put the tape on your anus, pull it off, and check for worms, which look like moving white threads. If you are checking one of your children, you can use the tape method or just look. Another cause of rectal itching is called pruritus ani, which can be caused by food sensitivities, contact with irritating substances (laundry detergent or toilet paper), fungi, bacterial infection, parasites, antibiotics, poor hygiene, or tight clothing. If you have hemorrhoids, you might find relief from the following suggestions.

Prevention

Explore all of the recommendations for constipation (earlier in this chapter).

Healing Options

- **Change your bathroom habits.** In many countries, people squat to relieve themselves. A squatting position on the toilet takes pressure off the rectum and can help during a flare-up of hemorrhoids. (You may feel a little silly, but who's watching?) Also, wipe gently with soft toilet paper. It may help to wash your anal area with warm water after each bowel movement, or if you have a bidet, now is the time to use it.
- **Use salves.** Salves can soothe inflamed tissues. Spread vitamin E oil, comfrey, calendula ointment, or goldenseal salve gently on the anus with your fingers. Witch hazel is also soothing to hemorrhoidal tissue. Put some on a cotton ball and press gently. Repeat treatments several times daily.
- **Take sitz baths.** Sitz baths are an old-fashioned remedy for hemorrhoids that are still in favor with the medical profession. Place three to four inches of warm water in the bathtub, and sit in it for 10 minutes several times daily. You can improve the results by adding 1/4 cup Epsom salts or healing herbs. Chamomile, chickweed, comfrey, mullein, plantain, witch hazel, and yarrow are all healing and soothing to mucous membranes. Most of these are weeds and may even be growing in your yard. (Comfrey is a very easy herb to grow; just put it in a place where it can spread. It helps with wound healing of any sort and is also soothing for colds and lung problems.) Bring a large pot of water to a boil. Steep 1 to 2 cups of fresh herbs or 1½ cups of dried herbs until cool; strain and add to bathwater.
- **Use horse chestnuts.** Horse chestnuts, also called buckeyes, help tone blood vessels, improve their elasticity, and reduce inflammation. They can also be used in a sitz bath. Chop up 2 cups of horse chestnuts, add to boiled water, strain, and

add infusion to bathwater. Sit in the bath twice daily for 10 to 15 minutes. You can also take 500 mg of the bark orally three times daily. Horse chestnut salves are also available.

- **Use butcher's broom.** Butcher's broom helps strengthen blood vessels and improves circulation. Take 100 mg extract three times daily.
- **Take vitamin E.** Vitamin E helps bring oxygen to the tissues and promotes healing. You can use it topically or take it internally. One small study used vitamin E as a rectal suppository. That makes sense—put it where you need it. Take 400 to 800 IU of d-alpha tocopherol and mixed tocopherols daily.
- **Take vitamin C and bioflavonoids.** Vitamin C and bioflavonoids increase capillary and blood vessel strength so that they don't rupture easily. Bioflavonoids are also essential to collagen formation and elasticity of blood vessels. Berries of all types and cherries have high amounts of protective bioflavonoids. Take 500 to 2,000 mg vitamin C daily plus 100 to 1,000 mg bioflavonoids, which can usually be purchased in a single supplement.
- **Use dimethyl sulfoxide (DMSO).** In the literature, there is one anecdotal study in which a physician used DMSO topically for hemorrhoids. By his report, a 70 percent solution of DMSO will dissolve blood-engorged hemorrhoids almost overnight. It may be worth trying.

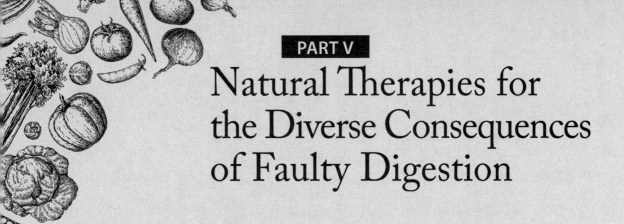

PART V

Natural Therapies for the Diverse Consequences of Faulty Digestion

"Disease bias means that we take health for granted, waiting to act when health is gone and disease emerges. Once we make this assumption, we can soon become so preoccupied that our horizon is filled with diseases to combat. Because disease looms so large, our sight is obscured to the possibilities of health."

—Russell Jaffe, MD

Part V discusses how digestion is linked to issues you would never imagine, including arthritis of all types; autoimmune diseases such as multiple sclerosis, scleroderma, and Behcet's disease; chronic fatigue syndrome; eczema; fibromyalgia; migraine headaches; obesity; psoriasis; schizophrenia; and women's health issues. When looked at through the lens of the DIGIN model and balanced pH, there can be significant improvements in these conditions. (Asthma, autism, attention deficit disorder, attention deficit hyperactivity disorder, and many other conditions have been included in *Digestive Wellness for Children*.)

For each health condition, you'll find general information about the disease, recommendations for functional laboratory testing, and healing options, with the most important ones discussed first. With careful investigation and patience, you may find the underlying conditions that influence how you feel. Many of the supplements and herbs can be found in combination products. You will note that although these health conditions are different, many of the healing options are the same. This goes back to the basic digestive principles presented in the DIGIN model and lifestyle changes from the first half of the book.

Of course, if at first you don't find major improvement, keep working at it. You may not have found the best remedy or combination of therapies on the first try. Patience and perseverance bring the best results. It takes time to resolve chronic illnesses.

Arthritis and Other Connective Tissue Disorders: Osteoarthritis, Rheumatoid Arthritis, Psoriatic Arthritis, Ankylosing Spondylitis, Scleroderma, and Sjögren's Syndrome Q DIGIN

Arthritis refers to more than a hundred diseases that cause inflammation of the joints. The old-fashioned term for arthritis is rheumatism, and today physicians who specialize in arthritis are called rheumatologists. Arthritis affects 40 million Americans and accounts for 46 million medical visits per year. It affects about 15 percent of our population and 3 percent of those severely, but it is severe in 11 percent of people ages 65 and older.

The two most common types of arthritis are osteoarthritis and rheumatoid arthritis (RA). Other common types include psoriatic arthritis, ankylosing spondylitis, gout, Lyme disease, Reiter's syndrome, lupus, and Sjögren's syndrome. Each of these diseases has its own characteristics, but they all share the symptoms of pain and inflammation in joints.

There are many causes of arthritis: genetics, infections, physical injury, nutritional deficiencies, allergies, metabolic and immune disorders, stress, and environmental pollutants and toxins. Several types of arthritis have well-documented associations with faulty digestive function. Osteoarthritis responds well to dietary changes. Rheumatoid arthritis, ankylosing spondylitis, lupus, Sjögren's syndrome, and Reiter's syndrome are all autoimmune conditions. As such, leaky gut probably plays a role, along with environment and genetics.

The current drugs of choice for mild to moderate arthritis pain are nonsteroidal anti-inflammatory drugs (NSAIDs). Although they may help with the pain, many NSAIDs also have a negative effect on the ability of cartilage to repair itself. They block our body's ability to regenerate cartilage tissue by lowering the amounts of heal-ing prostaglandins, glycosaminoglycans, and hyaluronan, and by raising leukotriene levels. NSAIDs block the production of healing prostaglandins, which stimulate repair of the digestive lining. This causes increased intestinal permeability. (See Chapter 4 for more information on NSAIDS and leaky gut.) Use of NSAIDs in children with rheumatoid arthritis showed that 75 percent had gastrointestinal problems caused by the drugs. And the more NSAIDs people take, the leakier the gut wall becomes; the leakier the gut, the more pain and inflammation follows, which sets up a continuously escalating problem. For rheumatoid arthritis and other autoimmune types of arthritis, disease-modifying, anti-arthritic drugs (DMARDS) are used. There is a wide variety of these, and they all have significant long-term unwanted effects.

Use of natural therapies and dietary change for arthritis can reduce the need for such medications and their accompanying side effects. Natural therapies can be used to help relieve pain, reduce inflammation, help regenerate cartilage, and slow the disease process. These natural therapies can be astonishingly effective. Look to all aspects of the DIGIN model if you have arthritis of any type. Balancing these can be the key to resolving your pain.

FOOD SENSITIVITIES, LEAKY GUT, AND ARTHRITIS

The dietary connection between rheumatoid arthritis and food sensitivities was first noted by Michael Zeller in 1949 in *Annals of Allergy*. He found a direct cause and effect by adding and eliminating foods from the diet. He joined forces with Drs. Herbert Rinkel and Theron Randolph to publish a book called *Food Allergy* in 1951.

Theron Randolph, MD was the father of a field of medicine called clinical ecology, which studies how our environment affects health. He found that people with rheuma-toid arthritis who were not reacting to foods had at least one sensitivity to an environ-mental chemical. Randolph sent questionnaires to more than 200 of his patients with osteoarthritis and rheumatoid arthritis to assess how well treatments were working. Their responses showed that when they avoided food and environmental allergens, there was a significant reduction in arthritic symptoms. Randolph also felt that other types of arthritis, including Reiter's syndrome, ankylosing spondylitis, and psoriatic arthritis, have an ecological basis. Dr. Randolph was a visionary and pioneer.

Since then, other studies have been done on the relationship between food sen-sitivities and arthritis. In a study of 43 people with arthritis of the hands, a water fast of three days brought improvement in tenderness, swelling, strength of grip, pain, joint circumference, function, and sedimentation (SED) rate (a simple blood test that determines a breakdown of tissue somewhere in the body). When some of these people were tested with single foods, symptoms recurred in 22 out of 27 people. In other studies, the foods most likely to provoke symptoms after an elimination diet were (in order of most to least) corn, wheat, bacon or pork, oranges, milk, oats, rye, eggs, beef, coffee, malt, cheese, grapefruit, tomato, peanuts, sugar, butter, lamb, lemon, and soy. Cereals were the most common food, with wheat and corn causing problems in more than 50 percent of the people.

Another study found that 44 out of 93 people with rheumatoid arthritis had elevated levels of IgG to gliadin. Among these 44 people, 86 percent had positive RA factors. In yet another study, 15 out of 24 people had raised levels of IgA, rheumatoid factor, and wheat protein IgG with a biopsy of the jejunum. Six of the wheat-positive people and one of the wheat-negative people had damage to the brush borders of their intestines. The researchers felt that the intestines play an important role in the progression of rheumatoid arthritis. Increased intestinal permeability allows more food particles to cross the intestinal mucosa, which triggers a greater sensitivity response.

Hvatut and colleagues measured IgG, IgA, and IgM antibodies in serum and intestinal fluid in 17 people with rheumatoid arthritis and 20 healthy controls. They concluded that measuring food antibodies in intestinal fluid gives a more "striking" result between rheumatoid arthritis, food sensitivities, and the immune activation of the mucosal lining (mucosal-associated lymphoid tissue, or MALT).

Kallikorm and Uibo reported that of 74 people admitted to the hospital with arthritic diseases, 12 percent had elevated antigliadin antibodies, indicating gluten intolerance; 1 person had celiac disease. Because people with one autoimmune disease are more susceptible to other autoimmune diseases, it's good to screen for celiac and gluten intolerance.

The concept of food sensitivity and increased intestinal permeability is gaining acceptance as more physicians see the clinical changes in their patients when they use this approach. Testing for food and environmental sensitivities, parasites, toxic metals, candidiasis, and intestinal permeability and performing a comprehensive digestive stool analysis (CDSA) often provide an understanding of an underlying cause of the disease.

DYSBIOSIS AND ARTHRITIS

Dysbiosis has been found to be a factor in many connective tissue diseases, including rheumatoid arthritis, systemic lupus, Sjögren's syndrome, and scleroderma.

Candidiasis frequently plays a role in "fungal" arthritis and is a possible aggravator in rheumatoid arthritis. While common in people who are on immunosuppressant drugs, it is beginning to be seen in people who have normal immune health. It has been found in the synovial fluid of knee joints, yet how often do physicians actually test synovial fluid for infection? Fungus in people with arthritis can be the result of using antibiotics, oral contraceptives, or steroid medications; increased use of alcohol or sugar; or a stressed immune system. Treatment of candidiasis in the digestive system has improved rheumatoid symptoms in many cases.

In many types of arthritis, known microbes trigger a molecular mimicry that then activates the disease. Genetics play a large role in these conditions. A total of 96 percent of people with ankylosing spondylitis have the HLA-B27 genotype, compared to 8 percent of the general population. In rheumatoid arthritis, 90 percent have the HLA-DR1 or HLA-DR4 gene. Rheumatoid arthritis is associated with *Proteus mirabilis* infection, *Porphyromonas gingivalis*, *Yersinia enterocolitica*, *Salmonella typhi*, *Shigella flexneri*, *Campylobacter jejuni*, *Klebsiella pneumoniae*, *Clostridium difficile*, *Candida albicans*, *Mycobacterium tuberculosis*, *Mycoplasma arthritidis*, *Borrelia burgdorferi*, Parvovirus, Epstein-Barr virus, and more.

Reactive arthritis is triggered by a gastrointestinal (GI) infection of several organisms, including salmonella, yersinia, campylobacter, and in the urinary tract, chlamydia and other microbes. Ankylosing spondylitis occurs in 20 percent of people who have reactive arthritis within a decade or two. Both of these conditions share the same HLA-B27 genotype. Ankylosing spondylitis has been associated with *K. pneumoniae, S. flexneri, and Y. enterocolitica*.

Infection can trigger arthritis and joint inflammation. Why they move to the joints or cause joint pain is unknown at this time. But the phenomenon is well documented. If candida, Lyme disease, chlamydia, klebsiella, salmonella, or another infection is present, your physician can recommend a variety of therapeutics, including both natural and pharmaceutical remedies.

NUTRITIONAL DEFICIENCIES

There is documentation in the literature about arthritis and deficiencies of nearly every known nutrient. When the needed nutrients are supplied, the body can begin to balance itself. Though many nutritional and herbal products help arthritis sufferers, no one thing works for everyone, so persist until you find the therapies that work best for you. Give each one at least a three-month trial before giving up on it. I remember Abram Hoffer, MD, speaking about a patient at a conference many years ago. He had recommended the man take 1,000 mg of vitamin C daily for his arthritis. The man took the vitamin C faithfully each day without any improvement. After a whole year, he suddenly became pain-free. So give whatever you try some time—maybe not a year, but at least a few months.

EXERCISE AND ARTHRITIS

Exercise and stretching are useful for all types of arthritic conditions. Yoga has been found to help with range of motion, pain, stiffness, and joint tenderness. Walking, swimming, physical therapy, and massage therapy may all play a role in reduction of symptoms. Movement is not optional. Even small amounts can give great relief.

OSTEOARTHRITIS

Osteoarthritis is the most common type of arthritis and the one we associate with aging, although nutritionally oriented physicians believe it has more to do with poor dietary habits and biochemical imbalances than age. Pain is usually the first symptom. The main characteristics are stiffness, aches, and painful joints that creak and crack. Stiffness may be worse in the morning and after exercise. Osteoarthritis begins gradually and usually affects one or a few joints, most commonly the knees, hips, fingers, ankles, and feet. As joints enlarge, cartilage degenerates. Eventually, hardening leads to bone spurs. You lose flexibility, strength, and the ability to grasp, accompanied by pain. Risk of osteoarthritis, especially arthritis in the knee, increases if you are overweight; losing weight helps. Acid-alkaline balance is also important in treating this illness.

RHEUMATOID ARTHRITIS (RA)

RA is characterized by inflammation of joints, most often in the hands, feet, wrists, elbows, and ankles, with symmetrical involvement. It can start in virtually any joint. The onset may be sudden, with pain in multiple joints; or it may come on gradually, with more and more joints becoming involved. Joints become swollen, feel tender, and can degenerate and become misshapen. Joints are often stiffest in the mornings and also feel worse after movement. RA is most common in women and in people who smoke. In a blood test, the rheumatoid factor (RF) will be elevated in most cases of rheumatoid arthritis. While it may get better or worse, once established RA is nearly always present to some extent. Treatment is aimed at lowering inflammation and TNF-alpha.

Many drugs are being used to treat rheumatoid arthritis, which can dramatically lessen pain and improve quality of life. Yet, all have complicating side effects. Natural therapies are an adjunct or replacement for medical intervention. For example, fish oils and curcumin lower TNF-alpha.

Rheumatoid arthritis has a genetic component, often running in families. It is believed to be triggered by a bacterial infection having the "right" genetics (HLA-DR1/4), and autoimmunity caused by a molecular mimicry. The infectious microbe disrupts the gut barrier. When genes meet the environment and a leaky gut, the illness is triggered. The gene marker HLA-DR1/4 is present in 50 to 75 percent of people with rheumatoid arthritis.

Many microbes are associated with rheumatoid arthritis, such as the following: proteus mirabilis, Epstein-Barr virus, mycobacteria, mycoplasma, chlamydia, yersinia, salmonella, shigella, campylobacter, staphylococcus, streptococcus, candida, clostridium, borrelia, leptospira, erysipelothrix, klebsiella, and oral bacteria.

P. mirabilis is a bacterium that can cause bladder and wound infections and bacteremia and trigger RA. *P. mirabilis* produces lipopolysaccharides (LPS) that inflame gut mucosa and increase permeability. It causes no problems in most people, but in people who have the HLA-DR1/4 genotype, it acts as a genetic mimic that cross-reacts with collagen XI and hyaline cartilage, breaking down the cartilage. It's postulated that incidence of RA is higher in smokers because smoking puts people more at risk of developing urinary tract infections. In one study, a decrease in antibodies to *P. mirabilis* was observed in subjects on a vegetarian diet. Proteus infections can be treated with either natural or pharmaceutical therapy.

Waldemar Rastawicki and colleagues in Poland studied 92 patients with RA. They were tested for bacterial genes in synovial fluid and blood. While bacterial genes weren't discovered, antigens to pathogenic bacteria were found: salmonella (8.6 percent), yersinia (20.7 percent), and enterobacterial common antigen (34.9 percent).

A 1973 study by Mardh and colleagues reported mycobacteria in synovial fluid. Just recently, a friend with chronic knee issues had her synovial fluid tested and discovered that she had Lyme disease.

Vegetarian, vegan, and raw-food diets have been shown in numerous studies to be successful at reducing the symptoms of rheumatoid arthritis. Vegetable-based diets help balance pH levels. They also provide an abundance of antioxidants, natural anti-inflammatory factors, vitamins, minerals, and phytonutrients. This diet also tends to be more hypoallergenic. Add fish oil to increase the benefits. Short-term fasting prior to beginning the vegetarian diet has also been shown to provide long-term benefits. Please work with a good nutritionist.

It's hard to generalize or predict which of these factors will be found in each person, but usually one or more is present. Each of them needs to be investigated. Leaky gut is probably not a primary cause of rheumatoid arthritis, but long-term use of medications used for the arthritis often makes it a factor.

PSORIATIC ARTHRITIS

Psoriatic arthritis affects 30 percent of people with psoriasis (the incidence used to be 3 to 7 percent), about 1.4 million Americans. People with severe psoriasis are more likely to develop psoriatic arthritis. In addition to the usual symptoms of psoriasis, they also have joint pain, tenderness, or swelling in the fingers, toes, or spine. Other symptoms include reduced range of motion, morning stiffness, redness and pain of the eye that is similar to conjunctivitis, and nail changes with pitting or lifting of the nail. Psoriatic arthritis is rarely found in people who do not also have psoriasis. Psoriatic arthritis is associated with bone erosion and deformities that affect half of the people with this disease. Skin and joint symptoms may flare up or improve simultaneously. Psoriatic arthritis closely resembles rheumatoid arthritis, although people with psoriatic arthritis usually have a negative rheumatoid factor. This disease can be mild, but it can also be severely deforming and disabling.

Like other types of autoimmune disease, psoriatic arthritis has genetic, environmental, and immunologic origins. The gene marker HLA-B27 is present in most people with this disease.

Inflammation of psoriatic arthritis is involved with arachidonic acid pathways and TNF-alpha. Biologic drug therapies, such as injectable infliximab and etanercept, aim at lower TNF-alpha levels. A healthy diet plus essential fatty acids help reduce and prevent further inflammation. Evening primrose, borage, and fish oils; turmeric; curcumin; bromelain; and quercetin all work on these pathways.

Li and Wang used traditional Chinese medicine (TCM) and integrative medicine in working with 47 people with psoriatic arthritis. In the study, 17 people were given TCM only, and 30 were given a combination of TCM and integrative medicine. Dosages of medications were reduced as symptoms were relieved, cured, or improved. They concluded that TCM and integrative medicine are effective for people with psoriatic arthritis with fewer negative effects than current medical treatment.

ANKYLOSING SPONDYLITIS (AS)

Ankylosing spondylitis (AS) is characterized by a progressive fusion of joints in and around the spine. Caucasian men constitute 90 percent of those with the illness, and it typically becomes evident between the ages of 10 and 30. It starts off as a low backache, which is often worse in the mornings. Symptoms get progressively worse and spread from the lower back to the midback and up to the neck. The spine gradually becomes fused. Later, shoulders, hips, and knees may be affected. Symptoms flare and subside.

The role of dysbiosis in ankylosing spondylitis is the most researched and best understood of all the arthritic diseases. Most researchers believe that AS is triggered by an inherited gene and interactions with the environment. Much research has been done on the role of infection as a primary trigger of AS. The gene implicated is HLA-B27, although others may still be found. HLA-B27 is present in 96 percent of people with ankylosing spondylitis. This marker is also present in 8 percent of the general population. Research shows 70 to 80 percent of people with ankylosing spondylitis have klebsiella bacteria in their stools. Yersinia, shigella, and salmonella bacteria are also associated with this process and may contribute to the disease in people who are not infected with klebsiella. These bacteria may not normally cause disease, but in people with the HLA-B27 gene marker, antibodies produced to kill the bacteria cross-react, causing pain and inflammation. This concept of autoimmune disease may explain why some people get certain illnesses and others don't. It's the presence not only of a specific gene, but also of a microbe or other environmental trigger that activates the disease process.

It is important to make an early diagnosis of ankylosing spondylitis so that progression of the disease can be slowed or halted. Because it usually appears as a low backache, many people will tend to seek chiropractic help or massage therapy or take anti-inflammatory medications. But such remedies can't correct dysbiosis in the intestinal tract. Because many men commonly have low-back pain, they often have irreversible damage before a correct diagnosis is made. Still, I have a friend who had ankylosing spondylitis that had progressed and affected his life greatly. He began working with a yoga therapist, eventually becoming a yoga therapist himself, and along with other natural therapies, he has made his issues a problem of the past.

In people with ankylosing spondylitis, also think about gluten intolerance. In a study by Togrol of 30 people, 36.7 percent were found to have antigliadin antibodies. Three of these people (10 percent) also had positive anti-endomysial antibodies. I personally know two men with AS who have experienced positive benefit from being on a gluten-free diet. Other studies have failed to show any significant difference in celiac disease rates in people with AS in comparison with control groups. There is no research on nonceliac gluten sensitivity (NCGS) or nonceliac wheat sensitivity (NCWS) in this population.

Leaky gut syndrome is present in people with ankylosing spondylitis. Unfortunately, NSAIDs are commonly used to treat ankylosing spondylitis, causing even greater intestinal permeability. This, in turn, causes more sensitivity to foods and environmental substances.

About half the people with ankylosing spondylitis experience dramatic improvement when they eliminate dairy products. In one study, 13 out of 25 people had good results, and another 4 had moderate improvements. Of the respondents whose results were good, 8 were able to discontinue NSAID medication, and 6 patients from this study remained dairy-free for more than two years because they were so satisfied with the results. The elimination of dairy products is a simple and effective treatment to try. Although the mechanism for this improvement is unclear, it is suggested that a dairy-free diet modifies the bacterial ecosystem of the gut, which may have benefits. Another hypothesis is that milk allergy causes chronic irritation to the gut as well as gut permeability.

Klebsiella and other disease-producing microbes that can contribute to ankylosing spondylitis use sugars and starches as their main food source. Some physicians are experimenting with a low-starch diet and are getting good results. Eliminate all breads, grains, pasta, cookies, candy, root vegetables, and legumes. Be patient: You may get amazing results, but you will need to stay on the diet for at least six months before you really reap the benefits.

I recently queried two friends with AS about what has been most helpful. They both responded that exercise and stretching have given the best response.

Functional Laboratory Testing
The letters following each list item indicate the illness that that test can be used to detect. Note that O = osteoarthritis, RA = rheumatoid arthritis, PA = psoriatic arthritis, and AS = ankylosing spondylitis.

- ELISA/ACT allergy testing for foods, molds, medications, and chemicals (O, RA, PA, AS)
- Organic acid testing (O, RA, PA, AS)
- Comprehensive digestive stool analysis (O, RA, PA, AS)
- Intestinal permeability screening; stop use of NSAIDs for three weeks prior to the test (O, RA, PA, AS)

- Candida testing, either separately or in CDSA (O, RA, PA, AS)
- Heidelberg capsule testing for hydrochloric acid (HCl) status (RA)
- Small intestinal bacterial overgrowth (SIBO) breath test (RA)
- Liver function testing; people with rheumatoid arthritis are also shown to have reduced function in the detoxification pathways (RA)

Healing Options

Some of these suggestions will significantly help your arthritis; others may not help at all. You can look for products that combine these nutrients and herbs. Be patient and give whatever you try time to work. Try one or two at a time until you find a program that suits your body's unique needs and your lifestyle. Recommendations work for all types of arthritis, unless I've specifically noted a type after the suggestion.

To Reduce Pain and Inflammation

- **Try one of the therapeutic diets mentioned in Chapter 14.** Unless you have symptoms similar to irritable bowel syndrome (IBS), begin with the elimination diet.
- **Exercise.** It's important to use your body as much as you can without aggravating the condition. Yoga, walking, swimming, stretching, water exercises, physical therapy, massage, and acupressure massage may all be helpful. Do something nearly every day.
- **Try the nightshade diet.** In the 1970s, Norman Childers, a horticulturist, popularized the nightshade diet. Elimination of nightshade foods helps only about 15 percent of people with arthritis, but the people who respond are usually helped a great deal. The nightshade foods are potatoes, tomatoes, eggplant, and peppers (red, green, yellow, and chili). Steven Gundry, in his book *The Plant Paradox*, has expanded on this approach, excluding all high-lectin foods with anecdotal success in arthritis. Thus far, no research on low-lectin diets has been published. An elimination diet of two weeks followed by a reintroduction of these foods provides a good test. Blood testing also picks up these sensitivities.
- **Try yucca.** Yucca has been used by Native Americans of the Southwest to alleviate symptoms of arthritis and improve digestion. It's a rich source of saponins with anti-inflammatory effects. Studies have been done with both rheumatoid and osteoarthritis with significant improvement in 56 to 66 percent of the people who tried it. People taking yucca for more than one and a half years had the additional advantage of improved triglyceride and cholesterol levels and reduction in high blood pressure, with no negative side effects. Take two to eight tablets daily.

- **Take cetyl myristoleate (CM).** Harry Diehl, a researcher at the National Institutes of Health, found that mice did not develop arthritis when CM was given. When he himself developed arthritis, Diehl took CM and his arthritis resolved. Jonathan Wright, MD, has found CM to be clinically valuable in about half of his patients. CM appears to actually cure arthritis in many instances. I was able to find two studies on CM that had astounding results. CM was found to be best used in combination with glucosamine sulfate, sea cucumber, and methylsulfonylmethane (MSM). Recommended duration of use is two to four weeks. Carbonated beverages, caffeine, chocolate, and cigarettes are not allowed while taking CM and its associated supplements.

- **Take vitamin C ascorbate.** Vitamin C is an essential nutrient for every anti-arthritis program. It is vital for formation of cartilage and collagen, a fibrous protein that forms strong connective tissue necessary for bone strength. Vitamin C also plays a role in immune response, helping protect us from disease-producing microbes. Many types of arthritis are caused by microbes, which vitamin C helps combat. It also inhibits formation of inflammatory prostaglandins, helping to reduce pain, inflammation, and swelling. Vitamin C is also an antioxidant and free radical scavenger; free radical formation has been noted in arthritic conditions. Take 1 to 3 grams daily in an ascorbate or ester form. For best results, try a vitamin C flush weekly for four weeks. (See Chapter 11.)

- **Increase omega-3 fatty acids and fish oils.** Fish oils come from cold-water fish and contain eicosapentaenoic acid (EPA) and docosahexaenoic acid (DHA). The fish with the highest levels are salmon, mackerel, halibut, sardines, tuna, and herring. These omega-3 fatty acids are essential because we cannot synthesize them and must obtain them from our foods. Fish oils inhibit production of inflammatory prostaglandin E2 series, cyclooxygenase, and thromboxane A2, all of which come from arachidonic acid. Fish oils shift the production to thromboxane A3, which causes less constriction of blood vessels and platelet stickiness than thromboxane A2. Research has shown fish oils are really helpful for some people with arthritis, reducing morning stiffness and joint tenderness. Fish oil capsules produce moderate but definite improvement in arthritic diseases at dosages from 8 to 20 capsules daily. Similar results can be obtained by eating fish with high EPA/DHA two to four times a week. Because fish oils increase blood clotting time, they should not be used by people who have hemophilia or who take anticoagulant medicines or aspirin regularly. High dosages in capsule form should be monitored by a physician.

- **Take gamma-linolenic acid (GLA) (RA).** In one study, patients with rheumatoid arthritis were given 1.4 grams of GLA from borage oil daily. It significantly reduced their symptoms: swollen joints by 36 percent, tenderness by 45 percent, swollen joint count by 28 percent, and swollen joint score by 41 percent. (Some people responded in more than one area.) Use of evening primrose oil in the study group and olive oil for the control group showed that both oils helped reduce pain and morning stiffness. Several people were able to reduce use of NSAIDs, but none were able to stop the medication. The modest results in this study were probably due to the use of NSAIDs with the evening primrose oil. The same results could be obtained by use of evening primrose or borage oil alone. Take 1,400 mg.

- **Take and/or eat ginger.** Ginger is an old Ayurvedic remedy that was given to people with RA and OA. In one study, it reduced pain and swelling in various amounts in 75 percent of the people tested, with no reported side effects over three months to two and a half years. Ginger can be used as an ingredient in food and tea or taken as a supplement. Take 2 ounces fresh ginger or 3,000 to 7,000 mg powdered ginger daily.

- **Take niacinamide.** Most of the B-complex vitamins have been shown to reduce inflammation and swelling associated with arthritis. Dr. Kaufman, MD, PhD, an expert on arthritis, recommended using niacinamide at a rather high dosage with excellent results. It doesn't cure the arthritis, but it really helps while you take it. If you are going to try this, do so with your physician's supervision. High levels of niacinamide can be liver toxic. Take 250 to 500 mg daily. Soft gel capsules are recommended. Make sure to get a brand without colors, preservatives, or solvents.

- **Take folic acid plus vitamin B$_{12}$.** In a recent study, those with osteoarthritis in their hands were given 20 mcg vitamin B$_{12}$ plus 6,400 mcg folic acid daily. They reported a significant reduction in symptoms. This is a tiny amount of vitamin B$_{12}$ and a large amount of folic acid, which is nontoxic even at these high levels.

- **Take superoxide dismutase (SOD).** SOD plays an important role in reducing inflammation and has been used alone, with copper, manganese or copper, and zinc for various arthritic conditions. Some physicians are using SOD in injections. Oral SOD doesn't seem to work as well, except when used in a copper-zinc preparation. Wheatgrass extracts of SOD can be purchased at health-food stores. Most people who try them experience benefits, but there is little scientific research to date. Some veterinarians are using wheatgrass SOD with arthritic animals with excellent results.

- **Take S-adenosylmethionine (SAMe).** A recent player on the scene is SAMe, a chemical that is found naturally in every living cell. Research in 10 studies that included more than 22,000 people has shown SAMe to have powerful antidepressant effects without the side effects of pharmaceutical antidepressant medications. SAMe has also been shown to be as potent an anti-inflammatory drug as indomethacin and other NSAIDs, with fewer negative effects. This product is expensive because it is difficult to stabilize. Use it with a good multivitamin that contains B-complex vitamins. Take 400 mg twice daily. Adjust up or down as needed.

- **Take methylsulfonylmethane (MSM) or dimethyl sulfoxide (DMSO).** DMSO is highly effective for reducing arthritis pain when used on skin. It has a distinct odor that prevents many people from using it, but MSM is odorless. MSM, a naturally occurring derivative of dimethyl sulfoxide, is now being used as a supplement. MSM has been found to be an antioxidant and anti-inflammatory in animal studies, probably because of its high sulfur content. It helps reduce pain and inflammation and gives the body the sulfur compounds necessary to build cartilage and collagen. It is also useful in allergies, blood sugar control, and asthma. Take 1,000 to 5,000 mg daily. It is best when taken with 1,000 to 5,000 mg of vitamin C for absorption. Or use DMSO topically on skin.

- **Take bromelain.** Bromelain is an enzyme derived from pineapple that acts as an anti-inflammatory in much the same way that evening primrose, fish, and borage oils do. It interferes with production of arachidonic acid, shifting to prostaglandin production of the less inflammatory type. It also prevents platelet aggregation and interferes with the growth of malignant cells. It appears to be as effective as NSAID medications at reducing inflammation. Bromelain can be taken with meals as a digestive aid, but as an anti-inflammatory, it must be taken between meals. Take 500 to 1,000 mg two to three times daily between meals.

- **Take quercetin.** Quercetin is the most effective bioflavonoid in its anti-inflammatory effects; others include bromelain, curcumin, and rutin. Bioflavonoids help maintain collagen tissue by decreasing membrane permeability and cross-linking collagen fibers, making them stronger. Quercetin can be used to reduce pain and inflammatory responses and for control of allergies. Take 500 to 2,000 mg daily. It appears to reduce inflammatory cytokines.

- **Take boswellia.** Boswellia is taken over the long term as a treatment for rheumatoid arthritis, not specifically for immediate pain. Boswellia serrata, an Ayurvedic remedy that has been traditionally used for arthritis, pain, and inflammation, has been shown to moderate inflammatory markers such as nitric oxide and 5-lipoxygenase. In a study, a specific preparation of boswellia called H-15 was given to 260 people and found to be effective in treating rheumatoid arthritis. Fifty to 60 percent of the subjects had good results. Take 1,200 mg two or three times daily.

- **Take turmeric or curcumin.** Four or five mornings each week, I add a hunk of fresh ginger and another of fresh turmeric to my morning smoothie. Turmeric has been shown to have powerful anti-inflammatory properties. Some of the mechanisms involved include its ability to block leukotrienes and arachidonic acid, both of which cause inflammation and pain. An effective dosage of turmeric is 10 to 60 grams daily. Curcumin, the active pain-relieving ingredient, can be taken in much smaller doses, 500 mg three times daily. Fresh turmeric can be found in some grocery stores and natural food stores, and in Indian grocery stores. If you live in a tropical area you can grow tumeric; it is a lovely flowering garden plant. Turmeric can be juiced, grated, used in stir-fry, and eaten freely.

- **Take devil's claw.** Devil's claw (*Harpagophytum procumbens*) is a South African root that is commonly used as an arthritis remedy. It reduces pain and inflammation. Several studies have shown it to work as well as phenylbutazone, a common NSAID medication. It is commonly used in low-potency homeopathic dilutions of 2X in Germany. This is a dilution of one part per hundred of devil's claw in a homeopathically potentized form. Devil's claw can also be found as an herbal supplement in capsules and as tinctures.

- **Use black cohosh.** Black cohosh (*Cimicifuga racemosa*) has long been used by European and American herbalists to reduce muscle spasm, pain, and inflammation. It can be used as either a tincture or in capsules.

- **Use capsicum (cayenne pepper).** Cayenne has been well studied for its temporary relief of arthritis pain. Creams with capsicum are used topically to relieve pain. (These creams may burn a bit when first applied.) In various studies, typically more than half of topical-cream users experience pain relief. The creams are available over the counter and by prescription.

- **Try DL-phenylalanine (DLPA) (RA).** DLPA is an amino acid that is used therapeutically for pain and depression. It is effective for treating rheumatoid arthritis, osteoarthritis, low-back pain, and migraines. "D" is the naturally found form, and "L" is its synthetic mirror. The combination of DL slows down the release of the phenylalanine. It appears to inhibit the breakdown of endorphins, our body's natural pain relievers. Take 400 to 500 mg three times daily.

To Nourish and Regenerate the Joints and Connective Tissue

- **Take a multivitamin with minerals.** People with arthritis are often deficient in many nutrients. Aging, poor diet, medications, malabsorption, and illness all contribute to poor nutritional status. At least 21 nutrients are essential for formation of bone and cartilage, so it's important to find a supplement that supports these needs. Look for a supplement that contains 500 to 1,000 mg calcium, 400 to 500 mg magnesium, 15 to 45 mg zinc, 1 to 2 mg copper, 10,000 IU vitamin A, 200 mcg selenium, 50 mg vitamin B_6, and 5 to 10 mg manganese in addition to other nutrients. Follow the dosage on the bottle to get nutrients in the appropriate amounts.

■ **Take glucosamine and chondroitin.** Glucosamine sulfate and chondroitin sulfate are nutrients used therapeutically to help repair cartilage, reduce inflammation, and increase mobility. Studies have consistently shown benefits of both glucosamine and chondroitin supplementation. Green-lipped mussels are a rich source of glycosaminoglycans. Use of glucosamine sulfate has no associated side effects, although anecdotally it may raise serum cholesterol levels. It either works or it doesn't. Give it a three-month trial. It's important to buy a product that has been broken down into a molecular size that your body can use. It's worth it to spend more on this product.

■ **Take vitamin E.** In one study, 29 participants with osteoarthritis were given 600 IU of vitamin E or a placebo daily. Out of 15 who received vitamin E, 52 percent reported improvement. Another study showed no improvement in those with osteoarthritis who were given vitamin E supplementation of 1,200 IU daily. Try 800 IU for two to three months. It is very safe and may help some people. Best is the "d-alpha" form of mixed tocopherols. Look for high levels of gamma-tocopherol.

■ **Use copper to treat RA symptoms.** Copper is involved in collagen formation, tissue repair, and anti-inflammatory processes. Rheumatoid arthritis sufferers often have marginal copper levels. Traditionally, copper bracelets have been worn to help reduce arthritic symptoms. W. Ray Walker, PhD, tested those who had benefited from copper bracelets by having them wear copper-colored aluminum bracelets for two months. More than half of the 40 participants reported that their arthritis worsened wearing the fake copper bracelets, and 14 of them deteriorated so much they couldn't finish the two months. Dr. Walker found that 13 mg of copper per month was dissolved by sweat, and presumably much of that was absorbed through the skin. Supplementation with copper increases levels of SOD. Wear a copper bracelet or supplement with 1 to 2 mg daily in a multivitamin preparation. If you are working with a physician, you may temporarily add a supplement of copper salicylate or copper sebacate until copper levels return to normal.

■ **Eat or take alfalfa.** Alfalfa is a tried-and-true folk remedy for arthritis. Many people attest to its benefits, but more research is needed on it. Alfalfa is an abundantly nutritious food, high in minerals, vitamins, antioxidants, and protein, and it may help because of its saponin content or its high nutrient and trace mineral content. It is widely used as a nutritional supplement in animal feed. Take 14 to 24 tablets in two or three doses daily, or grind up alfalfa seeds and take 3 tablespoons of ground seeds each day. You can mix them with applesauce, cottage cheese, or oatmeal or sprinkle them on salads. Another method is to cook 1 ounce of alfalfa seeds in 3 cups of water. Do not boil them, but cook gently in a glass or enamel pan for 30 minutes and strain. Toss away the seeds and keep the tea. Dilute the tea with an equal amount of water. Add honey if you like. Use it all within 24 hours. Yet another method is to soak 1 ounce of alfalfa seeds in 3 cups of water for 12 to 24 hours. Strain and drink the liquid throughout the day.

Diagnose and Treat Dysbiosis

- **Address hypochlorhydria and SIBO (RA).** Low levels of HCl were found in 32 percent of people tested with rheumatoid arthritis. Half of these people had SIBO; 35 percent of patients with normal levels of HCl had SIBO, compared with none of the control group. SIBO was found most in people with active arthritic symptoms. (See Chapter 2 for information on HCl and Chapter 7 on small intestinal bacterial overgrowth.)

Look for Environmental Triggers

- **Examine the side effects of breast implants.** Silicone breast implants may cause rheumatoid-like symptoms in some women, although research is divided on this point. If you have rheumatoid arthritis and silicone or saline breast implants, it would be smart to be tested for silicone antibodies or allergies on an annual basis. Many women feel remarkably better once breast implants have been removed.

SCLERODERMA (SYSTEMIC SCLEROSIS)

Scleroderma is an autoimmune connective-tissue disease characterized by a thickening and loss of elasticity in the skin, joints, digestive tract (especially in the esophagus), lungs, and thyroid; and scarring in the heart and kidneys. The most common initial complaint is loss of circulation in toes or fingers (Raynaud's syndrome), characterized by swelling and a thickening of skin. About 300,000 Americans have scleroderma. Like all autoimmune conditions, scleroderma is linked to genetics and your environment. Scleroderma has been linked to bacterial and viral infections as possible triggers that set up the molecular mimicry that causes cell damage. So far parvovirus B19, cytomegalovirus, Epstein-Barr virus, and retroviruses have been implicated.

There are two forms of the disease: localized, affecting one or two locations, and systemic (also called diffuse), which is found throughout the body. The systemic form can rapidly progress and can be quite serious. Generalized symptoms include fatigue, muscle pain, and arthritis.

People with the more limited form of scleroderma have less involvement, which is mostly confined to the skin on the fingers and face. Changes occur more slowly in this type of scleroderma but in a typical way that has been defined as CREST, which represents the initials of the symptoms. You may have only a few of these signs.

> **Calcinosis:** These are tiny calcium deposits in the skin. They look like hard, whitish areas and are most common on elbows, knees, and fingers. This is not as common as the other indicators.
>
> **Raynaud's phenomenon:** In Raynaud's, there are spasms of tiny arteries and your fingers, toes, nose, ears, and tongue can lose circulation. This is typically triggered by cold, heat, or dampness.
>
> **Esophageal issues:** The lower two-thirds of the esophagus are often affected by poor muscle function. This can lead to gastroesophageal reflux (GERD), which can lead to scarring and narrowing of the esophagus.
>
> **Sclerodactyly:** This is the thickening that occurs on the fingers and toes. It can look shiny and can limit your flexibility and ability to use your fingers and toes.
>
> **Telangiectasias:** These are tiny red areas that most often occur on your face and hands, inside your mouth, and inside your lips. If you press on them, they turn white.

TREATMENT

Medical treatment of scleroderma consists of dealing with symptoms and medical issues as they arise. Proton-pump inhibitors (PPIs) are used for GERD. SIBO is treated with antibiotics. If your lungs or kidneys are affected, those are treated as well. If blood pressure is high, that is also treated.

Integrative treatment consists of looking for underlying triggers and modulating inflammation, use of elimination diets and celiac testing, stress management, looking for and treating infections, looking for allergies and sensitivities to food and environmental chemicals, and anything else that may be of benefit in alleviating symptoms and slowing down the course of the disease.

In one study, use of vitamin B$_6$ and a Chinese medication called Xuefu Zhuyu Decoction were used in 33 people with localized scleroderma. Reductions in inflammation of interleukin-6 (IL-6) and TNF-alpha were similar in both groups. It is believed that the B$_6$ and herbal combination activated blood circulation.

DIGESTION AND SCLERODERMA

GI issues are present in 50 to 90 percent of people with scleroderma. There can be issues in any one of the DIGIN areas, so look at all of them carefully. The most common manifestations of scleroderma are in the esophagus with reflux and difficulty swallowing. If left untreated, this can lead to Barrett's esophagus. There can also be constipation or diarrhea, SIBO, and food sensitivities. SIBO occurs in 17 to 58 percent of people who have scleroderma. When treated, symptoms improve.

Delayed gastric emptying is found in 10 to 75 percent of people with systemic scleroderma. This correlates well with symptoms of early satiety, bloating, and vomiting.

Helicobacter pylori can be an issue in people who have scleroderma and GERD. Kanako Yamaguchi and colleagues tested 64 patients with scleroderma who had not been treated for GI imbalances. They found that 37 (57.8 percent) tested positive for *H. pylori*. Significantly more people without GERD had high *H. pylori* levels.

CELIAC, GLUTEN, AND SCLERODERMA

There is a high overlap of celiac disease in people with scleroderma. Eduardo Rosato and colleagues report that of 50 people studied, 5 had elevated tissue transglutaminase levels. When biopsied, four of the five had celiac disease, for an incidence of 8 percent. Remember that celiac disease is diagnosed only when there is serious erosion of the villi and microvilli. This study did not look at simple gluten intolerance.

DAMPENING INFLAMMATION

Free radical damage underlies the pathology of scleroderma. There are elevated levels of Th-2 cytokines (IL-6) in the early stages of scleroderma that lead to the thickening of tissues. Antioxidants are beneficial in people with scleroderma. Raynaud's causes a surge of free radicals that need to be quenched. Studies have shown that blood levels of vitamin C, vitamin E, selenium, and carotenoids are all lower in people with scleroderma, despite normal levels in their diets. G. Fiori and colleagues report that vitamin E used topically increases healing and reduces pain. It's also speculated that taurine can be used as an antioxidant. Supplementation with antioxidant nutrients and testing for antioxidant status to see if levels are adequate is advisable. Specific use of N-acetyl cysteine increases glutathione levels and is also advised. Use of several antioxidant supplements may be necessary for optimal results.

Homocysteine may be elevated in people with scleroderma. The higher the homocysteine level, the more progressive the disease. Screening for homocysteine can be extremely useful. Use of vitamin B_6, B_{12}, folic acid, and betaine (TMG) may be helpful in normalizing levels.

Low serum zinc levels have been found with frequency in people with scleroderma. In a recent study, 17 people with localized scleroderma were given 60 to 90 mg of zinc gluconate daily, and 53 percent saw benefits. Five people had partial remission, and four people had complete remission.

SCLERODERMA AND THE ENVIRONMENT

There is no single known cause of scleroderma. It is caused by a combination of genetics and environmental factors. Evidence suggests that prolonged exposure to silica, silicone, and chemical solvents significantly increases the risk of developing scleroderma.

In some individuals, solvents trigger the illness. An evaluation was made of 178 people with scleroderma, in comparison to 200 controls. People with scleroderma were more likely to have higher concentrations of and levels of exposure to solvents, especially trichloroethylene.

Silicosis has been well studied in scleroderma. People with silicosis from industrial exposure are 24 times more likely to be diagnosed with scleroderma. They are also two to eight times more likely to develop rheumatoid arthritis or systemic lupus erythematosus. Risk is greater in men. In a small study, 44 women and 6 men went through extensive testing and examination to see if there was a relationship between their work and autoimmune disease. They had been working for an average of six years in a factory that produced scouring powder with a high silica content. A total of 32 people, or 64 percent, showed symptoms of a systemic illness, 6 with Sjögren's syndrome, 5 with scleroderma, 3 with systemic lupus, 5 with a combination syndrome, and 13 who didn't fit into any definite pattern of disease. Further, 72 percent had elevated antinuclear antibodies (ANAs), an indicator of autoimmune connective tissue diseases. The conclusion was that workers who are continually exposed to silica have a high probability of developing an autoimmune problem.

The research on breast implants is mixed. Silicone breast implants may also play a role in some women with scleroderma, yet no relationship between autoimmune antibodies was found (for rheumatoid arthritis, ANA, and Scl-70 for scleroderma). In one study, 26 women with either lupus or scleroderma had breast implants, and 3 of them had complete remission of at least two years. Saline implants have a silicone casing that may also cause problems. If you have breast implants, being tested for silicone and chemical antibodies would help determine if you might benefit from their removal.

Natural therapies can work along with medical therapies for scleroderma. Infections must be treated and beneficial flora given. Nutrients that help with collagen maintenance and repair are essential to help prevent loss of elasticity in skin and organs. Consider supplementing with vitamin C, quercetin, zinc, glucosamine, and chondroitin. Foods and supplements that help reduce production of arachidonic acid will reduce inflammation and pain. Good-quality oils, fish, nuts, and seeds work in this way. It's also important to increase circulation and oxygen supply to the tissues. Finally, a nutrient-dense food plan must be developed that works to offset the problems of malnutrition, which are common.

Functional Laboratory Testing

- Breath test for SIBO
- Vitamin D levels
- Comprehensive digestive stool analysis
- Testing for food and environmental sensitivities
- Dehydroepiandrosterone (DHEA) and cortisol testing
- Liver function profile
- Testing for silicone antibodies (for women with breast implants)
- Nutrient testing, including homocysteine
- *H. pylori* testing
- Essential fatty acid testing

Healing Options

Scleroderma isn't one illness; it's many, and finding your own triggers and solutions will be a personal journey. Here are ideas that will help you on the journey. Very little research on using nondrug approaches has been done; you will be a pioneer.

- **Look for and treat infections.** *H. pylori*, esophageal and oral candidiasis, and other infections are associated with scleroderma. I could find only rare references to SIBO in association with scleroderma; however, my instincts tell me to at least explore the possibility. You may be able to keep the infections at bay with use of colloidal silver, berberine from goldenseal or Oregon grapes, grapefruit seed extract, oregano oil, garlic capsules, or combination herbs. Each of these substances has wide antimicrobial properties, low toxicity, and a low incidence of negative side effects. Your doctor may prescribe antibiotics or anti-fungal medications.

- **Test for HCl sufficiency.** See Chapters 3 and 11 for more information.
- **Try an elimination-provocation diet and make dietary changes.** Use one of the recommended therapeutic approaches from Chapter 14. Explore the relationship between your scleroderma and food and environmental sensitivities. While I cannot find any research on this, I have seen this approach work for several of my own clients who have scleroderma.
- **Check for food sensitivities and celiac.** Gluten sensitivity and food sensitivities are common in people with scleroderma. Try the elimination diet. (See Chapter 14.)
- **Check for high homocysteine levels.** Methylation issues can be demonstrated by checking homocysteine levels. High homocysteine levels are common in people with scleroderma. There are also labs offering methylation panels that delve deeper.
- **Check hormone levels.** In a case study with two women, estriol treatment provided considerable beneficial effects.
- **Check vitamin D.** Low levels of 25-OH D have been found in many studies of people with scleroderma. More than 80 percent were found to be vitamin D insufficient and 23 to 32 percent vitamin D deficient. As with other autoimmune diseases, bringing levels up to at least 50 ng/ml and possibly toward the upper normal range of between 80 and 100 ng/ml may be optimal. For maintenance take 2,000 IU vitamin D_3 daily; to bring levels up, take between 5,000 and 10,000 IU vitamin D_3 daily for 8 to 12 weeks and retest.
- **Test for essential fatty acids.** Supplement accordingly. People with scleroderma have oxidation of fats due to a lack of antioxidants.
- **Take zinc.** You can test for red blood cell zinc levels or do taste testing for zinc sufficiency with liquid zinc sulfate. People are often zinc deficient. Take 50 mg zinc daily. Try this for two to three months. Work with a clinician on this because you can take too much zinc and possibly deplete copper as a result.
- **Increase antioxidants.** The best food sources include fruits, vegetables, legumes, nuts, and seeds. Fresh vegetable and green juice is a concentrated source. Using green powders such as spirulina, blue-green algae, wheatgrass juice extract, or mixtures of powdered "reds" or "greens" can also give quite an antioxidant kick.

Think about taking several grams or more daily of mineral ascorbates (vitamin C). Consider adding 200 to 1,000 IU of vitamin E. Vitamin E can also be used topically on skin to soothe and soften it. Consider selenium at 200 mcg daily. Taurine has antioxidant properties; take 1,000 to 2,000 mg daily. Try N-acetyl cysteine or whey protein to boost glutathione levels; take 500 to 1,000 mg N-acetyl cysteine daily. Consider taking antioxidant supplements. Consult Susan Brown's website, https://betterbones.com, for more information.

■ **Detoxify.** A liver function panel can determine whether your phase one and phase two liver detoxification pathways are working normally. Because the risk of scleroderma increases with solvent exposure, a liver detoxification program may be of significant benefit. In the few people I've worked with who have scleroderma, this has proven to be an effective starting point.

■ **Check hormone levels.** People with scleroderma have been found to have low levels of the hormones: DHEA-sulphate, prolactin, and/or testosterone. Work with your doctor to determine if the level of any of these hormones are low and to find the correct therapeutic dosage for each hormone.

■ **Take a multivitamin with minerals.** Poor diet, loss of movement in the digestive tract, loss of elasticity of the organs, infections, and medications all contribute to the malabsorption of nutrients. Selenium and vitamin C deficiencies are common in people with scleroderma. At least 20 nutrients are essential for formation of bone and cartilage, so it's important to find a supplement that supports these needs. Look for a supplement that contains 10,000 IU vitamin A, 800 to 1,000 mg calcium, 400 to 500 mg magnesium, 400 IU vitamin E, at least 250 mg vitamin C, 50 mg vitamin B_6, 15 to 50 mg zinc, 5 to 10 mg manganese, 12 mg copper, and 200 mcg selenium in addition to other nutrients. Follow the dosage on the bottle to get nutrients in appropriate amounts.

■ **Take vitamin C.** Vitamin C is vital for formation of cartilage and collagen, which is a fibrous protein that forms strong connective tissue necessary for bone strength. Vitamin C also plays an important role in immune response, helping protect us from disease-producing microbes. It also inhibits formation of inflammatory prostaglandins, helping to reduce pain, inflammation, and swelling. If you have candidiasis or bacterial overgrowth, vitamin C can boost your body's ability to defend itself. Vitamin C is also an antioxidant, needed to counter free radical formation noted in sclerotic conditions. Take 1 to 3 grams daily in an ascorbate or Ester-C. For best results, do the vitamin C flush. (See Chapter 17.)

■ **Try gamma-linolenic acid (GLA).** In one study, 1 gram of evening primrose oil was given to four women with scleroderma three times daily for one year. They experienced a reduction in pain, with improved skin texture and healing of sores; red patches on skin due to broken capillaries were much improved. The researchers suggest that 6 grams daily may be of greater benefit. Take 3 to 6 grams of evening primrose oil, borage oil, or flaxseed oil daily.

- **Follow suggestions for GERD if it is present.** See Chapter 19.
- **Try nattokinase.** I have not seen research on this, but it makes sense to me. Protein-digesting enzymes taken on an empty stomach can help to break down fibrous tissues throughout the body. Nattokinase works to help break down blood clots, so I would probably begin with that. You could eat natto, a traditional Japanese food with an unusual flavor, at 2 to 15 ounces daily. Or you can purchase nattokinase in capsules. Products differ, so use as directed.

SJÖGREN'S SYNDROME

Sjögren's syndrome is an autoimmune disease in which moisture-producing glands are destroyed by white blood cells. Typically the first signs of Sjögren's syndrome are dry eyes and dry mouth. However, virtually all organs can be affected. More than 4 million people have Sjögren's in the United States; 90 percent are women. Venus Williams, champion tennis player, is likely the most famous person who has Sjögren's. Diagnosed in 2011, she came back to the sport with renewed vigor, competing globally. She has publicly stated that what enables her to compete and feel her best is getting enough rest, combined with a mostly vegan diet, smoothies, and fresh vegetable juice. Half of people with Sjögren's syndrome will have a second autoimmune disease, and it is often connected with rheumatoid arthritis, lupus, or scleroderma. Primary Sjögren's syndrome is when it occurs without other autoimmune illnesses; secondary Sjögren's is when you also have a second autoimmune disease. Like all autoimmune diseases, it can take on many forms and can flare up and improve.

Current medical treatments are aimed at symptom relief. People are told to chew gum, use artificial tears, and use bile stimulants to increase saliva production. Steroid and other immunosuppressive medications are also used. Several people with Sjögren's syndrome whom I have worked with have benefited from dietary changes, supplements, and exploration of the DIGIN model.

DIGESTIVE CONNECTION AND SJÖGREN'S

There is a high incidence of digestive distress in people with Sjögren's. People who have Sjörgren's are more likely to have IBS-like symptoms such as constipation, abdominal pain, diarrhea, fecal incontinence, and delayed gastric emptying. Although research is rare on the DIGIN model and Sjögren's, it's beginning to happen. In one study, 17 people with Sjögren's were found to have microbiome composition that is different than that of healthy people. A study in 35 people with Sjögren's were compared with controls for dysbiosis. A total of 21 percent of people with primary Sjögren's syndrome, compared to 3 percent in controls, had dysbiosis. Dysbiosis was associated with active disease at the time, as well as higher levels of calprotectin, a marker of inflammation in the gut. Interestingly, the dysbiosis did not show up as IBS, and incidence of IBS was not higher in the Sjögren's group than in controls. If you have Sjögren's, you are more likely to develop oral candidiasis. *H. pylori* infection also has been associated with Sjögren's syndrome.

FOOD SENSITIVITIES AND OTHER ALLERGIES IN PEOPLE WITH SJÖGREN'S

People with Sjögren's have a high prevalence of allergies to drugs (46 percent) and more skin contact allergies. People with Sjogren's have also been found to have food sensitivities. In 10 patients with IBS-like symptoms, endoscopies and colonoscopies were performed. One person was diagnosed with celiac-sprue, yet did not improve on a gluten-free diet. All had vitamin D deficiencies with levels below 20 ng/ml. IgG testing was performed to determine foods that might be issues in their health. It was found that 9 had reactions to wheat and dairy. Other common reactions were to eggs, beef, and corn, which are generally the most common allergenic foods. Further, 8 of the 10 completed an elimination diet for 6 months and reintroduced foods one at a time. All of them had complete resolution of abdominal pain, bloating, diarrhea, and joint pain while on the diet. If fatigue was a symptom, it improved while on the elimination diet but didn't entirely go away. When foods were reintroduced, symptoms reoccurred. Maria Liden and colleagues report that 20 percent of people with Sjögren's who also have the DQ1 gene type have mucosal inflammation when challenged with rectal gluten even though they don't have celiac disease. Dr. Liden labels them as gluten sensitive with a possible risk of developing celiac disease. Inflammation was measured by increases in nitric oxide and mucosal granules from neutrophils.

The same group gave rectal challenges of dried milk powder to 21 people (2 males, 19 females) with Sjögren's syndrome and 18 healthy controls. Eight of the 21 people with Sjögren's had a reaction two standard deviations above the mean of the controls, although IgG and IgA antibodies to casein, beta-lactoglobulin, and alpha-lactalbumin were similar in patients and controls. All people were also tested with a rectal challenge to soybean; none had any adverse reaction. Those with Sjögren's were also tested for the genetics for celiac. No association was seen between reaction to cow's milk and their genotypes. In fact, the two people who had the most inflammation had no reaction to gluten and were negative for the DQ2 and DQ8 genes associated with celiac. The researchers report that 2 out of 21 reacted to gluten only (one was subsequently diagnosed with celiac disease); 5 out of 21 were reactive to cow's milk; and 3 out of 21 reacted to both gluten and cow's milk. These patients also reported other allergies: 13 of 21 reported allergies to avocado, apple, peanut, strawberry, shellfish, pollen, dust, animals, or mold. GI symptoms were reported by 16 of 21 (76 percent), and 10 of 21 (48 percent) attributed their GI issues to food reactions from dairy products and wheat. A total of 13 out of 21 (62 percent) met the criteria for IBS.

Functional Laboratory Testing

- Celiac testing
- Breath test for SIBO
- Comprehensive digestive stool analysis
- Organic acid test
- Food sensitivity and allergy testing
- Fatty acid testing
- DHEA and cortisol testing
- Vitamins D, E, K, and A levels

Healing Options

- **Discover dysbiosis.** Do testing for SIBO, stool testing, and/or organic acid testing to discover whether these issues play a role in your illness.
- **Try an elimination diet.** I have seen an elimination diet work wonders in women with scleroderma. Also rule out celiac disease. See Chapters 11 and 22 for more information.
- **Increase good-quality omega-6 fats in your diet.** In a couple of studies, evening primrose oil was used at levels between 1,000 mg and 6,000 mg daily. Changes were seen in pain reduction, healing of ulcers, improved skin texture, and fewer attacks of Raynaud's. High omega-6 fats can also be found in nuts and seeds, borage oil, and black currant seed oil.
- **Check for HCl.** In six women who were tested for gastric acid sufficiency, four were deficient. Take the HCl self-test or Heidelberg capsule test or ask a gastroenterologist to test you for this.

- **Practice relaxation and stress management.** Stress plays a role in this illness, so relax as much as possible and do things that give you pleasure. See Chapter 16 for more on this topic.
- **Optimize fat-soluble vitamins.** Fat-soluble vitamins have anti-inflammatory effects. Get yours tested. In one study, people with more severe Sjögren's had lowered levels of vitamin A.

CHAPTER 26

Autoimmune Diseases
Overview ◌ D I G I N

Many autoimmune diseases were discussed in the previous chapters; we will look at more in the following chapters. They include type 1 diabetes, celiac disease, autoimmune hepatitis, cirrhosis, inflammatory bowel disease (IBD), rheumatoid arthritis, psoriatic arthritis, ankylosing spondylitis, Behcet's disease, fibromyalgia, scleroderma, and psoriasis.

This chapter gives you a general overview of autoimmune diseases. The definition of an autoimmune illness is one in which your body mistakes healthy cells for harmful ones and attacks them. The function of the immune system is to distinguish self from nonself. In these diseases, this goes awry. There are at least 100 known autoimmune diseases, and they can affect virtually every body tissue; many of these have overlapping symptoms, which makes them hard to diagnose. Typically, these conditions flare up and then go into remission so you may feel better for a while.

The most common autoimmune diseases include:

Addison's disease	Type 1 diabetes
Alopecia areata	Glomerulonephritis
Ankylosing spondylitis	Grave's disease
Antiphospholipid antibody syndrome	Guillain-Barré syndrome
Autoimmune hepatitis	Hashimoto's disease
Celiac disease	Hemolytic anemia
Crohn's disease	Multiple sclerosis
Dermatomyositis	Myasthenia gravis

Myositis

Parkinson's disease

Pernicious anemia

Polymyalgia rheumatica

Primary biliary cirrhosis

Psoriasis

Raynaud's disease

Rheumatoid arthritis

Scleroderma

Sjogren's syndrome

Systemic lupus erythematosus

Ulcerative colitis

Vitiligo

These illnesses affect 50 million Americans. You are most likely to get an auto-immune disease if you are female, have a family history of autoimmune conditions, work around solvents or other chemicals, and/or are African, Native American, or Latin in descent. Rheumatoid arthritis is two to three times more common in women. Ninety percent of those with lupus are women; lupus is also three times more common in African American women than in Caucasian women. Ankylosing spondylitis is one of the rare autoimmune diseases that is more common in men.

In autoimmune diseases, the immune system overreacts. There is increased inflammation and oxidative damage from free radicals. We need to dampen these reactions down so that our body doesn't see the world as unsafe. (Read Chapter 8 on inflammation and immunity, to get a deeper understanding.)

For an autoimmune illness to thrive, it needs the following conditions:

1. The right genetics
2. An environmental trigger (could be stress; sunlight; solvents; other chemicals; a virus, bacteria, or parasite; heavy metal; pesticide; or some other exposure)
3. Increased intestinal permeability
4. Dysbiosis has been found in all autoimmune diseases that have been studied. These include type 1 diabetes, inflammatory bowel disease, rheumatoid arthritis, systemic lupus, Sjögren's syndrome, autoimmune liver disease, Graves' disease, and multiple sclerosis. (For a larger list of diseases associated with leaky gut, see Chapter 4.)

These diseases can develop quickly or over a span of several years. Autoantibodies in the blood can typically be found years prior to the onset of the disease. Arbuckle reported that 88 percent of 130 patients who ultimately developed systemic lupus erythematosus (SLE) had elevated antibodies 9.4 years prior to the diagnosis. Ask your doctor to look for antinuclear antibodies (ANAs) antibodies or other more specific antibodies if you suspect you may have an autoimmune condition. Some of the regular tests that may be ordered include sedimentation rate, complete blood

Table 26.1   Association Between Viruses and Autoimmune Disease

EBV = Epstein-Barr virus CMV = cytomegalovirus VZV = Varicella zoster virus RA = rheumatoid arthritis ITP = idiopathic thrombocytopenic purpura (The double plus sign indicates that there is stronger research support for the finding.)

	EBV	CMV	herpes-1	herpes-2	herpes-6	VZV	measles
autism	+	+	+	+	++		++
RA	++	++					
thyroiditis	++						
Sjögren's syndrome	++				++		
myocarditis	+	+					
multiple sclerosis	+				++		++
type 1 diabetes	+	+					
Guillain-Barré syndrome	+	+					
uveitis		++	++	++			
keratitis			+				
autoimmune hepatitis			+			++	
Reiter's syndrome	+	+	+			+	
polymyositis	+						
pemphigus	+					+	
scleroderma		+					
psoriasis		+					
immune thrombocytopenic purpura (ITP)	+	+					
IgA nephritis	++	++					
glomerulonephritis	++						

Adapted and used with permission from Aristo Vojdjani, PhD, MT.

count, elevated C-reactive protein, 25-OH vitamin D testing, and looking for oxidative damage. Functional tests include organic acid testing, food allergy and sensitivity testing, lactulose/mannitol testing for leaky gut, and looking at methylation pathways through homocysteine or liver detoxification profiles. People with one autoimmune illness are more likely to develop additional autoimmune conditions. In Milan, Italy, in 2009, Bardella and colleagues reviewed 297 consecutive patients to determine the prevalence of autoimmune conditions in people with celiac and inflammatory bowel disease. They report that 25.6 percent of people with celiac had another autoimmune condition; 21.1 percent of people with Crohn's disease also had a second autoimmune condition; and 10 percent of people with ulcerative colitis had a second autoimmune condition. Various studies have reported the incidence of people with celiac disease who also have type 1 diabetes to be between 3 and 6 percent. Togrol reports that of 30 people with ankylosing spondylitis, 11 (36.7 percent) also had positive antigliadin antibodies; 3 of the 11 had positive antiendomysial antibodies (10 percent). People with autoimmune conditions can also display systemic inflammation. It has been reported that people with lupus have increased risk of developing atherosclerosis and osteoporosis.

In my own practice, I have seen people with autoimmune conditions improve significantly on an elimination diet. There is a lot of interest in intermittent fasting and fasting-mimicking diets and their role in the prevention and treatment of autoimmune conditions. More research needs to be done; thus far, animal research and early human research indicate improvements in quality of life and reduced disability. In people with rheumatoid arthritis, fasting for 7 to 10 days followed by a vegan diet for three and a half months reduced inflammation in lab testing (testing of C-reactive protein and sedimentation rates) and resulted in less pain.

People with autoimmune conditions can also have problems with gastrointestinal (GI) motility, causing constipation or IBS-like symptoms. Elderly people with Parkinson's disease were found to have lengthened stool transit time and some malabsorption, which was indicated by decreased mannitol absorption on intestinal permeability testing.

Conventional treatments for autoimmune diseases include medications to reduce inflammation and symptoms, eating well, getting as much exercise as you can without overdoing, getting rest, and using stress-management techniques. Rather than focusing on a single organ or system, using a broader view of the body will get you better results. Try chiropractic treatments, acupuncture, hypnotherapy, and chi gong. Meditate, listen to music, and cultivate methods of training your mind to feel safe and relaxed.

Whatever autoimmune condition affects you, look at the DIGIN model (discussed in Part II, Chapters 3 through 11) to discover whether you can reduce the severity of the illness and/or reduce the incidence of flare-ups. Reducing inflammation is key, so looking for what triggers your inflammation can be critical. While many people may need prescription medications to reduce inflammation, remember that food is typically our most inflammatory contact. So, trying elimination diets and discovering your specific dietary triggers are important.

The relationship between leaky gut and other autoimmune illnesses has also been demonstrated in autoimmune types of arthritis, multiple sclerosis, IBD, fibromyalgia, chronic fatigue syndrome, autism, primary biliary cirrhosis, psoriasis, Behcet's disease, and Parkinson's disease. (See Table 26.1 for details.) Healing a leaky gut, caused by your medications or other triggers, is another important step to keeping you healthy.

Dysbiosis is also found in every autoimmune condition that has been studied so far. Looking for dysbiosis and the competency of your digestive function can also give you significant information. Think about using probiotics to help modulate your immune system and to reduce inflammation. Consider using natural anti-inflammatory supplements and change your diet to enable you to reduce your reliance on prescription medications.

Selenium, magnesium, and zinc deficiencies have been associated with autoimmune diseases; low vitamin D levels are also seen in autoimmune conditions with frequency, so have these tested. The incidence of autoimmune conditions rises as you move away from the equator; less sunlight, more autoimmune disease. Vitamin D modulates immune function and inflammation when it is at normal or optimal levels.

CHAPTER 27

Behcet's Disease Q DIGIN

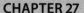

B ehcet's disease (BD) is an inflammatory autoimmune disease that affects blood vessels throughout the body, causing vasculitis, an inflammation of the blood or lymph vessel. It was first recognized in 1937 in the West by a Turkish doctor, Hulusi Behcet, although 1800 years earlier it was discovered by a Chinese physician, Zhang Zhongjing, who called it Huhuo disease. It is also known as Silk Road disease because the incidence is greatest in the Mediterranean, the Middle East, and the Far East, although there have been cases in people of all nationalities and descent. In the United States, it is more common in women than in men. In Middle Eastern countries, it is more common in men than women. Symptoms most commonly appear in one's 20s or 30s but can begin anytime. Statistics show that 15,000 to 20,000 Americans have been diagnosed, and many more are undiagnosed.

Symptoms vary depending on where the inflammation is in your body and are due to an overactive immune system. It is chronic, and the course is unpredictable. Some people are debilitated by the disease, while a lucky few may go into complete remission. The most common symptoms are recurrent sores in the mouth and genitals, skin lesions, and eye inflammation. The sores often have a white or yellow center with redness at the edges and are very painful. There may be additional symptoms, including skin lesions, painful joints, bowel inflammation, and meningitis. Symptoms may involve the nervous system, causing Parkinson-like symptoms; memory loss; impaired speech; hearing loss; loss of balance; blindness; headaches; stroke; and digestive complications, such as bloating, gas, bloody stools, and diarrhea. About 15 percent of people with BD also have heart disease complications. Sufferers sometimes experience a profound sense of fatigue. BD usually presents itself in a rhythm of remissions and flare-ups of disease activity. It may be worsened by extremes of hot and cold climates or menstrual cycles.

There is no known cause for Behcet's disease. It is suspected that an environmental exposure, such as a viral or bacterial infection, can trigger the illness in people who are already genetically susceptible. There are dozens of genes that are both associated with increased risk of developing Behcet's and protective against that risk. *Streptococcus sanguinis* and herpesvirus are suspected infectious triggers. Dysbiosis and low levels of butyrate are found in people with Behcet's.

A large body of research focuses on the insufficiency of antioxidant nutrients and enzymes in people with BD. Glutathione peroxidase levels are lower in people with BD. Glutathione is an enzyme that depends on vitamin E and selenium for optimal function. Superoxide dismutase (SOD) activity is also diminished. It appears that production of nitric oxide is excessive in people with BD. Use of antioxidant nutrients can bring nitric oxide under control.

One recent study examined levels of vitamin C and malondialdehyde in people with BD. Malondialdehyde is a metabolite that is produced when there is lipid peroxidation, which is a chain reaction requiring antioxidant nutrients. Vitamin C levels were lower in people with BD than in controls, and malondialdehyde levels were higher than in controls. Vitamin C levels were low in people with BD, even when the illness was in remission. Different researchers looked at vascular health and found that 1 hour after intravenous (IV) vitamin C was given, there was improved function in the blood vessels.

Another study looked at vitamin E supplementation in BD. It was found that vitamins A and E, beta carotene, and glutathione levels were lower in people with BD than in controls. When given vitamin E supplementation for six weeks, levels of blood antioxidants rose in the treatment group and were higher than in the untreated control groups.

BD sufferers have significantly increased intestinal permeability. Leaky gut syndrome can be aggravated by use of certain foods. Use of dairy products, gluten-containing foods (see section on celiac disease in Chapter 23), and other foods may trigger an immune response and symptoms. Testing for food and environmental sensitivities and allergies makes sense. Use of nutrients such as glutamine, quercetin, probiotics, and antioxidants can be helpful.

No specific diagnostic test exists for Behcet's disease. Diagnosis is made by elimination of other possibilities and through symptom analysis, and is best done by a physician experienced in the treatment of Behcet's patients. A list of patient-recommended physicians is available at the American Behcet's Disease Association website (http://www.behcets.com). BD may begin gradually at first, with sores that come and go, and may be undiagnosed for a long time; it may also be misdiagnosed as herpes. Like patients with chronic fatigue syndrome, people with BD are often told it's "all in your head" because they look so healthy. Most of the inflammations are internal and not readily apparent to family and friends. To be diagnosed with BD, a person must have had recurrent oral ulcers at least three times in a year. They must also meet two of four additional criteria: recurrent genital ulcers, eye lesions, skin lesions, or a positive "pathergy test." The pathergy test is simple. The forearm is pricked with a sterile needle and if a small red bump or pustule occurs, the result is positive. This is very useful in Middle Eastern populations, where 70 percent of people with BD test positive, but less so in Europe and the United States, where the majority test negative.

Conventional treatments are similar to those for other autoimmune conditions and involve the use of immunosuppressive medications such as steroids, interferon alpha 2A and B, Levamisole, cyclosporine, Cytoxan, colchicine, Trental, and thalidomide. This is not a group to be dealt with lightly.

This is a perfect condition in which to use the DIGIN model to try to find underlying imbalances and triggers.

Functional Laboratory Testing

- Intestinal permeability testing
- Organic acid testing
- Lactose intolerance test
- Testing for gluten and antigliadin antibodies
- IgE, IgG, IgM food and environmental sensitivity testing

Healing Options

After testing, you'll have a better idea of any underlying problems. Look up related sections in this book to help you with the specifics. Then detoxify if necessary, clean up your diet, take probiotics, and increase your intake of vitamins, minerals, and other antioxidants.

- **Try metabolic cleansing.** Metabolic cleansing involves going on a hypoallergenic food plan for one to three weeks and taking a nutrient-rich protein powder designed to help restore your liver's detoxification capacities. For a thorough discussion of metabolic cleansing, see Chapter 17.
- **Take and eat antioxidants.** You'll find fruits and vegetables to be great natural sources of antioxidants. Make sure you eat 5 to 12 servings daily, if not

more. They probably won't give enough protection by themselves, so add nutritional supplements. Vitamin C, vitamin E, glutathione, trace minerals, and other antioxidants may be helpful in decreasing the incidence and severity of flare-ups. Research shows that BD patients have an increased need for antioxidants. Therefore, supplementation with trace elements involved in the antioxidative processes may increase scavenger enzyme activities, and consequently, an improvement in clinical symptoms may be expected. While much more research is needed in this area, there is no reason not to add them to your daily routine. Take an antioxidant combination with carotenoids, selenium, glutathione, or N-acetyl cysteine, and that may contain lipoic acid, grape seed extract, Pycnogenol, or other antioxidant nutrients.

- **Take vitamin E.** Take 800 to 1,000 IU d-alpha tocopherol with mixed tocopherols daily. Look for a product with a high gamma-tocopherol or high tocotrienol content.
- **Take vitamin C.** Take a minimum of 2,000 mg of vitamin C daily. To maximize effects see the section on vitamin C flush in Chapter 17.
- **Try BG-104.** BG-104 is a Chinese herbal supplement. One study looked at the effectiveness of BG-104 in people with BD and Sjögren's disease. The main ingredients in BG-104 include panax ginseng, *Rhizoma coptidis*, which contains berberine, and bitter melon. Both BG-104 and vitamin E were found to have an anti-inflammatory effect. They enhance antioxidant activity to reduce sedimentation rates (a measure of tissue breakdown) and the number of neutrophils (white blood cells) and lower C-reactive protein levels, which is a measure of inflammation.
- **Try *Glycyrrhizae* decoction for purging stomach fire (GDPSF).** According to a 2018 paper by Chen, published in *Medicine (Baltimore)*, Chinese history and modern treatment in BD has utilized GDPSF. Chinese studies report remission rates of 22 to 81 percent, and typically above 70 percent, and a current placebo controlled study is underway. The GDPSF formula contains seven herbs: *Glycyrrhiza uralensis* Fisch (licorice root), panax ginseng, *Scutellaria baicalensis* Georgi (skullcap), *Pinellia ternate* (BanXia), *Coptis chinensis* (HuangLian), ginger, and jujube. No dosage is given.
- **Try acupuncture.** There is limited research in this area, but one study showed a positive effect on improving immune function and trace mineral status; however, a 2002 letter in the *British Journal of Ophthalmology* (Murray and Aboteen, 2002) discussed a BD patient who developed pathergy-like pustules at the sites of acupuncture needle placement, indicating caution in the use of this treatment.

- **Investigate allergies and sensitivities.** Although more research needs to be done in this area, one study indicated an immune response when patients were given cow's milk. Eliminate dairy products for two weeks. See if you have improvement in symptoms. Then add back cultured dairy, such as yogurt, kefir, and cottage cheese. See how you feel. It may be necessary to avoid dairy products altogether. Rule out other food sensitivities with an elimination-provocation diet and/or food-allergy or food-sensitivity blood testing.

    Cigarettes, toothpaste, mouthwash, and flavored dental floss can cause irritation. In a conversation I had with Joanne Zeis, the author of several books on Behcet's disease (http://www.behcetsdisease.com), she said, "ironically, according to some research studies, people who quit smoking cigarettes sometimes develop excessive oral ulcers, which can be a real problem for BD patients who quit—some go right back to smoking again. This is a paradox but will vary from person to person.

    "Toothpastes containing sodium lauryl sulfate may create aphthous ulcers in some BD patients and should be avoided."

- **Take probiotics and eat probiotic-rich foods.** *Lactobacillus acidophilus* is often beneficial in prevention and treatment of canker sores and may be useful in BD. No clinical research has been done in this area, but it makes sense. Take one to two capsules or ⅛ to ¼ teaspoon of the powder three times daily; take it between meals.

- **Practice stress-management skills.** Stress can contribute to a flare-up of the disease. Development of a strong support system is vital. This is a lifelong illness, and you can greatly benefit from support groups, many of which are available on the Internet. Exchange of information and dialogue with others who understand what you are going through can expedite recovery. Take time for yourself, rest, and relax.

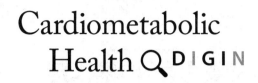

CHAPTER 28

Cardiometabolic
Health Q DIGIN

"Gaining 20 pounds between the ages of 21 to 65 is the difference between 4 to 5 calories a day, or less than half of a potato chip. No one has that much willpower."

– Lee M. Kaplan, MD, PhD, at the Diet and Microbiota
in Health and Disease Symposium, Harvard University, July 2015

As research unfolds about the microbiome, it appears that the drivers of liver disease, diabetes, and obesity are tied closely back to gut health. (See Chapter 20 for more information on the gut in fatty liver disease.) This is a mutual relationship that goes in both directions. As dysbiosis increases, we also see increases in gut permeability and bacterial lipopolysaccharide (LPS), inflammation, weight gain, insulin resistance, and metabolic syndrome. This increases appetite, as well as the risk of type 2 diabetes, heart disease, and other inflammatory and autoimmune conditions. As we improve health by changing diet and lifestyle, losing weight, and rebalancing the gut and microbiome through the DIGIN model, balance is improved and risk is lessened.

Metabolic syndrome affects about 47 million Americans. If you have more than three of these factors, you may be diagnosed with metabolic syndrome: large waist size, triglyceride levels higher than 150 mg/dl, low high-density lipoprotein (HDL) cholesterol levels, high blood pressure, and fasting blood sugar levels of over 100 mg/dl. It's characterized by insulin resistance and difficulty in handling glucose. Most people with metabolic syndrome are overweight and often apple-shaped as well, but it also occurs in people who are thin. If left unchecked, metabolic syndrome often leads to type 2 diabetes and increased risk for cardiovascular disease.

Research in the FINRISK study associated increases in bacterial endotoxins (LPS) with obesity, metabolic syndrome, diabetes, heart attack, and stroke. This was independent of whether the participants had elevated C-reactive protein (CRP),

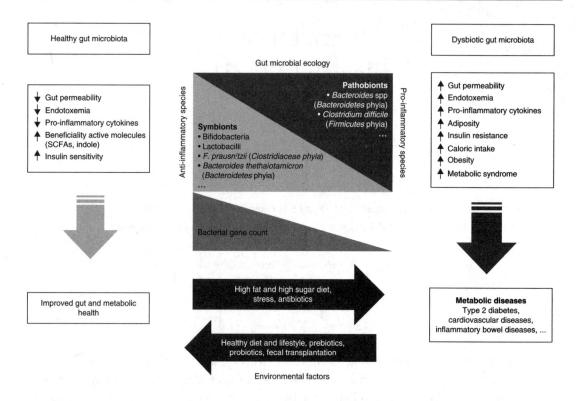

nutrient, or calorie intake; or preexisting obesity, metabolic syndrome, or diabetes. As stated in Chapter 21, the drivers of cardiometabolic syndrome and disease resemble those of a disrupted microbiome:

- Obesity
- Changes in food supply
- Too little physical activity
- Chronic stress
- Medications
- Toxins
- Hormone imbalances
- Microbial LPS and increased intestinal permeability (leaky gut)
- Circadian cycle disruption
- Disrupted microbiome/dysbiosis
- Being bottle fed as an infant

Using the DIGIN model can help you restore cardiometabolic health and prevent disease.

OBESITY

Obesity is a complex issue—you could fill a small library with what has been written on it. Here, I'm going to introduce you to new research on the connection between obesity and your digestive system. There is a growing consensus in research that obesity has several defining characteristics:

- Alterations in gut bacteria
- Low-grade inflammation
- Subsequent leaky gut
- Elevated levels of LPS and endocannabinoids

If obesity is left unchecked, it can lead to metabolic syndrome, type 2 diabetes, high serum lipids, and cardiovascular disease.

ALTERATIONS IN GUT BACTERIA

The gut microbiome is responsible for maintaining our metabolism and determining how much fat we store. Repeated use of antibiotics in early childhood has been linked to a greater risk for obesity later in life, with higher rounds of antibiotics associated with higher body mass index, overweight, and obesity. Antibiotics are used in animal husbandry to put weight on them before they are slaughtered. Early repeated use of antibiotics in infants and toddlers also increases risk of asthma, allergy, autoimmune disease, and behavioral issues.

People who are obese have a different balance of gut microorganisms than people who are thin. This much is known, and yet we don't really know yet exactly which bacteria are involved. While research is mixed, Million (2013) reports that lean people have a greater number of Bacteroidetes and Bacteroides, and protective microbes such as *Akkermansia muciniphila*, Bifidobacterium, and *Lactobacillus animalis*, while people who are obese have higher levels of Firmicutes, Enterobacteria, *Staphylococcus aureus*, *Faecalibacterium prausnitzii*, and *Lactobacillus reuteri*. As people lose weight, the microbiota come into a more normal balance. Other researchers have not found this to be the case; for instance, Duncan and colleagues found no differences in the amount of

Bacteroidetes in the stool of people who were obese, and levels didn't change when people dieted. Firmicutes levels went down when people dieted, which is the opposite of the finding from Ley's group. It appears that research looking at specific species of bacteria will yield better results than just looking at the main phyla.

High-fat, high-glycemic diets worsen all of this, increasing leaky gut, inflammation, immune activation, and obesity. Probiotics and prebiotics help to normalize these imbalances, while antibiotics make it worse. Probiotics that have helped with weight loss in humans and animals include *Lactobacillus acidophilus LA-5, B. animalis subsp. lactis BB-12, Lactobacillus salivarius (which also helps with gum health), Lactobacillus gasseri, Lactobacillus plantarum, Lactobacillus rhamnosus, Bifidobacterium* spp., *Streptococcus thermophilus,* and *Streptococcus boulardii. Lactobacillus plantarum* is one of the main microbes found in fermented vegetables, such as kimchee and sauerkraut. *S. thermophilus and B. animalis* are found in some yogurts. For example, *B. animalis sub sp. Lactis BB-12* is utilized in the yogurt brand Proviact; Dannon's Activia yogurt is also *B. animalis lactis* but a different subspecies.

HIGH ENDOCANNABINOIDS IN GENETIC AND CENTRAL OBESITY

If you have every smoked pot or used CBD, did you get the "munchies?" Well, marijuana is an external cannabinoid, but we also make our own internal cannabinoids in our brain, muscles, liver, digestive system, and fat cells. When turned on, food tastes amazing. Endocannabinoids help to regulate appetite, perception of pain, and heart rate; affect mood; protect the nervous system and neurons; control certain phases of memory processing; act as a feedback loop that signals our neurons to stop secreting neurotransmitters and to regulate heart rate, blood pressure, and bronchial function; and affect the fat cells, liver, muscles, and pancreas. This system, called the endocannabinoid system (eCS), is comprised of lipids (fats) and receptors (CB1 and CB2). Along with the hypothalamus, it stimulates production of ghrelin, and we feel hungry. It also regulates energy balance. In people who have central adiposity (are apple shaped), the eCS is overactivated, and levels are high. Endocannabinoids slow gastric emptying and intestinal transit, reduce vagal function and gastric acid, and (as mentioned previously) make food taste great. The eCS also aids in nutrient transport and storage of fat.

When we eat more calories than we need at any given time, our body converts those extra calories to fat. When we have eaten enough, cholecystokinin is secreted in our duodenum and leptin is secreted, which lowers our appetite and turns off the eCS. Levels of endocannabinoids drop as leptin is secreted, and we no longer feel hungry. In obese people, levels of endocannabinoids stay chronically high. If we keep the eCS activated continually, it leads to high triglyceride levels, which in turn can lower our protective HDL cholesterol, increase LDL cholesterol, and lead to atherosclerosis (plaque buildup in our arteries). High levels of eCS also decrease adiponectin, which in turn decreases insulin sensitivity. This leads to increased weight gain and ultimately can lead to metabolic syndrome and/or type 2 diabetes. This constant inflammation contributes to increased gut permeability. The increased permeability leads to more inflammation and food sensitivities. If the inner lining of our duodenum is inflamed, we may not release cholecystokinin, and our eCS stays activated. When active, eCS stimulates our liver to make fatty acids.

FOOD SENSITIVITIES

Clinicians working with food sensitivities have noticed that when people deal directly with their food sensitivities, they begin to lose weight. Although there is little research to support this, it makes sense. Food can be inflammatory, and obesity is an inflammatory condition, so going on an anti-inflammatory diet can help lower inflammation and help normalize function. Cell Science Systems, maker of the ALCAT food sensitivity testing process, has sponsored a couple of studies that verify that by avoiding foods you are sensitive to, you can facilitate weight loss.

In clinical practice, when working with someone who is obese, I often begin by putting the person on an elimination diet. I'm not the only person who finds this useful: Elson Haas, MD, wrote a book called *The False Fat Diet* (Ballantine Books, 2001), which utilizes an elimination diet for weight loss; and Mark Hyman, MD, wrote *The Ultra Simple Diet* (Pocket Books, 2007) to express how an elimination diet plus detoxification could jump-start weight loss as well. Food sensitivities are tightly linked with leaky gut. So, it makes sense that if leaky gut is associated with obesity, food sensitivities will follow. By avoiding inflammatory foods and choosing one of the therapeutic elimination diets in Chapter 14, you may find that it's easier to lose weight.

Testing for All Cardiometabolic Issues 🔍 D I G I N
Here are some tests that you may want to consider for cardiometabolic issues. These will help you define where your key issues may be.

Functional Laboratory Testing

- **Comprehensive digestive stool testing:** This test will give an indication of microbial balance and probiotic levels.
- **Fasting glucose:** Fasting glucose is typically run-on metabolic panels and can be ordered by any clinician.
- **Hemoglobin A1C and Oral Glucose and Insulin Tolerance Test:** The hemoglobin A1C test gives a three-month average of glucose and is often utilized to diagnose diabetes and insulin resistance.

   Research presented by Maria Mercedes Change Villacreses, MD, and Elena Christofides, MD, at the 2019 Endocrine Society meeting challenges this. They report diabetes is missed in 73 percent of people using the Hemoglobin A1C test. They suggest confirming a high level with an oral glucose tolerance test. I also recommend measuring insulin levels each time glucose is measured. An oral glucose tolerance test is also utilized to determine transient low blood glucose levels, known as hypoglycemia.
- **Food sensitivity testing:** Delayed food sensitivities can predispose a person to obesity.
- **Vitamin and mineral testing:** There are often micronutrient deficiencies in people with metabolic syndrome.
- **Measure CRP and fibrinogen levels, test for the Apo E-4 gene and look at family history to determine risk.** CRP is a general level of inflammation in the body. Fibrinogen looks at how well your blood coagulates. The Apo E-4 gene is associated with higher risks of having heart attacks, strokes, and Alzheimer's disease. These tests can be easily run by any clinician through local labs.
- **Advanced Testing:** The Cleveland Heart Lab and Quest Labs offer advanced panels to assess your cardiovascular risk. The panels include the following tests which can give a much more complete picture of your cardiovascular risks than basic lipids, blood pressure, and CRP levels. These include F2-Isoprostanes, adiponectin, insulin C-peptide, oxidized LDL cholesterol, Lp-PLA2, myeloperoxidase, and Glycomark.

Healing Options

- **Use the DIGIN model to reduce inflammation, heal leaky gut, and balance dysbiosis and the microbiome.** Cardiometabolic issues begin in the gut.
- **Move more.** Probably the most potent regulator of energy, stress, mood, and weight is exercise. Find an exercise program that you enjoy and do it routinely.
- **Eat probiotic and prebiotic-rich foods; perhaps take a probiotic supplement.** (See Chapter 6 for more information on this subject.)

- **Try one of the therapeutic dietary approaches in Chapter 14.**
- **Eat bitter melon.** Bitter melon is available in Asian stores. Research repeatedly reports that it helps to stabilize blood sugar levels.
- **Reduce carbohydrates and increase protein.** Trade some grains, starches, and sugars for protein foods such as legumes, fish, chicken, and bison.
- **Take a blood sugar support supplement.** There are many products on the market that are designed to help reduce blood sugar and increase insulin sensitivity. Look for products that contain magnesium, B-complex vitamins, bitter melon, holy basil, cinnamon, fenugreek, green tea, *Gymnema sylvestre*, chromium, vanadium, and lipoic acid. There may also be some ginseng, prickly pear, banaba, manganese, biotin, zinc, vitamin C, bilberry, and additional antioxidants. Use as directed.

CHAPTER 29

Myalgic Encephalomyelitis/ Chronic Fatigue Syndrome ℚ D I G I N

Fatigue is one of the most common complaints that bring people into a physician's office. Fatigue can be caused by nearly every illness and is part of the natural healing process. Excessive fatigue that lasts and lasts may be a sign of illness or of myalgic encephalomyelitis/chronic fatigue syndrome (ME/CFS). Also called chronic fatigue and immune dysfunction syndrome (ME/CFS), CFS, myalgic encephalomyelitis (ME), chronic Epstein-Barr virus (CEBV), and yuppie flu, ME/CFS is a long-lasting, debilitating fatigue that is not associated with any particular illness. Although people have been fatigued for millennia, the term *chronic fatigue syndrome* was only coined in 1988. This condition is considered to be an autoimmune disease. According to the Institute of Medicine in 2015, 836,000 to 2.5 million Americans have ME/CFS. According to the Centers for Disease Control and Prevention (CDC), 90 percent of people with ME/CFS have not yet been diagnosed because there isn't a unique test to diagnosis it. About 50 percent return to normal health within five years. The rest may be affected for decades.

The CDC has provided the following criteria for diagnosis of ME/CFS. By definition, individuals with ME/CFS have been extremely tired for at least six months for no obvious reason. First, the fatigue is not eliminated by rest, and the fatigue substantially reduces the person's ability to function normally. Second, at least four of the following symptoms have been present for a period of at least six months: loss of ability to concentrate or short-term memory function; sore throat;

swollen and tender lymph nodes; muscle pain; multiple-joint pain without swelling or redness; headaches of a new type, pattern, or severity; sleep disturbances; and exercise-caused fatigue that lasts more than 24 hours.

People with ME/CFS share many common symptoms, but not everyone has all the same ones. ME/CFS often begins with an infectious flu-like disease accompanied by fevers that come and go, joint stiffness and pain, sore throat, cough, sleep disturbances, light sensitivity, night sweats, and extreme exhaustion after the slightest exertion. Commonly, a short walk or bit of exercise will wipe out your energy for days afterward. The causes of ME/CFS are not really known. In about 10 percent of cases where people have an illness caused by the Epstein-Barr virus (known for causing mononucleosis), Ross River virus, or *Coxiella burnetii*, people will have continuing symptoms that warrant a diagnosis of ME/CFS. Other infections that have been associated with the condition include herpesvirus 6, enterovirus, rubella, *Candida albicans*, bornaviruses, mycoplasma, and human immunodeficiency virus (HIV). Sometimes healthy people have high blood antibodies for these viruses and have no symptoms of ME/CFS. It's possible that these viruses trigger ME/CFS, but it's also possible that the low immune function in people with ME/CFS increases their chances of catching a wide variety of infectious illnesses. Although you can chase the virus, it's often just the trigger, not the ultimate cause of the illness. As with many illnesses, there is speculation on the part of researchers that there may be an autoimmune mimicry that gets triggered by a virus. In some people, there is a disregulation in the hypothalamus/pituitary/adrenal (HPA) axis. Stress may play a large role in triggering ME/CFS. There is some literature associating so-called type A behavior with development of the disease, suggesting that being an overachiever may increase risk. Other issues that have symptoms similar to ME/CFS include high levels of D-lactic acid, mold/biotoxin issues, or Lyme and coinfections.

Many with ME/CFS cannot hold down a job and become depressed because the fatigue is so extreme. Those who do work come home exhausted and immediately go to bed so they can generate enough energy for work the next day. Because there isn't any apparent cause and no observable symptoms, and because people often look healthy, people with ME/CFS are often confronted by people and doctors who just don't believe they are sick.

In 1990, the CDC began to keep records and study people with ME/CFS to understand more about possible causes and therapies. We now know that ME/CFS is multifactorial and affects many biochemical systems. Cytokine production of interleukin-2 (IL-2) is low and causes poor immune function. Other immune parameters appear to be overstimulated. Although this seems paradoxical, it's probably not. According to Hans Selye, an expert on stress, our systems initially react to stress by overproducing. If working harder doesn't eventually solve the problem, they underproduce. Many people with ME/CFS have exhausted adrenal glands and produce low amounts of cortisol and other adrenal hormones. They often have thyroid insufficiencies and may require thyroid hormone replacement. Other hormones, such as estrogen, progesterone, dehydroepiandrosterone (DHEA), and testosterone, may also be out of balance.

To find relief for ME/CFS, use the DIGIN approach discussed in Part II. In some people there is a disregulation in the hypothalamus/pituitary/adrenal (HPA) axis. Stress may play a significant role in triggering ME/CFS. There is some literature associating the so-called type A behavior with development of the disease, suggesting that being an overachiever may increase risk. Other issues that have symptoms similar to ME/CFS include high levels of D-lactic acid, mold/biotoxin issues, or Lyme and coinfections. There is often malabsorption. The liver is overburdened and overworked, so the toxic by-products of life accumulate in tissues, and the cycle deepens.

Eventually, the mitochondria are affected. Mitochondria are the energy factories inside our cells, creating adenosine triphosphate (ATP) from glucose in a complicated process called the citric acid cycle, or Krebs cycle. Mitochondrial DNA is extremely susceptible to environmental damage from nutritional deficiencies, infection, disrupted sleep, pregnancy, changes in pH balance in the cell, magnesium status, hormonal deficiencies, and stress. Mitochondrial function can be inhibited by magnesium insufficiency, changes in cellular pH, and abnormal products of metabolism. These can be interpreted by the body as toxins. Magnesium is essential for mitochondrial functioning and is part of the matrix. Mitochondria also require vitamins B_1, B_2, B_3, B_6, lipoic acid, manganese, zinc, coenzyme Q10 (CoQ10), glucose, fatty acids, and amino acids. Mitochondrial function can be tested with an organic acid test, which has provided evidence that mitochondrial DNA is damaged much more easily and is more susceptible to environmental toxins and other stressors. As ME/CFS symptoms progress, the mitochondria often need nutritional support of their own.

Jacob Teitelbaum, MD, a specialist in chronic fatigue syndrome and fibromyalgia, speculates that this is a mitochondrial and hypothalamic disorder. Viral infections can disrupt hypothalamus and mitochondrial function. The hypothalamus controls sleep, autonomic nervous system function, body temperature, and hormone balance. When energy stores in the hypothalamus are depleted, all of these systems become imbalanced.

With the blood pressure test used with a tilt table, researchers have found that many people with ME/CFS have low postural blood pressure. Complementary medicine physicians have long used reclining and standing blood pressures to detect poor adrenal function. Individuals with healthy adrenal function experience only a five- to ten-point rise in blood pressure when they move from a reclining to a standing position. In people with poor adrenal function, blood pressure remains the same or drops. So, is the tilt-table hypotension the primary culprit or an indicator of poor adrenal function? In any case, some people with low blood pressure respond to an increase in salt intake to at least 1,000 mg daily or by taking medication to increase blood pressure.

There aren't any panaceas for ME/CFS, but there are therapies that can gradually help restore people to health. It's important to address detoxification, viral load, digestive function, dysbiosis (including candida and parasites), mitochondrial function, intestinal flora, environmental contaminants, heavy metals, underlying allergies, and hormone imbalances (especially thyroid and adrenal), as well as to restore functioning of the immune system. If this seems daunting, it can be. The causes and specifics are different for each person. Careful partnership between practitioner and patient will give the very best results. ME/CFS is one area in which conventional, mainstream medicine has little to offer. If you've tried everything that your doctor has recommended and still aren't any better, you need to broaden your approach.

Restoration of digestive competency and nutrition go a long way toward normalizing ME/CFS. Work with a nutritionally oriented health professional to design a program that meets your specific needs. The first steps are discovering any underlying problems that aggravate and drive the condition using the tests listed. It's important to check carefully for parasites; one study found giardia in 28 percent of subjects with ME/CFS. Develop and follow a diet based on foods that are healthy for you and a nutrient-rich program designed to boost immune, brain, and cellular function. When you are ready, add exercise, a little bit at a time. People with ME/CFS often feel worse after exercise, so go slowly. Several researchers link elevated cytokines and TNF-alpha and low levels of antioxidants and heat shock proteins in people with chronic fatigue. Increasing anti-inflammatory nutrients and antioxidants could be really beneficial. (See Chapter 8 on inflammation and the immune system.)

Physical therapy, counseling, occupational therapy, acupuncture, chi gong, Emotional Freedom Technique, and mind-body techniques can all be of great benefit.

The biological, rather than medical, approach to ME/CFS saves money and works better. In one study of cost-effectiveness, it was determined that a nutritional approach costs $2,000, compared to $10,000 for a medical approach. The patients on nutritional programs reported greater improvements in function and subjective well-being. They were able to significantly reduce the amount of medication they used.

Resources

- Institute of Medicine and Board on the Health of Selected Populations, *Beyond Myalgic Encephalomyelitis/Chronic Fatigue Syndrome: Redefining an Illness*
- Kasia Kines, *The Epstein-Barr Virus Solution*
- Jacob Teitelbaum, *The Fatigue and Fibromyalgia Solution*

This is a condition where testing is warranted. Begin with regular medical testing for infection and hormone balance. Look for parasites, such as giardia. Then, consider doing these additional tests.

Functional Laboratory Testing
- Comprehensive digestive stool analysis with parasitology
- Testing for food, environmental, mold, and chemical sensitivities
- Food allergy testing
- Intestinal permeability screening
- Organic acid testing
- Blood analysis for nutrients
- Fatty acid analysis

Healing Options
After testing, you'll have a better idea of any underlying problems. Look up related sections in this book to help you with the specifics.

- **Work with a therapist on mental health/shift your energy.** Cognitive behavior therapy and other counseling has helped many people with ME/CFS. Consider acupuncture, chi gong, or other energetic therapy to bring your systems into balance.
- **Investigate food and environmental sensitivities.** Try an elimination diet. Use shampoos, soaps, and toiletries that are hypoallergenic for your specific needs and natural household cleaning products that are healthier for you, your family, and the environment. Some people are sensitive to their mattresses, gas stoves, carpeting, and upholstery. If you are, you may need to wear 100 percent cotton or other natural fiber clothes and use 100 percent cotton sheets and blankets. Cotton is one of the largest genetically engineered crops, and some people are so sensitive to artificial substances that they can tolerate only organic cotton. Work with a health professional who can help you thread your way through the details.

- **Supplement with probiotics.** Supplemental use of beneficial bacteria can make a tremendous difference in your ability to digest foods. Beneficial flora can help reestablish the normal microbial balance in your intestinal tract. A recent study of people with ME/CFS found that 6 of the 15 participants reported cognitive improvements in the four-week study.
- **Try digestive enzymes.** Pancreatic or vegetable enzymes supply the enzymes that your body needs to digest fats, proteins, and carbohydrates. Products differ. See Chapter 3 for more information. Take one to two capsules with meals.
- **Take a multivitamin with minerals.** Because people with ME/CFS have difficulty with absorption and utilization of nutrients, a highly absorbable, hypoallergenic nutritional supplement is necessary. Although products that contain herbs, bee pollen, spirulina, and other food factors are good for many people, people with ME/CFS often feel worse after taking food-based supplements. Make sure you buy the supplements that are herb and food free. Choose a supplement that contains the following nutrients: 25 to 50 mg zinc, 5,000 to 10,000 IU vitamin A, 10,000 to 25,000 IU carotenes, 200 or more IU vitamin E, at least 200 mcg selenium, 200 mcg chromium, at least 25 mg of most B-complex vitamins, 400 to 800 mcg folic acid, and 5 to 10 mg manganese.
- **Take vitamin C.** Vitamin C boosts immune function, helps detoxification pathways, and has been shown to have antiviral effects. Clinicians, including me, have found it useful in people with ME/CFS. Take 3,000 to 5,000 mg daily. Do a vitamin C flush (detailed in Chapter 17).
- **Increase magnesium.** Magnesium is found in the ATP complex. Found in green leafy vegetables and whole grains, magnesium is involved in more than 300 enzymatic reactions in the body. It is essential for energy production, nerve conduction, muscle function, and bone health. People with ME/CFS are often deficient in magnesium. Supplemental magnesium can improve energy levels and emotional states, while decreasing pain. Most people improve with use of oral magnesium supplements, but some need intravenous injections. Physicians can give 1,000 mg magnesium sulfate by injection. In one study, magnesium injections improved function in 12 out of 15 people, compared to only 3 receiving the placebo. Magnesium can be hard for many people to use. Adding 1 teaspoon of choline citrate daily for each 200 mg of magnesium taken can significantly improve magnesium uptake. Take 500 to 2,000 mg magnesium glycinate, potassium aspartate, malate, or ascorbate. Caution: Too much magnesium causes diarrhea.
- **Try coenzyme Q10 (CoQ10).** CoQ10 is necessary for energy production, immune function, and repair and maintenance of tissues. It also enhances

cell function. CoQ10 is widely used in Japan for heart disease and has been researched as an antitumor substance. Take 60 to 300 mg daily.

- **Take essential fatty acids.** Several studies have shown people with ME/CFS to have fatty acid imbalances. In a recent study, a combination of evening primrose oil (primarily omega-3) and fish oil (primarily omega-6) or a placebo of olive oil was given to 70 people with ME/CFS. Of the people taking fish and evening primrose oils, 74 percent showed improvement at 5 weeks, and 85 percent showed improvement at 15 weeks. In comparison, the placebo group showed 23 percent improvement at 5 weeks and 17 percent at 15 weeks. Another study of the use of supplemental fatty acids showed improvement in 27 out of 29 people with ME/CFS over 12 to 18 weeks. It also showed that 20 people who had previously been unable to work full time for an average of more than three years were able to go back to work full time after an average of 16 weeks. Further, 16 months later, 27 out of 28 remained improved, and 20 were still progressing. Do fatty acid testing, and then adjust doses to match your needs.

- **Add methionine.** Methionine, an essential sulfur-containing amino acid, is commonly deficient in people with ME/CFS. It acts as a methyl donor for transmethylation reactions throughout the body, especially in the brain. It also helps sulfoxidation for liver detoxification pathways and is a precursor for other sulfur-containing amino acids such as cysteine and taurine. People with ME/CFS probably have an increased need for methionine. Some people find improvement with a general amino acid supplement that supplies methionine, lysine, and carnitine simultaneously. Take 500 to 1,000 mg daily.

- **Try SAMe.** S-adenosylmethionine (SAMe), a compound that is naturally found in every cell in our body, is made from methionine. Research on SAMe shows it to have powerful antidepressant effects without the side effects of pharmaceutical antidepressant medications. SAMe has also been shown to be as potent an anti-inflammatory drug as indomethacin without the negative side effects in people with arthritis.

- **Try acetylcarnitine.** The vast majority of people with ME/CFS have low levels of acetylcarnitine, although their levels of free carnitine are normal. Carnitine, vital for the conversion of fats into energy, also plays some role in detoxification and is believed to be essential for heart function. Finally, carnitine helps transport long-chain fatty acids into the mitochondria. Carnitine deficiencies result in muscle weakness, aches, and poor tone. Take 500 mg of carnitine two to four times daily for three months. For those on a budget, L-carnitine will also work.

- **Try D-ribose.** Ribose is a structural sugar that helps provide energy. Dr. Jacob Teitelbaum did a pilot study with 41 people with either fibromyalgia or chronic fatigue syndrome. Overall, two-thirds reported benefits, with 45 percent reporting improvements in energy, and 30 percent reporting improvements in overall well-being after about 20 days; several also reported pain reduction. Take 5 grams three times daily, for three weeks, and then reduce to 5 grams twice daily. Mix in a cold, cool, or room temperature beverage.

- **Try lysine.** Often people with ME/CFS also have herpes infections. Some people find good results with a general amino acid supplement, which supplies carnitine, lysine, and methionine as well as other amino acids. Take 1 to 2 grams lysine daily at the first sign of an outbreak; 500 mg daily for prevention.

- **Try malic acid.** Malic acid comes from apples and is important in energy production at a cellular level. Several physicians have found malic acid supplementation reduces fatigue and pain of fibromyalgia. Take 6 to 12 tablets daily, decreasing dosage over time. Each tablet contains 300 mg malic acid–magnesium hydroxide.

- **Use immune-modulating herbs and mushrooms.** Echinacea, goldenseal, astragalus, phytolacca (pokeweed), licorice, and lomatium all have immune-stimulating properties. Immune-balancing mushrooms, such as maitake, shiitake, or reishi, can also be eaten. They can help prevent secondary infections while you are in a susceptible state. Take them preventively or therapeutically as directed.

- **Provide adrenal support.** People with ME/CFS often need adrenal support. Think first about rest and nurture. Then also consider supplements, such as adrenal glandular supplements or herbal supplements, such as licorice and Siberian ginseng. Vitamin C and pantothenic acid (vitamin B_5) are also needed for proper adrenal function. If your blood pressure is low, you can use whole licorice; if not, use DGL, which will not affect blood pressure. It's best to take adrenal support in the morning and at lunch. If taken too late in the day, adrenal support can stimulate energy when you want to be winding down.

- **Consider nicotinamide adenine dinucleotide (NAD).** In a study monitoring the effect NAD has on people with ME/CFS, 26 subjects were given the reduced form of it for four weeks and a placebo for an additional four weeks. In the results, 31 percent showed improvement when on NAD, while only 8 percent improved when taking the placebo. Subjects were less fatigued and had improvement in quality of life. NAD is integral to the citric acid cycle of energy production. Once again, we are reminded that each person has unique needs. While most people did not benefit, NAD may be a useful treatment for some people. More research needs to be done to see if 10 mg daily, the amount given in the study, is the proper dosage; if a longer treatment program would be of additional benefit; and what, if any, the long-term benefits are.

- **Try Meyer's cocktail.** Intravenous (IV) nutrients, given by a physician, can quickly help revitalize your nutrient status. Nutrients can be absorbed and used at higher concentrations. Meyer's cocktail is a combination of magnesium, calcium, vitamins B_{12} and B_6, pantothenic acid, and vitamin C. It has been used successfully in people with a variety of ailments.
- **Exercise.** People with ME/CFS find exercise to be totally exhausting and draining. It is common for one period of exercise to be followed within 6 to 24 hours by 2 to 14 days of exhaustion and muscle aches. Paradoxically, exercise is helpful for restoring function in people with ME/CFS, so it's advisable to begin with simple walking, swimming, or biking for 5 minutes daily. If you can, increase the time by 1 or 2 minutes a day each week. If you feel that you are at your maximum, maintain your present length of exercise time until your fatigue decreases. Don't push yourself too hard. Slow and steady wins the race. Studies have shown that two-thirds of people with ME/CFS benefit through exercise, although it is critical to not overdo.

  A new hypothesis suggests that those with ME/CFS are functioning in an anaerobic state, so light anaerobic exercise may be most beneficial. Working with light weights, leg lifts, and weight machines without causing fatigue may be more beneficial than aerobic exercise. As you begin to feel better, incorporate aerobic exercise—walking, biking, swimming, and dancing. Prioritize, so you have energy for what's most important. Be patient, kind, and loving to yourself.
- **Practice stress-management skills.** Development of a strong support system is vital. People with ME/CFS often have the illness for a long time and can greatly benefit from support groups. Exchange of information and dialogue with others who understand what you are going through can expedite recovery. Take time for yourself, rest, and relax.

CHAPTER 30

Fibromyalgia Q D I G I N

Fibromyalgia is characterized by long-term muscle pain and stiffness. According to the American College of Rheumatology, fibromyalgia affects 3 million to 6 million Americans, 85 to 90 percent of whom are women. It affects about 2 to 4 percent of the general population and 20 percent of people with arthritic disease. It used to be called fibrositis, which implies an inflammation of fibrous and connective tissues such as muscles, tendons, fascia, and ligaments. Myofascial pain syndrome is similar but is characterized by just a few painful and achy places, most often in the jaw, that are tender when trigger points are touched.

Fibromyalgia is characterized by generalized aching, pain, and tenderness throughout the body. People complain of neck, shoulder, lower back, and hip pain that seems to move around from place to place. People often report fatigue and changes in sleep patterns. They often wake up during the night with a feeling of achiness or stiffness. About 40 to 70 percent of people with fibromyalgia also report irritable bowel symptoms: abdominal pain, constipation, diarrhea, gas, or bloating. Other symptoms that occur with frequency include cognitive decline, extreme sensitivity to touch, fatigue, bladder syndrome, tooth grinding, headaches, jaw pain or temporomandibular joint (TMJ) problems, and depression. Symptoms that occur less often are heightened sensitivity to chemicals; intolerance to cold, heat, or bright lights; bladder problems; Raynaud's phenomenon; difficulty concentrating; mood changes; dry eyes, skin, and mouth; painful menstruation; chest or pelvic pain; dizziness; nasal congestion; and numbness or swelling in the hands or feet.

According to the American College of Rheumatology, fibromyalgia is diagnosed by ruling out other conditions, based on a few simple criteria.

Other medical conditions that can masquerade as fibromyalgia include hypothyroidism; anemia; rheumatoid arthritis; lupus; polymyalgia rheumatic; Lyme disease; other rheumatic disorders, such as ankylosing spondylitis, multiple sclerosis, and Sjögren's disease; and cancer.

Dysbiosis, postviral immune suppression, mold exposure, and blood sugar imbalances can also contribute to muscle tenderness.

Fibromyalgia shares many symptoms with myalgic encephalomyelitis/chronic fatigue syndrome (ME/CFS), though it is classified as its own disease. One way to distinguish fibromyalgia from ME/CFS is that in fibromyalgia you won't usually find low acetylcarnitine levels or an underlying viral infection.

Once all of the other possible conditions have been ruled out, if you have pain in many areas in your body, experience fatigue, wake up unrefreshed, and have cognitive issues that have lasted over three months, and you have no other diagnosable condition, you will be diagnosed with fibromyalgia. It's a catch-all phrase and not very specific. Giving it this name doesn't really help you to determine why you are having these issues.

CAUSES OF FIBROMYALGIA

There are many hypotheses as to the cause or causes of fibromyalgia, but no consensus has been reached yet. It's likely that it's a cluster of symptoms that has many root causes. I remember a woman who had debilitating fibromyalgia. The medical team she was working with had looked at dysbiosis, food reactions, infection, and so forth. She diligently tried every recommendation. One day, her next-door neighbor recommended a multivitamin. She recovered fully and within a week was out dancing. I wish it were this simple, but in my experience, it typically isn't.

Fibromyalgia responds well to the DIGIN model presented in this book. Diligently look to discover the underlying issues for your fibromyalgia. Find the levers that will help you rebalance. These will be different for each person.

Fibromyalgia can be a physical manifestation of emotional trauma. Statistically people with fibromyalgia have a higher history of chronic stress and emotional, physical, and/or sexual trauma than people without fibromyalgia. People with fibromyalgia often report a traumatic event that triggered initial symptoms: emotional or physical stress, an accident, or a severe infectious illness. This is often accompanied by insomnia due to hypervigilance of the immune system (see Chapter 8).

Lack of sleep is associated with a dysfunction of the hippocampus, which can manifest as short-term memory loss and cognitive impairment. These are also classic fibromyalgia symptoms.

Intestinal permeability is markedly increased in people with fibromyalgia. There is a large overlap in people who have both fibromyalgia and irritable bowel syndrome (IBS). In these cases, research reports a small incidence between 1.1 and 7 percent of undiagnosed celiac disease in people diagnosed with fibromyalgia. There are also case reports and a couple of studies on nonceliac gluten intolerance in people with fibromyalgia. Therapeutic dietary approaches, discussed in Chapter 14, are a good starting point.

Dr. Mark Pimentel, MD, reported in a 2004 study that out of 42 people with fibromyalgia, all of them had abnormal hydrogen breath tests, indicating small intestinal bacterial overgrowth (SIBO). I'm not certain why this study has not been repeated, and yet I cannot find more in the literature on this topic.

Nutrient deficiencies play a role in fibromyalgia. Without proper nutrients, energy production in the mitochondria doesn't work correctly. Doing nutritional testing and organic acid testing can help you to optimize your nutritional status.

It's important to be checked for vitamin D status. About half of all people with fibromyalgia are deficient in this nutrient. Vitamin D deficiencies affect about one-third of Caucasians, two-thirds of Hispanics, and 90 percent of people of African descent. Sometimes, just optimizing vitamin D levels can "cure" fibromyalgia. Ask your doctor to check your 25-OH vitamin D level. Normal levels are between 32 and 100 ng/ml. Optimal levels are probably between 60 and 100 ng/ml. Our bodies make vitamin D from sunlight, but in northern climates, or if people aren't outdoors, we can become deficient. The best food source is coldwater fish, such as salmon, sardines, mackerel, and herring. Vitamin D also helps facilitate magnesium absorption. An increased need for magnesium is found in most people with fibromyalgia.

Use of a single supplement may bring some relief, but a total program is necessary to bring dramatic relief and true healing. Taking coenzyme Q10 (CoQ10); vitamins B_1, B_6, and arginine; 5-hydroxytryptophan (5-HTP); S-adenosylmethionine (SAMe); essential fatty acids; antioxidants; niacin; and magnesium malate (magnesium plus malic acid), in addition to a hypoallergenic diet, has been shown to have positive effects. Acupuncture has been proven useful in treating fibromyalgia. Chiropractic or osteopathic adjustments and massage treatments may also be of help.

People with fibromyalgia have an increased need for antioxidants. Use of antioxidant supplements and increasing fruits, vegetables, nuts, seeds, and whole foods can reduce inflammation and free radical damage.

People with fibromyalgia are generally put on anti-inflammatory drugs and antidepressants. One study showed that 90 percent of people treated with anti-inflammatory drugs were still symptomatic after three years. Conventional medical therapies for fibromyalgia usually are unsuccessful in the long term because they fail to address possible underlying causes of the illness. Food and environmental sensitivities, candida, toxicity, unresolved emotional issues, and/or parasites can be causal factors in fibromyalgia. A stool test may be useful in diagnosing the cause of fibromyalgia. When the underlying problem has been identified and treated, fibromyalgia resolves.

A small but promising study was done with 32 people who had fibromyalgia for 5 to 10 years. There were 25 active participants and seven controls. The participants were tested for food and environmental sensitivities with the ELISA/ACT test and given dietary restrictions. They were put on a detoxification program and personalized nutritional therapies to meet their needs and stimulate repair of cells and tissues. The final component was stress management, with recommendations for relaxation training, exercise, and biofeedback. In 6 to 12 weeks, these people showed a reduction of 80 to 90 percent in their symptoms. They also showed a significant reduction in the number of foods and environmental sensitivities in repeated testing. More research needs to be done in this area.

Nutritional therapies have been successful in the reduction of symptoms. In a study, 50 people with either Myalgic Encephalomyelitis/Chronic Fatigue Syndrome or fibromyalgia were given products made by Mannatech, a multilevel supplement company, including freeze-dried aloe, plant-derived saccharides with freeze-dried fruits and vegetables, and a wild yam product with multivitamins and minerals. Although all subjects in this study had undergone previous unsuccessful medical treatment, a remarkable reduction in symptoms was noted, with continued improvement over the nine-month test period. Although this was a small, preliminary study, it shows promise.

Resources:

- David Brady, *Fibro Fix.*
- Ginevra Liptan, MD, *The FibroManual: A Complete Fibromyalgia Treatment Guide for You and Your Doctor.*

Functional Laboratory Testing
- Breath test for SIBO
- Organic acid testing
- Nutritional analysis

- Adrenal stress testing (salivary DHEA and cortisol)
- ELISA/ACT food and environmental sensitivity testing
- Oxidative stress evaluation
- Provocation testing for heavy metals
- Hormone testing

Healing Options

- **Look for the underlying cause.** Use the DIGIN model to correct digestive imbalances, look for food reactions, and look for hormone imbalances and nutritional deficiencies. With fibromyalgia there is almost always an emotional/spiritual component; use therapies such as counseling, acupuncture, cranial sacral therapy, or homeopathy to unblock emotional stress and trauma. Rule out infection and mold toxicity. Do your best to get a good night's sleep. Look until you discover underlying root issues.
- **Take vitamin D.** Vitamin D deficiency is often diagnosed as fibromyalgia. About half of people with fibromyalgia have low serum vitamin D levels. We make vitamin D in our skin from exposure to sunlight. So, get outdoors more. It's difficult to get enough vitamin D from our foods. Have your vitamin D level tested. Optimal levels in people with fibromyalgia are likely to be between 80 and 100 ng/ml. Dosages range from 2,000 IU daily as a maintenance dose to 10,000 IU daily if vitamin D levels are extremely low.
- **Detoxify and cleanse.** Metabolic cleansing involves going on a hypoallergenic food plan and taking a nutrient-rich protein powder designed to help restore your liver's detoxification capacities. Use this protocol for one to three weeks. See Chapter 17 for more information on this topic.
- **Investigate food and environmental sensitivities.** Eliminate all foods and chemicals that you are sensitive to for four to six months. (See Chapters 9 and 17 for an elimination diet.) Get tested to find the specifics. Work with a health professional who can help you with the details.
- **Try ascorbigen and broccoli powder.** A study of 12 patients with fibromyalgia was done with ascorbigen and broccoli powder. Ascorbigen is the most common indole found in cooked cabbage, broccoli, brussels sprouts, and other cabbage family foods. In one month, symptoms improved by nearly 20 percent. After the supplements were discontinued, symptoms returned to usual levels within two weeks. Take 100 mg ascorbigen plus 400 mg broccoli powder daily.
- **Take a multivitamin with minerals**. A high-quality, hypoallergenic nutritional supplement is necessary. Although products that contain herbs, bee pollen, spirulina, and other food factors are good for many people, it's best to buy

supplements that are herb and food free. Look for the following levels of specific nutrients: 50 to 100 mg vitamin B_1, 50 to 100 mg vitamin B_6, 200 to 400 IU vitamin E, 10,000 IU vitamin A, 10,000 to 25,000 IU carotenes, 200 mcg selenium, 200 mcg chromium, 5 to 10 mg manganese, glutathione, cysteine, or N-acetyl cysteine (NAC), plus additional nutrients. Antioxidant nutrients—carotenes, vitamins C and E, selenium, glutathione, CoQ10, cysteine, and NAC—have been shown to be needed in larger quantities in people with fibromyalgia.

- **Take vitamin B_1 (thiamin).** People with fibromyalgia have lower levels of red blood cell transketolase, which is a functional test for thiamin status. Researchers found that supplemental thiamin pyrophosphate worked better than other forms. This suggests a metabolic defect rather than a true deficiency. This may also reflect a magnesium deficiency because thiamin-dependent enzymes require magnesium. Take 25 to 100 mg daily.

- **Take vitamin C.** Vitamin C boosts immune function, helps detoxification pathways, and has antiviral effects. Take 3,000 mg daily. Once a week, do a vitamin C flush (see Chapter 17).

- **Take magnesium.** It is very common for people with fibromyalgia to be deficient in magnesium. Serum magnesium levels often appear normal, but if more sophisticated tests such as red blood cell magnesium are done, magnesium levels are often low. Supplemental magnesium can improve energy levels and emotional states while decreasing pain. Most people improve by using oral magnesium supplements, but some need an intravenous injection of 1,000 mg magnesium sulfate by a physician (for more on magnesium, see discussion on chronic fatigue syndrome). Choline citrate can greatly enhance oral magnesium utilization (available from Perque, listed at http://www.digestivewellnessbook.com). Take 500 to 1,000 mg magnesium citrate or magnesium glycinate.

- **Try arginine.** People with fibromyalgia have been shown to have lower levels of arginine than other people. Take 500 to 1,000 mg or a mixed free amino acid supplement.

- **Try 5-hydroxytryptophan (5-HTP).** People with fibromyalgia have lower tryptophan levels than controls. Studies have shown 5-HTP to be of benefit with fibromyalgia. Tryptophan is a precursor to serotonin, a neurotransmitter that helps us sleep and prevents depression. Passionflower, an herb with high levels of tryptophan, has been used historically for depression, anxiety, and insomnia, all of which are symptoms of fibromyalgia. Tryptophan is also found in cashews, cheddar cheese, eggs, halibut, peanuts, salmon, sardines, shrimp, turkey, and tuna. In addition, our body produces it when we eat starchy foods. Take 200 to 600 mg daily of 5-HTP. Doses can be divided between morning and bedtime.

- **Try capsaicin (cayenne pepper cream).** The prescription drug capsaicin was used in a study of 45 people with fibromyalgia. It was found to improve grip strength and reduce pain over a two-week period. Capsaicin cream burns temporarily, but this diminishes over time.
- **Try SAMe.** A recent study of 47 people with fibromyalgia showed that injections and oral supplementation of SAMe significantly reduced muscle tenderness and the number of tender points, lowered pain severity, and benefited depression and anxiety. SAMe is produced in our bodies from methionine. It is the active methylating agent for many enzyme reactions throughout the body, especially in the brain. It is probably the sulfur that is needed. People with fibromyalgia can probably make this conversion, so oral methionine may be useful clinically (1,000 to 2,000 mg). Other sulfur-containing supplements are dimethylsulfoxide (DMSO), taurine, glucosamine or chondroitin sulfate, and reduced glutathione. In the study, the dose was 200 mg given daily as intramuscular injection, plus 400 mg taken orally twice daily.
- **Try Meyer's cocktail.** Intravenous (IV) nutrients, given by a physician, can quickly help revitalize your nutrient status. Nutrients can be absorbed and used at higher concentrations. Meyer's cocktail is a combination of magnesium, calcium, vitamins B_{12} and B_6, pantothenic acid, and vitamin C. It has been used successfully in people with a variety of ailments.
- **Try traditional Chinese medicine.** Acupuncture has been established as giving benefit to people with fibromyalgia. A 2010 multicentered study of 186 people with fibromyalgia reported that 65 percent of those who received acupuncture combined with cupping and Western medicine had benefits. This produced better effects than either just acupuncture with cupping or use of Western medicine alone. A 2010 review study of 1,516 people with fibromyalgia (from 25 combined studies) reports that acupuncture reduced the number of tender points and reduced pain scores when compared with conventional medications. When combined with cupping, results improved for pain reduction and improving depression scores. On the other hand, a Cochrane Review in 2009 reported that there was no change in pain intensity when compared to a placebo. Acupuncture and cupping may or may not be of benefit to you, but the possible benefits coupled with low risk make it worth trying.
- **Try malic acid.** Malic acid, found in apples, is important in energy production at a cellular level. Several physicians have found malic acid supplementation reduces fatigue and the pain of fibromyalgia. It also helps alkalize. Take 6 to 12 tablets of 300 mg malic acid–magnesium hydroxide daily, decreasing dosage over time.

- **Take quercetin.** Quercetin is the most effective bioflavonoid in its anti-inflammatory effects, and it can be used to reduce pain and inflammatory responses and control allergies. Take 500 to 1,000 mg three to four times daily.
- **Take glucosamine sulfate.** Glucosamine sulfate is used therapeutically to help repair cartilage, reduce swelling and inflammation, and restore joint function, with no reported side effects. Take 500 mg two to four times daily.
- **Try digestive enzymes.** Take one to two tablets or capsules with meals.
- **Supplement with probiotics.** Use of supplemental beneficial bacteria can help reestablish the normal microbial balance in your intestinal tract. The supplement you purchase may have additional microbes as well. Take as directed on label as products vary. Mix powdered supplement with a cool beverage.
- **Try coenzyme Q10 (CoQ10).** CoQ10 is necessary for energy production, immune function, repair and maintenance of tissues, and enhanced cell function. Take 60 to 100 mg daily.
- **Try glutamine.** Glutamine, the most abundant amino acid in our bodies, is used in the digestive tract as a fuel source and for healing stomach ulcers, irritable bowel syndrome, ulcerative bowel diseases, and leaky gut syndrome. Begin with 8 grams daily for four weeks.

CHAPTER 31

Migraine Headaches Q DIGIN

Migraines usually begin with a throbbing pain on one side of the head, which may spread to the other side. About 60 percent of people experience symptoms 24 hours prior to the actual migraine, which include mood changes, food cravings, repetitive yawning, thirst, fluid retention, stiff neck, irritability, fatigue, numbness or tingling on one side of the body, lack of appetite, diarrhea, constipation, a feeling of coldness, lethargy, changes in vision, or seeing bright spots. These symptoms, referred to collectively as an aura, could signal that a migraine is on the way; they may disappear when the headache appears, or they may remain. Medications and other techniques work best if used at this point. Although symptoms vary from person to person, the pattern is consistent in each individual. Migraine attacks may last from hours to days and may be accompanied by nausea, vomiting, and extreme sensitivity to light.

Migraine headaches cause periodic disruption in the lives of 28 million Americans, affecting 6 percent of men and more than 18 percent of women every year, averaging just over 10 percent of our population and making it the most prevalent neurological illness. Costs to society are $13 billion annually, which includes 157 million workdays that are lost each year. Migraines have genetic, hormonal, immune, and environmental components.

Migraines usually come on in response to a trigger. Common triggers are foods and beverages, alcohol, stress, emotions, hormone changes, medications such as estrogen therapy, visual stimuli, or changes in routine. A recent study of 494 people with migraines cited the following triggers: stress (62 percent), weather changes (43 percent), missing a meal (40 percent), and bright sunlight (38 percent). Cigarettes, perfumes, and sexual activity also provoked migraines in some people. Other triggers are red wine, exhaustion, and monosodium glutamate (MSG). Tobacco, birth control pills, and ergotamine (a drug used to treat migraines) increase the frequency of migraines in some people.

Hormone fluctuations in women can worsen, improve, or trigger migraines. Many women experience migraines only at specific times in their menstrual cycle, from ovulation through menstruation. Birth control pills and other estrogen-containing medications are widely recognized to trigger migraines in susceptible women. When women stop taking the medications, their migraines typically disappear. When I was in my teens, I was put on birth control pills for severe menstrual cramps. I developed migraines, but because the relationship between hormones and migraines wasn't yet established, my doctor did not feel this was the cause. I was put through brain scans and neurological tests. When all was said and done, going off the pill stopped the migraines, and I've never had another. Unfortunately, this took several years to figure out.

Jean Munro, MD, an English doctor who specializes in working with people with multiple chemical sensitivities, breaks migraines into four types. The first type is a classic migraine, which begins with a visual disturbance of some sort—flashing lights, blackening, or blurred vision. It usually involves one side of the head, and people often vomit. The migraine usually lasts one to three days and can be quite severe. The second type is called a common migraine and is almost identical to the first, except that there is no visual warning. It begins on one side, sometimes progressing to the other, and there may be vomiting. The third type is called a basilar migraine, when the blood vessels at the base of the head dilate. It can be quite frightening and often causes a panicky feeling, accompanied by a sense of doom. A generalized headache is accompanied by a pins-and-needles sensation around the mouth, nausea, and tingling hands. The fourth type, called a motor migraine, is a variation on the basilar and may be quite severe. Half the body feels weak, head pain centers around the eye, and vision is distorted.

A 2010 paper in *Headache* looked at comorbid conditions in 1,348 people with migraine: 88 percent were women; 31 percent had myalgic encephalomyelitis/chronic fatigue syndrome (ME/CFS) chronic fatigue syndrome; 25 percent had arthritis; 15 percent had endometriosis; 14 percent had uterine fibroids; 10 percent had fibromyalgia; and 6.5 percent had interstitial cystitis. Maltreatment in childhood was reported in 58 percent. Interestingly enough, abuse and neglect were associated with different diseases along with migraine. Emotional abuse was associated with IBS, ME/CFS, and arthritis; physical neglect was associated with arthritis in the entire group and with uterine fibroids in women; physical abuse was associated with endometriosis.

Using medications for migraines is the standard medical approach. The main drugs to treat acute migraines are those that increase serotonin (sumatriptan, naratriptan, and zolmitriptan), opiate pain medications, and dihydroergotamine. Drugs that help prevent migraines from occurring include valproic acid, beta blockers, and methysergide. According to Alan Gaby, a prominent nutritionally oriented MD and the author of *Nutritional Medicine*, the most effective medications reduce frequency only by half and have significant side effects. In his book, Dr. Gaby writes, "In my experience at least two-thirds of patients who comply with an appropriate regimen of dietary modification and nutritional supplements experience a substantial reduction in, or a complete cessation of, migraine headaches."

PREVENTING MIGRAINES BY CHANGING WHAT YOU EAT

One common trigger of migraine headaches is dysregulated blood sugar levels: hypoglycemia, diabetes, and/or high insulin levels. It's one of the first things that I consider and why I always ask my clients to keep track of what they have eaten or if they have eaten prior to a migraine. If migraines appear early morning or late afternoon when glucose levels are typically lowest, hypoglycemia is a likely suspect.

Avoiding caffeine or salt can help others. One study reports that people had significant improvement on a low-fat diet. Whether the results were from eating healthier foods or from the low-fat aspect of the diet is unknown to me. Virtually any food can be a migraine trigger. Figuring out which ones can be of great personal benefit.

The relationship between food sensitivities or allergies and migraines was studied during the 1930s. In 400 people, complete or partial relief was achieved 50.8 percent to 78 percent of the time. True IgE food allergies trigger some migraines; IgG sensitivities can also play a role. Since the 1930s, many studies have been done that replicate these results. Here are a few of those studies.

Of 282 patients with migraines whom Dr. Munro studied, 100 percent had food allergies or sensitivities; more than 200 of them were sensitive to wheat and/or dairy products. Other common trigger foods were tea and coffee, oranges, apples, onions, pork, egg, and beef. Dr. Munro found that foods eaten daily provoked more reactions than chocolate, alcohol, and cheese, which are thought to be the most common triggers. Dr. Munro also found that people who eliminated these foods from their diet and cleared their homes of environmental contaminants had the best results in prevention of migraines. Using mild household cleaners, getting rid of gas appliances, removing house plants with molds and fungus, frequent cleaning, and making a bedroom an oasis by removing carpets and curtains resulted in fewer migraines. Although these people were still exposed to smoke, perfume, and other environmental triggers outside, changing the home environment and their diets lowered their total load enough so that they became more tolerant.

In a 1979 issue of *Lancet*, E. C. Grant published a study in which 60 adults were put on a strict elimination diet for five days in an inpatient setting. They then added foods back into their diets. Migraines were triggered by wheat (78 percent of the time); orange (65 percent); eggs (45 percent); tea and coffee (40 percent each); chocolate and milk (37 percent each); beef (35 percent); and corn, sugar, and yeast (33 percent each). Headache rates dropped 85 percent. A quarter of people who had high blood pressure had normalization of the hypertension.

Dr. J. Egger and colleagues put 78 children on an elimination diet that included lamb or chicken, rice or potato, banana or apple, one vegetable, water, and vitamin and calcium supplements for three to four weeks. Children who did not improve were given a second elimination diet. On the first or second diet, 88.6 percent recovered completely. A total of 55 foods provoked migraines. The most common were cow's milk (31 percent); egg (27 percent); chocolate (25 percent); orange and wheat (24 percent each); benzoic acid (16 percent); cheese and tomato (15 percent each); tartrazine and rye (14 percent each); pork and fish (10 percent each); beef and corn (9 percent each); soy and tea (8 percent); oats, goat's milk, and coffee (7 percent each); and peanuts (6 percent). In the study, 40 of these children participated in blinded food testing; this confirmed that food allergies provoked migraine.

John Diamond, MD, of the Diamond Headache Clinic in Chicago, reports that foods high in amines also provoke migraines in some people. Dietary amines, which promote constriction of blood vessels, are normally broken down by enzymes, but some people with migraines have lower than normal amounts of the appropriate enzymes. The amines that provoke vasoconstriction are serotonin, tyramine, tryptamine, and dopamine. They are found in the greatest quantities in avocados, bananas, cabbage, eggplant, pineapple, plums, potatoes, tomatoes, cheese, canned fish, wine (especially red), beer, aged meats, and yeast extracts.

Nitrates, phenylethylamine, histamine, phenolic compounds, and monosodium glutamate can be triggers of migraine in certain people. Artificial sweeteners have also been implicated in migraines in some people. Aspartame (NutraSweet) was found to trigger migraine in 8.2 percent of people by Lipton and colleagues. Others speculate about the use of sucralose (Splenda). M. E. Bigal and A. V. Krymchantowski report about one woman whose migraines were consistently triggered by sucralose. Dr. R. M. Patel suggest that it's important for doctors to recognize sucralose as a potential trigger of migraines.

PREVENTING MIGRAINES WITH NUTRIENTS AND HERBS

Taking oral magnesium daily can be excellent for preventing migraines. This has been well studied. Magnesium is used in more than 300 enzymatic reactions in your body. Its main role is to relax muscles, nerves, and in this case, blood vessels. Dr. E. Koseoglu and colleagues found that when people were given magnesium, there was increased blood flow to the cortex, frontal, temporal, and insular regions of the brain. Many women have migraines triggered by menstruation. Others have reported that high levels of estrogen and progesterone decrease cellular magnesium levels and also have direct effects on smooth muscles in the brain. People with migraines often have impaired mitochondrial production; magnesium is needed for energy production. It's also used in neurotransmitter production. Various studies report benefits of 0 to 80 percent reduction in severity and frequency of migraine with magnesium supplementation.

Riboflavin (vitamin B_2) was first studied for prevention of migraines in the 1940s and 1950s. More recently, 49 people with recurrent migraines were given 400 mg of vitamin B_2 daily with breakfast for three months. The number of migraines declined by 67 percent and the severity diminished by 68 percent. Its maximum effect is reached after two or three months, so be patient and give it a good try. In another study, 55 people were given either a placebo or 400 mg of riboflavin daily. Over three months, 59 percent of the people on riboflavin improved by at least 50 percent. There were minor side effects in two people—one had diarrhea and the other had frequent urination. If you experience either of these side effects, decrease the dosage. In some people more modest doses can be effective.

Fish oil supplements contain high levels of docosahexaenoic acid (DHA) and eicosapentaenoic acid (EPA) oils. They have been shown in many studies to reduce the severity, duration, and frequency of migraine headaches. Most of us can produce EPA and DHA by using flaxseed oil, borage oil, or evening primrose oil, or by taking alpha-linolenic acid (ALA) and gamma-linolenic acid (GLA) supplements. However, this conversion requires that we have not only the genetic ability to complete the conversion, but also adequate vitamin B_6 and magnesium. One study gave subjects 1,800 mg of GLA and ALA in six capsules daily, plus 3 mg of niacin,

20 mg of vitamin C, 25 IU of vitamin E, 20 mg of soy phosphatides, 50 mg of magnesium, 1.3 mg of beta-carotene, and 0.3 mg of vitamin B_6. Of the 128 people who participated in the study, 86 percent had a reduction in the severity, frequency, and duration of their migraine headaches, 22 percent became migraine-free, and 90 percent had reduced nausea and vomiting. Further, 14 percent of the subjects were able to reduce their medication to simple pain relievers. Stress reduction and relaxation are also recommended.

In another study, 20 people with a history of migraines for more than one year and with a frequency of two to eight per month were given 1 mg vitamin B_{12} daily for three months in a nasal spray. Half of the people had a 53 percent reduction in migraines. In these people, there was a reduction from 5.2 to 1.9 attacks on average per month. In the other half, there was virtually no improvement. Vitamin B_{12} is nontoxic, inexpensive, and widely available in sublingual and nasal sprays. Oral forms are not well absorbed.

Supplementing with vitamin B_6, B_{12}, and folic acid can be useful in people with genetic typing that allows for easy use of folic acid. One study found that in people with the CC and CT MTHFR 677 C to T genotypes, supplementing with 2 mg folic acid, 25 mg of B_6, and 400 mcg of B_{12} significantly lowered the severity and frequency of headaches. Severity decreased from 75 percent to 28 percent. People with the TT genotype of MTHFR, which makes utilizing folic acid difficult, did not have these improvements. It's possible that taking easily utilized folic acid, such as methyltetrahydrofolate, could have helped even these people.

Melatonin has been tested in several studies for migraines in children and adults. Melatonin levels have been demonstrated to be lower in people who have migraines than in people who don't. Melatonin was given to 32 people with migraines at a dose of 3 mg given 30 minutes before bed, for three months. Headache frequency decreased 60.5 percent, intensity by 51.4 percent, and duration by 55.6 percent. The mechanism is unknown. Many of the medications used for migraines modulate serotonin, and serotonin is converted into melatonin. Perhaps that's why this works. In another study, 22 children were given 3 mg of melatonin before bed. In two-thirds of the children, headaches decreased by half, and four children had no headaches at all. One child dropped out of the study because of daytime sleepiness.

Butterbur (*Petasites hybridus*) is a European herb that has been used for centuries for such diverse problems as plaque, cough, asthma, and skin wounds. It works by lowering inflammatory markers that cause pain. Most recently, it has been shown to be effective for hay fever. In its natural state, it contains liver toxins, but a patented product, Petadolex, has removed these substances. In a 2004 study of 60 people with migraines, 33 were given 25 mg Petadolex twice daily and 27 were given a placebo twice daily. After three months, the average incidence of migraines decreased from 3.4 per month to 1.8 per month in the Petadolex group. Forty-five percent of the people responded really well and accounted for most of the results. In another study, 108 children demonstrated benefits from butterbur: 91 percent of the children felt substantially or slightly improved after four months of treatment, 77 percent had at least a 50 percent reduction in the frequency of headaches, and 63 percent noted at least some reduction in frequency.

Numerous studies have shown the herb feverfew (*Tanacetum parthenium*) to be effective in preventing and minimizing the severity of migraines. Others show no effectiveness. You can try it for yourself and see if it works for you. In one study by Drs. R. Shrivastava, J. C. Pechadre, and G. W. John, feverfew was given to 12 people with migraine without aura. They were given 300 mg feverfew twice daily, plus 300 mg white willow bark twice daily for 12 weeks. There was a significant reduction in frequency, severity, and duration of migraines.

Dr. Alan Gaby has given Meyers cocktail, an intravenous combination of magnesium, calcium, B-complex vitamins, and vitamin C, during migraine in six or more patients. Gaby reports that when given during a migraine, he has found complete or marked improvement within two minutes, with sustained improvement over 24 hours. One patient was treated more than 70 times in six years and responded well nearly all the time.

CHECK FOR DYSBIOSIS

This is an emerging area of research that is worth exploring. Several studies have explored the link between *Helicobacter pylori* infection and migraine. Dr. K. G. Yiannopoulou and colleagues studied 49 people aged 19 to 47 for migraines without aura. In people who had migraines with menstruation or family members who also had migraines, the incidence of *H. pylori* from gastric mucosal biopsy was 36 percent and 37 percent, respectively. In people who had no predisposing factors, prevalence of *H. pylori* was 81 percent in men and 87 percent in women. Dr. I. Ciancarelli et al. report that of 30 people with migraine, 16.7 percent had *H. pylori* IgA and IgG antibodies. Dr. A. Gasbarrini and colleagues report that of 225 people with migraine with and without aura, 40 percent tested positive for *H. pylori* with 13-urea breath testing. Another study by the same group reports higher levels of *H. pylori* in people with aura than without aura. Dr. L. Hong and colleagues report that when *H. pylori* was treated in people who had both migraine and cirrhosis, incidence, duration, and severity of migraines was reduced significantly.

I haven't seen any studies on small intestinal bacterial overgrowth (SIBO) or fungal overgrowth in people with migraine. There is a large overlap among people who have IBS, chronic fatigue syndrome, fibromyalgia, allergic rhinitis, and migraine. I look forward to seeing further studies on this.

HYPOTHYROID AND MIGRAINE

Many years ago, I worked with a woman who had severe migraines that decreased her quality of life. We discovered that she was hypothyroid. When her physician regulated her thyroid, her migraines were minimal. In 2007, A. J. Huete and colleagues reported in *Headache* the story of a person whose Hashimoto's thyroiditis resulted in symptoms that looked exactly like a migraine headache with an aura. Her thyroid tests were within a normal range, yet she had elevated antithyroid antibodies. While the incidence of hypothyroidism, subclinical hypothyroidism, or autoimmune thyroid disease and migraines has not been well studied, it seems worth looking into.

MOOD AND MIGRAINE

People with migraine often have mood and anxiety problems as well. Using strategies that address these at the same time is warranted: psychological counseling, biofeedback, acupuncture, chiropractic manipulation, emotional freedom technique, meditation, relaxation skills, and other mind-body modalities. Some of these modalities will also help with the neck pain that accompanies migraine so often.

Functional Laboratory Testing
- Intracellular magnesium, either red blood cell (RBC) or lymphocytes
- *H. pylori* testing
- Homocysteine levels (will give an indication about folate, B_6, and B_{12} status)
- ELISA/ACT testing for food and environmental allergies or sensitivities—IgG, IgE, and if possible, IgA and IgM
- Thyroid testing
- Organic acid testing

Healing Options
Migraines have many triggers that vary from person to person. Finding your triggers and the treatments that work best for you is the key. Begin by looking

at hormones, the DIGIN model, and food reactions. You certainly won't need all the therapies listed here, but hopefully you'll find relief from some of them:

- **Make dietary changes.** Remove all sugars, alcohol, salty foods, refined carbohydrates, and caffeine. Try to figure out what works best for you personally. Simply avoiding caffeine can dramatically reduce the incidence and severity of migraines. Similarly, Dr. Gaby reported on a 1930 study on the effects of salt in migraine incidence, in which 12 people avoided all salted snack foods before meals. At a six-month follow-up, migraines resolved completely in 3 people, and 7 more had fewer attacks. Another study found that a low-fat diet of less than 20 grams daily lowered the incidence of headache from nine each month to three. Headache intensity and the need for medications also dropped substantially. This information shows the importance of the diet and the quality of fats. In combination with good-quality omega-3 fatty acids, this could give great results for many people.

- **Examine effects of caffeine.** Caffeine plays a mixed role in migraines. For some people, it significantly reduces the number and severity of headaches; for others, it triggers them. Find out what works for you.

- **Be sure to eat often.** Low blood sugar levels often trigger migraines, so don't skip meals. You may find that eating five to six small meals each day works better for you than three main meals.

- **Try an elimination diet.** This may be the most significant thing you can do to discover what is triggering your migraines. Avoid foods you are sensitive to.

- **Make your home environmentally safe.** Use only natural cleaning supplies, remove gas appliances, clean out mold and mildew, use a dehumidifier, and make your bedroom into a safe harbor by removing unnecessary items, such as carpeting and drapery.

- **Avoid monosodium glutamate (MSG).** MSG can provoke migraine headaches, asthma, diarrhea, vomiting, and gastric symptoms. These problems can occur immediately after eating or may be delayed up to 72 hours, which makes their relationship to MSG more difficult to discover. Food product labels may be misleading, with MSG labeled as "natural coloring"; in addition, some hydrolyzed vegetable protein contains MSG. You can challenge yourself with MSG to see if it brings on a migraine. The ELISA/ACT blood test includes tests for MSG and glutamate sensitivity.

- **Begin with a multivitamin and mineral supplement.** Since so many nutrients have been demonstrated to help with migraine prevention, taking four to nine pills a day of multiple vitamin and mineral supplements may be a simple way to approach this with broad nutritional support.

- **Take magnesium.** Try 400 to 2,000 mg magnesium glycinate, ascorbate, keto-glutarate, malate, or other well-absorbed magnesium daily for at least three months. When you've reached saturation, you'll get diarrhea. I use this with my clients to figure out the correct dose. If you need more than 1,000 mg daily before your stools loosen, add 1 teaspoon choline citrate to facilitate the magnesium absorption.

- **Use riboflavin (vitamin B$_2$).** Studies used 400 mg daily. You may have good results on a lower dose. There have been reports of benefit using between 15 and 30 mg daily.

- **Take vitamin B$_{12}$.** Take 1,000 mcg B$_{12}$ nasally or sublingually. Use for at least three months to see the best effect.

- **Try niacin.** David Velling and colleagues report on a woman who began taking niacin to help lower cholesterol. Her migraines stopped for a month at 375 mg of sustained release niacin twice daily. When she reduced the dosage, she had two migraines the following month. There are reports of physicians using niacin intravenously during a migraine to decrease the severity and duration of headaches. The dose contains at least 100 mg niacin, which is infused slowly.

- **Try CoQ10.** You can have your CoQ10 levels tested. In 1,550 children with migraines, nearly 33 percent had low levels of CoQ10. Of those who came back for follow-up, CoQ10 levels increased and incidence and headache disability were reduced. In another study, 42 people with migraines took 100 mg of CoQ10 three times daily; another group took a placebo. In the CoQ10 group, 47.6 percent had their frequency of headaches reduced by half. Two other studies have demonstrated about half of people respond to CoQ10 supplements. Take 100 mg three times daily.

- **Increase consumption of omega-3 fatty acids, olive oil, and polyunsaturated fats.** Take 1,800 mg GLA/ALA and 2,000 to 3,000 mg of fish oil daily.

- **Try feverfew.** Feverfew needs to be taken on a daily basis as a preventive measure rather than as a treatment. There is a difference between fresh and dried feverfew and between various samples. If you don't get relief from one type, try another. Fresh feverfew seems to work best. It is easy to grow, so you could just eat a few leaves each day. Tinctures are available and would best approximate fresh leaves. It also comes in a freeze-dried form that seems to be effective. Twice daily, take 15 to 20 drops tincture, or take one to three capsules or one to three fresh leaves daily.

- **Try butterbur (Petadolex).** If you are one of the lucky, this could be a great remedy for you. Take 25 mg twice daily.
- **Take antioxidants.** Migraines are often triggered by substances that promote free radicals, such as cigarette smoke, perfume, hair spray, pollution, and household chemicals. One researcher found lower levels of superoxide dismutase (SOD) in platelets of people with migraines than in people with tension headaches. More research needs to be done in this area, but taking adequate antioxidants in a multivitamin with minerals may help prevent migraines.
- **Check for *H. pylori*. *H. pylori*** infection has been linked to migraines.
- **Explore possible candida infection.** A recent study of the relationship between candidiasis and migraines found that 13 out of 17 migraine sufferers responded to a three-month program of diet and medication with fewer and less severe headaches. Blood testing showed a lowering of candida antibodies as well. The four people who did not respond well didn't stick to the program. Test for candida. (See Chapter 11 for more information.)
- **Try acupuncture.** Acupuncture has been shown to reduce the incidence and severity of migraine headaches in some people. Study results vary. You may find great benefit or none at all.
- **Explore behavioral techniques.** Many studies have been done and biofeedback, hypnotherapy, and stress-reduction techniques have all proven useful to some migraine sufferers. They may be 35 to 50 percent effective. Plus, you'll have better stress-management skills to use in all areas of life. Behavioral techniques help us better understand stressors and how to cope more effectively.
- **Try chiropractic manipulation and massage.** Chiropractic manipulation and massage can help blood and lymphatic supply and relax muscle tension.

CHAPTER 32

Mental Health: Depression, Anxiety, and Schizophrenia ⭘ D I G I N

In the United States, we have an epidemic of mental health issues. According to the National Institutes of Mental Health, 18.1 percent of us have anxiety issues, 6.9 percent have major depression, 2.6 percent are diagnosed with bipolar disorder, and 1.1 percent of us have schizophrenia. Mental illness and depression are higher in Native American; native Alaskan; and lesbian, gay, bisexual, transgender, and questioning (LGBTQ) populations than in the general population. Furthermore, 20 percent of American children and teens currently have or will have a serious mental illness during their lifetime. Mental illness begins in 50 percent of people by the age of 14 and 75 percent by the age of 24. Prevention of some mental illness can be enhanced by establishing a healthy microbiome in the first two to three years of life. Mental health issues overlap and contribute greatly to addiction disorders, school dropout rates, and homelessness. A total of 26 percent of people who utilize homeless shelters have serious mental health issues.

We see overlaps in people with gastrointestinal (GI) illness and mental illness. In people with celiac disease, 35 percent reported a history of psychiatric disease. Also, 70 to 90 percent of people who have irritable bowel syndrome (IBS) have mood or anxiety disorders, including schizophrenia, major depression, and panic disorder. According to Gerakani et al. (2003), with people in treatment for mental health issues, IBS is prevalent: 46 percent of people with panic disorder, 29 percent of people with major depression, and 19 percent of people who have schizophrenia also have

IBS. Hausteiner-Wiehele and Henningsen (2014) reviewed the link between mental health issues and IBS and reported that over 90 percent of people with mental health issues also have IBS. These rates vary from study to study, and yet overall, they report that half of people with IBS also have concomitant mental health issues, which can include anxiety, panic disorder, depression, and trauma. Other research has shown increased rates of bipolar disorder in people with IBS.

This leads us to clinical practice: How often do mental health workers ask their patients about their bowel habits? In practice, I saw over and over that once the digestive system began coming back into balance, depression, anxiety, and obsessive thoughts often also came back into balance. As discussed in Chapter 10, the relationship between behavior and gut health is unfolding. It appears that using psychobiotics, eating elimination diets, healing leaky gut, balancing the gut microbiome, and engaging in mind-body therapies can optimize mental health. It's beyond the scope of this book to go deeply into mental illness therapeutics; this chapter will focus specifically on the intersection between the brain and gut. Look at Chapter 10 for information on the enteric nervous system and the gut-brain connection. Read Chapters 13 and 14, focusing on changes in diet. Utilize the DIGIN model to find the underlying brain-gut connections that can give the greatest possibility for change.

DEPRESSION AND ANXIETY

Depression

Depression is a chronic mood disorder characterized by brain inflammation and oxidative stress. It has many causes, including social and psychological issues; hormonal, blood sugar, neurotransmitter, and mineral imbalances, toxins; molds; poor nutrition; feelings of loneliness; and trauma. As with any other condition, it's important to look for each individual's contributing factors and work to optimize function on all levels.

Depression can set in at any age. Being depressed affects all parts of your life. According to the National Institute of Mental Health, depression can be categorized in many ways, but they all have similar signs, including the following:

We've probably all described ourselves as "depressed" from time to time. Situational depression happens to all of us, but typically it resolves either as things change or we get used to our new situation. Yet for many, the cloud of depression doesn't lift and lingers for months or years. This can be due to a loss of some sort, health issues, aging, and medications that can increase depression. Depression leads

- Persistent feelings of sadness, anxiety, or empty mood
- Feeling hopeless or pessimistic
- Irritability
- Guilt, worthlessness, or helplessness
- Loss of interest or pleasure in life
- Fatigue
- Moving or talking more slowly

- Restlessness; inability to sit still
- Difficulty concentrating, remembering, or making decisions
- Sleep issues
- Changes in appetite or weight
- Suicidal thoughts or actions
- Aches and pains, or digestive problems with no clear cause

Adapted from NIMH.NIH.gov

to suicide in 15 percent of people it affects and is the leading cause of disability in adults. Some people get the blues from lack of sun in the winter, and this is called seasonal affective disorder (SAD).

Some families have depression and mental health issues that pass from generation to generation of family members. Although this can be due to many contributing social issues, there are also genomic ones. Methylation, which is a process requiring B-complex vitamins and methionine, is often compromised in people with mental health issues. Researchers are exploring the genetics of major depression and have discovered genes in 44 areas associated with it. These genes affect weight and body size, nervous system functioning, inflammation in the brain, the functioning of synapses, how we handle stress and govern immune responses, how our cells communicate, and the functioning of dopamine and glutamate receptors.

Anxiety

Anxiety can be defined as excessive worry about the future or ruminating about the past. It often goes hand in hand with depression, but it also can stand on its own. We've all experienced anxiety, yet according to the National Institutes of Mental Health, 19.1 percent of adults in the United States experience mild to severe anxiety disorder. The incidence is higher in women at 23.4 percent, 14.3 percent in men, and 31.9 percent in adolescents.

With anxiety our muscles feel tight and tense, and we typically avoid situations that may potentially make us feel anxious. Anxiety is a story we are telling ourselves and can include fear. We all have worries, but when the level of stress about our life situation is disproportional to the actual issues, that is a problem. Mark Twain said, "I've had a lot or worries in my life, most of which never happened." Yet when someone has an anxiety disorder, these worries dominate.

Anxiety disorder has many forms: fear of just about anything, obsessive-compulsive behavior, social anxiety disorder, panic attacks, post-traumatic stress disorder (PTSD), specific phobias, and/or generalized anxiety. Some of the signs of anxiety include sweating, rapid heart rate or palpitations, inability to focus or concentrate, difficulty remembering, shallow breathing, trembling, mental vigilance and feeling constantly on guard, and feeling like you are frozen in place. It can be due to nearly any stressor, including life and relationship issues, finances, job or family stress, and other problems.

As with depression, looking for the underlying issues helps to balance anxiety. Chronic Lyme disease and co-infections, mold, chemicals, hormone imbalances, and feeling unsafe may all be root issues. Anxiety can also be associated with virtually any health issue, and sometimes there is good reason for it. No matter what, it is a real concern and needs to be addressed. Caffeine is a common, yet often unrecognized, cause of anxiety. Stopping its use can greatly help with anxiety and sleep issues. Low blood sugar from late or skipped meals can trigger anxiety and panic attacks, so eating regularly is an important habit to establish if you think that might fit your pattern.

Depression and Anxiety: The DIGIN Connection

Research is mushrooming about the gut-brain connection to mental health. GI motility is often altered in people with depression and anxiety. Bruce Stevens et al. (2018) reported that increased intestinal permeability was much more evident in people with people with depression and anxiety. Markers of bacterial liposaccharides (LPS), zonulin, and intestinal fatty-acid binding protein 2 (FABP2) were all elevated. These molecules increase an inflammatory response as they (and other substances) get released into the bloodstream.

The gut-brain connection works both ways: Having a diagnosis of GI disease can be a cause of anxiety and depression in children and adults alike. For example, in preschool-age children, celiac disease is associated with depression, anxiety, sleep issues, and aggressive behavior. Often, this is seen prior to the diagnosis of celiac disease. Common symptoms in adults with untreated celiac disease can include depression and anxiety. In people with inflammatory bowel disease (IBD), there is also an increased incidence of depression and anxiety. One study reported the incidence of depression in people with IBD to be 25.8 percent, anxiety in people who have IBD was evident in 21.2 percent, and 30.3 percent of people with IBD experienced both anxiety and depression. A study of Asian people with IBD reported that 27 percent of the participants had depression and/or anxiety. A review of over 158,371 people and 171 papers said that in people with IBD,

20.5 percent had anxiety disorders, and 15 percent experienced depression. Higher levels of anxiety and depression were noticed in people with active Crohn's or ulcerative colitis versus people whose IBD was well controlled.

There are many animal studies reporting dysbiosis being related to depression and anxiety, but thus far, there are few human studies. Those that have been done report that probiotic supplementation with Lactobacilli and Bifidobacteria helps reduce general depression, postpartum depression, and anxiety. So far, most studies report a benefit in people with mild to moderate depression and anxiety with the use of probiotics. These findings are promising, but there are many questions about which probiotics will work best, for whom, at what dose, and for how long they work. We have theoretical papers on how fermented foods can help reduce depression and anxiety, but there are no human studies yet. The science in all of these areas is budding but not currently blooming.

As discussed in Chapter 10, 70 to 90 percent of people with IBS experience some sort of mood or anxiety disorder. This could present as schizophrenia, depression, and/or panic disorder.

Lyme and coinfections, such as Bartonella, can cause brain inflammation that sometimes results in severe anxiety and depression. If you have tried everything else, consider doing testing for Lyme disease. If you don't find it on a Western blot test, do DNA testing.

Psychologists and other professionals working in the area of mental health will benefit from exploring GI issues in their patients. Family physicians, internal medicine physicians, and gastroenterologists will benefit from exploring the relationship between mental health issues and GI issues. The two go hand in hand, but in current practice settings, this is often ignored.

Resources:

- Bongiorno, P. *Holistic Solutions for Anxiety and Depression in Therapy: Combining Natural Remedies with Conventional Care.* W. W. Norton.
- Brogan, K. & Loberg, K. *A Mind of Your Own: The Truth About Depression, and How Women Can Heal Their Bodies to Reclaim their Lives.* Harper Wave.
- Kharrazian, D. *Why Isn't My Brain Working?* Elephant Press.
- Ross, J. *The Mood Cure: The 4-Step Program to Take Charge of Your Emotions—Today.* New York: Penguin Books.
- Scott, J. *The Anti-Anxiety Food Solution.* New Harbinger Publications.
- Walsh, W. *Nutrient Power: Heal your Biochemistry and Heal Your Brain.* Skyhorse Publishing.

Functional Laboratory Testing

These tests can be widely varied but can include the following:

- Vitamin D testing
- Amino acid testing
- Organic acid testing
- Neurotransmitter testing or a questionnaire
- Stool testing
- Nutritional testing
- Lyme and coinfections. Western blot often misses chronic Lyme. Use more sophisticated testing, such as DNA Connections or Igenex.

Healing Options

- **Begin by exploring lifestyle, nutrition, hormone imbalances, metals, infections, toxic exposure and the DIGIN model to find underlying issues.** Mental health symptoms can stem from a wide variety of root issues. Looking at your overall lifestyle, balancing your microbiome, and healing leaky gut are a great starting place. I've seen depression and anxiety improve simply by eliminating sugar from one's diet. If the answer isn't simple, explore chronic infections such as Lyme and Bartonella, environmental or metal toxicity, and hormone balance.
- **If you need medication to feel better, use it.** Sometimes this can be temporary.
- **Spend time in nature and get regular exercise.** Study after study reports that movement is equal to medication for people who experience depression. Spend time in your garden, walk in the woods or on the beach, or do other activities that please you.
- **Engage in talk therapy.** Cognitive behavior therapy (CBT) is an effective therapy for depression and anxiety. Either go to a therapist for counseling, find a support group, or spend time with friends.
- **Improve your diet.** The standard Western diet increases inflammation throughout the body. It also increases dysbiosis and intestinal permeability. Depression and anxiety have both been associated with processed food, high sugar intake, gluten sensitivity, and food additives. Read Chapters 13 and 14 for more information.
- **Control your blood sugar levels.** Remember to eat at least three meals a day and snack when needed. Low blood sugar levels can make you feel tired, anxious, and depressed.

- **Limit or avoid certain substances.** These include cigarettes, alcohol, and caffeine.
- **Test your vitamin D levels.** Low vitamin D levels are associated with SAD, depression, and anxiety. Optimal 25-OHD levels are between 60 and 100 ng/ml. Retest in 3 months. Dosage: 2000–10,000 IU daily.
- **Take a great multivitamin with minerals, plus omega 3 fatty acids.** Low levels of virtually *all* nutrients have been associated with depression and anxiety. B-complex vitamins, essential fatty acids, chromium, zinc, magnesium, and similar substances are all essential nutrients to reduce inflammation and balance your body. To be specific, do nutrient testing to see which ones are most important.
- **Try amino acid therapies:** Leaders in the field, such as Datis Kharrazian and Julia Ross, utilize amino acid–supporting therapies to balance brain biochemistry.
- **Try electrophysiology (functional electroencephalogram [EEG] or neurofeedback training).** Many health centers and mental health centers utilize EEG or neurofeedback to retrain and rewire the brain.
- **Take St. John's wort for depression and anxiety.** St. John's wort has been shown in many studies to help with depression, anxiety, and sleep. Dosage: 300 mg daily of a standardized extract.
- **Take ashwagandha for anxiety and nonrestorative sleep.** Dozens of studies have reported improvement in anxiety by taking standardized extracts of ashwagandha. Dosage: These vary by product and range from 125 mg daily, to 250 mg twice daily, to 300 mg twice daily.
- **Use lavender oil for anxiety.** Taking lavender oil as an oral supplement has decreased anxiety and improved sleep quality in over a dozen studies and works as well as medications. Many people find that putting lavender oil on their temples, feet, or forehead also relieves anxiety. I keep a lavender oil spritzer by my bed in case I wake up at night. I just spritz it a couple of times on my forehead and rub it in. I make it by putting 20 to 30 drops of lavender oil and a 3 to 4 oz. of water into a spray bottle. Lavender oil also has antimicrobial properties, so look for changes in your digestion. Begin with a low dose and build up slowly if needed. Dosage: Take Silexan, Lavela WS 1265, or other products at 80 or 160 mg daily.
- **Take other natural substances that have been found to be useful.** These include hops dry extract supplement for depression, anxiety, and stress; magnesium supplementation for anxiety; and saffron for treatment of anxiety and depression. Other herbs that have strong evidence include passionflower and kava.

SCHIZOPHRENIA

Schizophrenia is a chronic, disabling brain disease. People with schizophrenia experience altered realities, including hallucinations, hearing voices, delusions, and confused or paranoid thoughts. Speech and behavior of people with schizophrenia can be very disorganized, which can be disturbing or confusing to those around them. During acute periods, people with schizophrenia experience a loss of energy, sense of humor, and interest in living. It affects one million Americans each year, and 1 percent of us will have it during our lifetime. It's one of the top 10 worldwide causes of disability. It can be progressive or episodic. Schizophrenia has an autoimmune component, which may be a result of the disease itself. A large number of studies find correlation between prenatal and postnatal infections, including flu, herpes, polio, German measles, toxoplasmosis, and respiratory infections, and increased incidence of schizophrenia.

Research is beginning to emerge that indicates dysbiosis in people who have schizophrenia. Because the gut plays such a huge role in immune response, researchers are looking to the microbiome as an essential trigger in the development of schizophrenia. Toll-like reactors (TLRs) are activated, and tryptophan and glutamate pathways are disordered, with subsequent changes in kynurenine levels and N-methyl-D-aspartate (NDMA) receptor activity. Medication is useful for many people with schizophrenia, but some are not greatly helped by it. Fortunately, there are other therapies.

This is definitely an illness where a complete approach must be taken to get the best results. An entire field of nutritional medicine, called orthomolecular medicine (named by Linus Pauling), is based on treatment of schizophrenia and other mental illnesses, although its original definition was broader. Specific testing of amino acids, food sensitivities, fatty acids, heavy metals, and gut health will reveal information relevant to each person. Often, studies of schizophrenia using nutritional models have been disappointing because all patients are lumped into one group. When groups are broken into subtypes or patients are treated individually, improvements are seen.

Deficiencies in vitamin C, niacin, and folic acid have been found in people with schizophrenia.

Abram Hoffer, MD, and Humphry Osmond, MD, were pioneers in the field. Their protocols are based around 3,000 mg daily of niacin (vitamin B3), 3,000 mg daily of vitamin C, and loving care. Niacin therapy works best when used early after the diagnosis. Be patient: it can take months before it begins to work. Niacin causes a skin flush brought on by the release of prostaglandins in the skin; in people who don't flush, that probably indicates a fatty acid deficiency. A niacin challenge offers a simple way to test for this group of people. Loving care expedites the healing process.

Carl Pfeiffer, MD, PhD, found that some people with schizophrenia had faulty metabolism of specific B-complex vitamins. He once stated, "For every drug that yields a beneficial result, there is a nutrient that can produce the same effect."

Fatty acid metabolism is faulty in people with schizophrenia, and schizophrenics have shown altered fatty acid panels. Levels of arachidonic acid and the omega-3 fatty acids eicosapentaenoic acid (EPA) and docosahexaenoic acid (DHA) are often low. Schizophrenics are found to have high levels of interleukin-2, an inflammatory substance known to have the potential to cause symptoms similar to schizophrenia. Fish oils can help reduce levels of interleukin-2 and cytokines. Doing a fatty acid test would make sense.

People with schizophrenia have an increased need for antioxidant nutrients. Other antioxidants have also been found to be deficient. Poor free radical protection can damage fat-dependent membranes, the nervous system, and the brain. Testing for specific antioxidants would be advised.

Gluten and Schizophrenia

It appears that having a leaky gut and being undernourished are connected to a higher-than-average incidence of gluten intolerance in people with schizophrenia. Review studies indicate that between 2.6 and 4.2 percent of people with schizophrenia also have celiac disease, whereas the incidence of celiac disease in a normal population is about 1 percent. Further, the incidence of people who have schizophrenia and nonceliac gluten sensitivity (NCGS) is high; although numbers vary, it's expected to be more than 10 percent. A total of 57 percent of people with neurological issues of unknown origin test positive for antigliadin antibodies. Many papers have documented that people with schizophrenia improve on a gluten-free diet.

In some people, proteins in wheat that are not fully digested act like opioids, changing thinking, behavior patterns, and gut motility. The earliest reports were published by Lauretta Bender, MD, in 1953, who noticed that 4 out of 37 boys admitted that year for schizophrenia also had celiac disease.

F. C. Dohan noted less schizophrenia during World War II in five countries when wheat was scarce, while in the United States both wheat consumption and schizophrenia increased. Dohan also used anthropological data from the South Pacific islands to show that as wheat, barley, beer, and rice consumption increased, so did schizophrenia. He subsequently compared two groups of schizophrenic males; 47 were assigned a grain-free diet; 55 ate a high-grain diet. According to the findings,

62 percent of those on the gluten-free diet were released to a nonlocked ward within seven days, compared to 36 percent on the high-gluten diet. Wheat sensitivity can stimulate the production of chemicals in the brain that resemble opiates and cause hallucinations and behavior disturbances.

M. M. Singh and S. R. Kay studied 14 people with schizophrenia who were in a locked research ward. They followed a gluten-free diet for six weeks and were rated on 33 psychopathology measures and 6 social measures of social avoidance and participation. Treatment was blinded from the people who did the outcome measurements. There was significant improvement on 30 of 39 measures.

It appears that for the most part, people with schizophrenia and gluten intolerance have different genetics than people with celiac disease. As per the recent findings in a paper, people with schizophrenia, both new onset and recurrent, had high levels of IgG and IgA antigliadin antibodies but no elevated markers of celiac disease.

Although gluten intolerance and celiac disease are not present in all people with schizophrenia, it is important to screen for it.

Casein and Food Sensitivities

Checking for additional food allergies and sensitivities can be useful. Elevated IgA antibodies to the dairy proteins beta-lactoglobulin and casein have been reported. Casein can have opioid-like effects in the brains of people with schizophrenia and autism. There are four specific types of casein in milk and 13 genetic variations of beta-casein. It is believed that the A1 variant leads to the type of bioactive peptide beta-casomorphin 7 (BCM-7). High levels of BCM-7 have been found in the urine of people with schizophrenia and autism. This peptide crosses the intestinal mucosa, gets absorbed into the blood, and passes through the blood-brain barrier, causing an opioid-like response.

Other classic food offenders in schizophrenia include dairy products, food additives, and chocolate, although nearly any food can cause problems.

Could a Low-Carbohydrate Diet Help?

In 2009 Bryan D. Kraft and Eric C. Westman reported on a schizophrenic woman whose auditory hallucinations resolved on a ketogenic diet. A ketogenic diet, such as the Atkins Diet, is very low in carbohydrates. The woman's hallucinations resolved by day 19 of the diet and remained so over the next 12 months, even though she had a couple of lapses during the winter holidays. Dohan and colleagues previously have noted an association between schizophrenia and consumption of grains. Others have noted an association specifically with gluten-containing grains. Still others have noted an increased incidence of psychotic episodes immediately after eating a carbohydrate load.

Schizophrenia and the Gut

People with schizophrenia have an increased risk of developing stomach and duodenal ulcers. Others have found that when there is an ulcer, *H. pylori*–associated gastritis, or motor disorders of the upper gastrointestinal tract (GI), schizophrenic episodes are less severe.

Functional Laboratory Testing

- Celiac testing
- Food allergy testing—IgE and IgG, plus IgM and IgA if possible
- Nutrient testing
- Essential fatty acid testing
- Urinary amino acid testing
- Genetic testing for methylenetetrahydrofolate reductase gene (MTHFR)
- Homocysteine testing

Healing Options

Schizophrenia is a complex illness. Digestive issues do not play a role in all people with schizophrenia, but for the subset of those whom it does affect, resolving these issues can be life changing.

- **Rule out celiac disease and food sensitivities.** Do blood testing for food allergies and sensitivities. Try an elimination diet. See Chapter 14 for more information.
- **Look for nutritional deficiencies.** Checking for specific nutrients and supplementing will give the best results because each person's needs will be different. Beginning with a good multivitamin and mineral supplement can help but probably won't fill in the gaps if there are severe deficiencies in specific nutrients.
- **Take niacin.** Abram Hoffer, MD, long used niacin therapy for schizophrenia. It is believed that there is faulty niacin metabolism in this condition, because people with schizophrenia often do not experience the intense flushing that usually occurs with niacin ingestion. Take up to 3,000 mg daily.
- **Increase intake of 5-hydroxytryptophan (5-HTP).** In 14 patients tested, dietary restriction of tryptophan worsened their symptoms. Tryptophan can easily be converted to niacin, which may be one reason why it is of benefit. Tryptophan is also a precursor to serotonin, which affects mood, behavior, sleep, and carbohydrate cravings. At a recent conference Bill Walsh, PhD, medical director at Great Plains Laboratory, expressed concern about possible negative effects of

tryptophan and recommended using only 5-HTP. To err on the side of caution, I recommend taking 300 to 600 mg 5-HTP.

- **Increase consumption of good fats.** Schizophrenics often have low omega-3 fatty acid levels, low arachidonic acid levels, and low levels of polyunsaturated fatty acids. Benefit would be found by increasing good fats in the diet from sources such as nuts, seeds, whole grains, unprocessed vegetable oils, and cold-water fish, including salmon, halibut, tuna, mackerel, sardines, or herring. Twenty hospitalized patients were given 10 grams of fish oil daily. There were significant improvements in psychological symptoms, behavior, and tardive dyskinesia (uncontrollable movements) after six weeks. Another study used a smaller dose: 180 mg EPA, 120 mg DHA, plus 400 IU vitamin E and 500 mg vitamin C twice daily. There was improvement in lab testing and also in schizophrenic symptoms.

- **Try serine.** Research indicates that high-dose glycine is beneficial for schizophrenia. Concern has been posted as to the possible long-term neurological effects of high-glycine supplementation, however. The mechanism of the response was believed to be the effect on the receptor sites for NMDA, a neurotransmitter. NMDA function is low in people with schizophrenia. Newer research by Toru Nishikawa shows that the positive effects of enhancing NMDA function can be achieved by taking serine, without the risks of high-dose glycine. Dosage in one study was 0.8 grams of serine per kilogram of body weight daily. It would be advisable to do a urine amino acid test before using this type of therapy. Work with a physician.

- **Check your MTHFR gene and homocysteine levels.** Homocysteine levels are often high in people who have schizophrenia. There are many studies looking at genetic variations in the MTHFR gene in people with schizophrenia. These studies have mixed results. Nonetheless, if you do have a genetic variation of this gene, you are less able to utilize folic acid from food and supplements. People with this genetic variation (MTHFR gene 677 C>T) benefit from supplements that have preformed folic acid, called methyltetrahydrofolate. People who have this genetic variation and schizophrenia are more likely to develop metabolic syndrome.

- **Take magnesium.** Magnesium deficiency can produce depression, agitation, confusion, and disorientation. In one study, 20 schizophrenic patients were evaluated for serum magnesium levels. The results found that 25 percent were found to be magnesium deficient. Serum magnesium is not a sensitive test of magnesium deficiency, so if red blood cell magnesium had been analyzed, the results would probably have been much higher. Half of the magnesium-deficient patients were exhibiting psychotic behavior, including hallucinations. In drug-treated schizophrenics, magnesium levels have been found to be consistently low. Supplementing with magnesium does not always show improvement in symptoms. Magnesium injections or use of choline citrate may be necessary at first to "prime the pump." Because so many enzymes are dependent on magnesium, a deficiency could affect other nutrients, including vitamins B_1, B_6, E, and C and minerals such as zinc, copper, and selenium.

Osteoporosis: The GI Connection Q D I G I N

Osteoporosis is a disease where bones are porous and tend to break easily. It affects about 20 percent of women over the age of 50. It also affects men but, due to their higher initial bone mass, less often. Osteoporosis contributes to more than 1.3 million fractures a year. Twenty percent of people who have a hip fracture die within a few weeks, and many others end up needing long-term care.

You are more likely to develop osteoporosis if you are fair skinned, thin, underdo or overdo exercise; smoke or use corticosteroids; if one of your parents has broken a hip; or if you are being treated for an autoimmune disease such as diabetes, rheumatoid arthritis, inflammatory bowel disease (IBD), or lupus. Aluminum-containing antacids, diuretics, overuse of thyroid hormones and antibiotics, and the use of acid blockers, proton pump inhibitors (PPIs), and chemotherapy drugs can all increase bone loss. High salt intake, low mineral intake, and a high-phosphorus diet (including such items as soft drinks that contain phosphorus, meat, poultry, fish, eggs, and cheese) have also been associated with bone loss.

While hormonal changes and aging play a large role in bone loss, these do not explain the entirety of bone health. A new body of evidence ties bone loss to digestive health through multiple mechanisms, some of which are described here. Most of the research is in mice at this time, but clinical studies are under way.

The microbiome produces B-complex vitamins, vitamin K, and bile acids. B-complex vitamins and vitamin K are nutrients that support bone health; bile helps with calcium absorption.

People with small intestinal bacterial overgrowth (SIBO) were treated with antibiotics. When measuring bone health in these patients compared to healthy controls, there was significantly lower bone density in the SIBO group than in the controls, after looking at other possible variables.

Another mechanism of bone loss is systemic inflammation. Inflammation from impaired barrier function is implicated in bone loss. Different mechanisms have been explored. When there is leaky gut, there are higher levels of inflammatory markers, including higher levels of TNF-alpha and IL1-beta. Insulin-like growth factor (IGF-1) enhances synthesis of new bone cells and bone remodeling. Mice given antibiotics had lower levels of IGF-1. Yet when the mice were given dietary fiber to increase short-chain fatty acids (SCFAs), bone metabolism normalized.

Prebiotics decrease inflammatory markers, improve barrier function, and have been shown to enhance bone density and calcium, magnesium, and zinc absorption. All three of these minerals have been shown to increase bone density in women. The probable mechanism is enhancing SCFAs in the colon.

Probiotics have been shown to enhance bone health in both human and mouse studies. *Lactobacillus helveticus*–fermented milk given to 20 postmenopausal women increased serum calcium levels and reduced serum parathyroid hormone, showing a benefit to calcium metabolism. Probiotics given to surgically induced menopausal mice protected them from bone loss. *Bifidobacterium longum* administered over 16 weeks enhanced bone formation and slowed bone turnover. Lactobacillus reuteri also protected mice from bone loss.

At least 20 nutrients are needed to build healthy bone. Most of the spotlight falls on calcium, phosphorus, and vitamin D, but an Israeli study reported increases in bone mass from 250 to 750 mg of magnesium taken daily for two years. The group taking magnesium had increases of 1 to 8 percent in bone mass compared to the control group, who lost between 1 and 3 percent of bone mass. Other nutrients needed for proper bone formation include protein, fluoride, silica, zinc, manganese, copper, boron, potassium, strontium, vitamin K, and virtually all other vitamins. Getting enough protein is also essential.

BONE LOSS AND CELIAC DISEASE

It has been widely reported that people with celiac disease have a higher prevalence of osteoporosis. A recent study done in Manitoba reported that of women who had bone density testing within six months prior to being diagnosed with celiac disease, 67.6 percent had osteoporosis compared with 44.8 percent of the controls.

In 2004, the National Institutes of Health (NIH) stated that osteoporosis was associated with the nutritional deficiencies caused by untreated celiac disease. The NIH consensus statement and subsequent research state that there isn't an increased rate of celiac disease in people with osteoporosis. However, Legroux-Gerot and colleagues report that 8 percent of 140 people with osteoporosis had elevated IgG antigliadin antibodies and 11 percent had elevated IgA antigliadin antibodies. This suggests gluten intolerance.

OUR GUT TALKS TO OUR BONES

It has long been thought that the only mechanism linking osteoporosis and the digestive system was malnutrition due to celiac disease. Now another mechanism has been discovered that seems even more compelling.

Ninety-five percent of the serotonin in the body is produced in the gut in the enterochromaffin cells in the small intestine and duodenum. The other 5 percent is produced in the brain. It's been known for a long time that serotonin modulates peristalsis. Newer research indicates that high levels of serotonin in the gut lower bone density by lowering formation of new bone (osteoblasts) and increasing destruction of old bone (osteoclasts). This is regulated by various genes: Wnt, Lrp5, and Tph1. The Wnt genes regulate how we develop bone, muscle, and nervous system tissues. Genetic research has discovered that there are variations in the Wnt gene that predispose us to having either really strong bones, medium bone density, or bones that are weak from early on in life (causing an early onset of osteoporosis called osteoporosis pseudoglioma).

Inflammation in the gut, such as in Crohn's disease, increases the production of serotonin, which in turn activates the Wnt system. Most people are continually eating foods that cause low-grade inflammation in the gut. The standard American diet is basically an inflammatory diet. Inflammatory cytokines have been shown to increase after eating a high-fat, high-sugar meal. This increases serotonin and activates the Wnt system, reducing bone cell production.

Functional Laboratory Testing
- Vitamin D levels
- Possible celiac and/or food sensitivity testing
- **FRAX Index Assessment Tool.** This was developed by the World Health Organization to assess the risk of breaking bones due to osteoporosis. It's free and available at: shef.ac.uk/FRAX/tool.jsp?country=9.

- **Dexa-Scan.** Urine testing for cross-linked pyridinium proteins can be utilized to monitor whether your program for bone health is aggressive enough. The test doesn't measure bone density, as a Dexa-Scan does, but it can indicate whether you are currently losing bone. These are available from regular commercial labs and also from Functional Labs.
- Hydrochloric acid (HCl) self-test or Heidelberg capsule test
- Nutritional testing for vitamins and minerals

Healing Options

- **Get exercise.** Exercise builds muscle and bone. Exercise is not optional. Find something you like to do and do it regularly.
- **Balance pH.** When cells are in a low level of chronic acidosis, we pull minerals from bone to balance blood pH levels. Susan Brown, at www.betterbones.com, offers excellent information on acid-alkaline balance and its effect on bone health.
- **Optimize vitamin D levels.** Get your vitamin D level tested. Bringing vitamin D to optimal levels works as effectively to build bone as medications do. Aim for 60 to 100 ng/ml of 25-0H vitamin D. For maintenance, take 2,000 IU daily. For optimizing levels, take 5,000 to 10,000 IU daily.
- **Decrease inflammation.** Eat more fruits, vegetables, nuts, seeds, and beans. Lower your intake of processed foods, salt, low nutrient-density foods, caffeine, and alcohol. Stop smoking. Use herbs and spices in cooking. Eat a rainbow of foods. If this still isn't enough, use anti-inflammatory herbs and nutrients such as fish oil, vitamin D, and curcumin.
- **Practice stress-management skills.** See Chapter 16 for techniques for lowering stress.
- **Take bone-building supplements.** Take a multivitamin plus a bone-building supplement that contains calcium, magnesium, vitamin D, vitamin K, and other nutrients.
- **Explore HCl adequacy.** Do the self-test in Chapter 11 or get tested for achlorhydria.

CHAPTER 34

Skin Conditions Q DIGIN

ECZEMA

Eczema, or atopic dermatitis, is a chronic skin condition characterized by redness, itching, and sometimes oozing, crusting, and scaling. The itch makes us scratch, which causes redness and inflammation. It affects 30 million Americans. Approximately 1 to 3 percent of the population has eczema, and it affects 10 to 20 percent of all infants. A total of 50 percent of children outgrow it by age 15; the rest may have mild to severe eczema throughout their lives. It can first appear at any age but most often during the first year of life. Babies can have eczema on their faces, scalp, bottom, hands, and feet. In children and adults, it may be more localized. Eczema is on the rise in industrialized countries. The causes are multifactorial and include imbalanced intestinal flora; leaky gut syndrome; food allergies; environmental contaminants, such as air pollution and tobacco smoke; and genetic predisposition.

The red patches are itchy, scaly, and dry, which encourages people to use lotions and creams to which they are often allergic. This complicates the problem further. Eczema varies over time, flaring up and calming down, at times better and worse. Emotional stress, heat, increase in humidity, bacterial skin infections, sweat, peuts, hormone fluctuations, dust, molds, pollens, toiletries, cosmetics, and wool clothing commonly aggravate eczema. As children age, they may continue to have eczema; it may disappear; or they may develop other allergies, including asthma. People with eczema have high levels of IgE, secretory IgA, and eosinophils, all allergy signs.

Strong connections exist between eczema and food, microbial, and inhalant allergies. The word *atopy*, which is often used by physicians synonymously for allergy, refers to inflammations of the skin, nasal passages, and lungs. People with eczema often have allergies to dust, mold, dander, pollens, and foods.

Food allergies diagnosed through IgE and skin testing are apparent in most children with eczema. In a study of 165 children between the ages of 4 months and 22 years, researchers found that 60 percent had at least one positive skin-prick test for food allergies. When they challenged these results with a double-blind, placebo-controlled study, 39 of 64 subjects had a positive test, with milk, egg, peanut, soy, wheat, codfish, catfish, and cashews accounting for 89 percent of the positive food-allergy challenges. Undoubtedly, many more would be borne out by IgG, IgA, and IgM testing. Another study of children with eczema showed that eczema improved in 49 out of 66 children after elimination of the particular foods. Foods that aggravated eczema in this particular study, in descending order, were eggs, cow's milk, food coloring, tomatoes, fish, goat's milk, cheese, chocolate, and wheat.

A study was made of 122 children, aged four months to six years, with food intolerance. Of them, 52 children had eczema; the rest had chronic diarrhea. The allergies caused damage to the intestinal lining, and there was a decrease in the body's ability to defend itself because of lactose intolerance and dysbiosis. This, in turn, caused leaky gut syndrome, leading to more food antigens and sensitivity. Children with eczema had more intestinal damage than those with chronic diarrhea.

Research on the use of probiotics during pregnancy and in the first three to six months of infancy is mixed. Some studies report that eczema can be prevented in about half of children who have allergic family histories when probiotics are given at birth to both the mothers and the nursing babies. Other papers have shown no benefit at all. When my son, Kyle, was 10 days old he began getting eczema on his bottom. By the time he was three months old, he looked like a burn victim despite my attempts to heal him. I took him to Andrea Rentea, MD an anthroposophic pediatrician in Chicago, who recommended that I give him *Bifidus infantus* and that I take it myself. After 10 days, his eczema had completely healed. So had his cradle cap, and his fussiness also had ceased. He's just one baby, but my personal experience showed me that at least in some children, probiotics make an enormous difference.

Breast-feeding dramatically reduces a baby's risk of developing eczema and allergies. Babies with eczema, and probably most babies, should not be given cow's milk, milk products, eggs, or wheat before one year of age. As their digestive system matures, they can better handle these complex foods. Babies with eczema who drink formula should be tested by skin prick to determine which formulas are most suitable for them. Because babies are born without intestinal flora in their digestive tracts, giving supplemental flora to the baby (and the mother, if she's nursing) can quickly alleviate baby eczema.

Elimination of foods, stress, and allergens can significantly alter the course of the disease. Even though you cannot control all factors, controlling enough of them will allow you to stay under the symptom threshold.

Helicobacter pylori, a bacteria most often linked with ulcers, gastritis, and stomach cancer, has also been strongly associated with acne rosacea. Yet, this relationship has been controversial because when people are treated for *H. pylori*, their rosacea doesn't always improve. This makes sense because acne rosacea is a condition with many possible underlying causes. A 2018 review study concluded that people who have acne rosacea ought to be tested for *H. pylori*. If they are positive, they ought to be treated to eradicate the infection. There is more information on *H. pylori* in Chapter 19, in the section on ulcers.

Jonathan Wright, MD, had success in 39 out of 40 patients with eczema who followed this combined program: 50 mg zinc three times daily for six weeks, plus 2 mg copper daily, 5 grams omega-6 fatty acids (evening primrose or borage oil) twice a day for three months, and 1 to 2 grams omega-3 fatty acids (EPA/DHA fish oils) three times daily for four weeks.

Many people with eczema have low HCl levels. See Chapter 3 for more information and to take the HCl self-test.

It's commonly believed that use of steroid creams doesn't have effects outside of the skin. Research disagrees. There can be systemic effects to the eyes, increased susceptibility to infection, delayed wound healing, skin damage, and changes to the hypothalamic pituitary adrenal (HPA) axis. Also, it may trigger latent diabetes, make skin worse, or other effects. Years ago, I worked with a woman in her early twenties who had severe eczema on much of her body. She contacted me when lab tests revealed that her cortisol levels were sky high. Medical treatments for eczema focus on symptomatic relief. Steroids can become addicting because when you stop using them, the eczema flares up even worse. Looking for underlying root issues can bring relief and even cure the condition.

Exercise may be especially beneficial for people with eczema. A recent study indicated that exercise reduced the inflammation associated with eczema by increasing the body's adaptability to stress.

To cut down on allergens in the home, vacuum fastidiously and use air purifiers in bedrooms and other rooms you are in frequently. One recent study attributed a reduction in eczema severity to a reduction in mattress dust and carpet mites by using a high-filtration vacuum cleaner and mattress covers. Keep your bedroom clean and clutter free.

Functional Laboratory Testing

- Test for *H. pylori* infection
- Allergy testing for IgE, food, mold, dust, and inhalants
- ELISA/ACT testing for food, chemical, mold, and pharmaceutical sensitivities
- Comprehensive digestive stool analysis
- Heidelberg capsule test for adequacy of hydrochloric acid production

Healing Options

- **Investigate food and environmental sensitivities.** For more information, see Chapter 9. An elimination-provocation diet can significantly reduce eczema. We don't yet have research on low-histamine diets in people with eczema, but as eczema is an allergic condition, it logically follows that they may be beneficial. Often, foods that you are sensitive to will make you itch. The itching may start soon after the meal, but it can be delayed up to 48 hours, which makes tracking down the foods a bit tricky. Food allergy and sensitivity testing can help you determine which foods to eliminate from your diet. Eliminate all foods and chemicals that you are sensitive to for four to six months. Use natural household cleaning products and shampoos, and select soaps and toiletries that are hypoallergenic. If you are sensitive to mattresses, gas stoves, carpeting, and upholstery, you may need to use cotton and other natural fiber clothing and sheets that allow the skin to breathe naturally. Work with a health professional who knows how to help you meet your needs.

- **Supplement with probiotics.** Restoring the normal balance of flora in your intestinal tract can help reduce eczema. Use of supplemental beneficial bacteria can make a tremendous difference in your ability to thoroughly digest foods.

- **Check for hypochlorhydria.** Dr. Alan Gaby in his 2018 book, *Nutritional Medicine, 2nd edition* discusses a 1929 study in which nearly two-thirds of people with eczema had low stomach acid. Taking HCl with meals resolved their eczema. See Chapter 3 for more details.

- **Check for candida infection.** Fungal infections are a common cause of eczema. In a study of 115 men and women with eczema, 85 were sensitive to fungus; after they were treated with fungal creams, oral ketoconazole, or a yeast-free diet, there was much improvement. Take the yeast self-test and do blood testing or Comprehensive Digestive Stool Analysis (CDSA) to determine if yeast is contributing to your eczema. (See Chapter 11 for the quiz.)

- **Try black cumin seed oil.** In four human studies, black cumin seed oil (*Nigella sativa*) has been shown to alleviate the symptoms of eczema and other allergies. It also moderately helps to normalize serum triglycerides and cholesterol. Black cumin seeds are a food, so there is low toxicity. Take 20 to 40 mg daily per pound of body weight. A 150-pound adult could take 3,000 to 6,000 mg. This is about ½ teaspoon to a bit more than a teaspoon of black cumin oil daily. Take internally or drizzle on food. It can also be mixed with lotion and put on the skin.

- **Use natural eczema creams.** Herbal creams can be as effective as cortisone creams in reducing eczema, and they don't have the negative side effects. Licorice root stimulates production of healing and anti-inflammatory prostaglandins. Use of a 2 percent licorice cream is recommended. Chamomile creams are widely used in Europe. A recent study compared a chamomile product, Kamillosan, against 0.5 percent hydrocortisone cream. After two weeks, the Kamillosan was reported to give slightly better results than the hydrocortisone cream. Look in health food stores or ask your health professional to find a product that works for you.

- **Try Jonathan Wright's protocol.** This is outlined earlier in the chapter.

- **Take vitamin C.** A study of 10 young people with severe eczema showed that supplementation with vitamin C significantly improved eczema and immune function. They needed only half as many antibiotics for treating skin infections as the control group. Take 1,000 to 3,000 mg mineral ascorbates or Ester-C daily. Do a vitamin C flush once a week. (See Chapter 17.)

- **Try evening primrose, flaxseed, and borage oils.** Studies show that people with eczema generally have low levels of both omega-3 and omega-6 fatty acids. The first step in metabolism of linoleic acid, which allows for the conversion into gamma-linolenic acid (GLA), is often impaired in people with eczema. Taking GLA directly in evening primrose, flaxseed, or borage oil circumvents blockage. GLA has an anti-inflammatory effect and benefits immune function. Take 1 to 2 grams three times daily of any of these oils or a combination.

- **Increase fish oil consumption.** One recent study on people with eczema showed a 30 percent improvement in a four-month trial of eight capsules of fish oil per day. Though the placebo group was given corn oil, which gave an improvement of 24 percent, results suggest that people with eczema have a generalized need for essential fatty acids. Eating coldwater fish—salmon, halibut, sardines, herring, tuna—two to four times each week can provide you with the omega-3 oils you need. If you use fish oil capsules, do so under the supervision of a physician. They cause a significant increase in clotting time and should not be used by people with hemophilia or those on aspirin or anticoagulant drugs.

- **Try quercetin.** Quercetin, the most effective bioflavonoid for anti-inflammation, can be used to reduce pain and inflammatory responses and control allergies. Take 500 to 1,000 mg three to four times daily.

- **Use turmeric.** For eczema, turmeric can be used in combination with neem, an Ayurvedic remedy for parasites and infections.
- **Try a nickel-restricted diet.** The relationship between nickel sensitivity and eczema has appeared recently in scientific literature. Nickel is an essential nutrient that is found in many enzymes. However, excess nickel is an irritant to the GI lining. You can be tested for nickel sensitivity through skin testing or an oral challenge. Nickel is used as an alloy in jewelry, so if jewelry irritates your skin or turns it gray, you may be sensitive to nickel. If you are, a low-nickel diet should be followed for a limited period of time. High-nickel foods are chocolate, nuts, dried beans and peas, and grains.
- **Neutralize reactions.** There are many ways to minimize the effects of food sensitivities. Clinical ecologists can provide neutralization drops to counteract your reaction to particular foods. These drops work like allergy shots—a small amount of what you are sensitive to helps stimulate your body's natural immune response. Malic acid can also curtail sensitivity reactions.

PSORIASIS

Psoriasis is a chronic skin rash characterized by scaling, patchy, or silvery-looking skin. It has a cyclic nature, flaring up and simmering down. It can affect just knees, elbows, or scalp or can spread over most of the body. It often occurs at the site of a previous injury. Psoriasis often runs in families and usually develops gradually. It affects about 1 percent of the American population as a whole (4.5 million) but 2 to 4 percent of Caucasians.

Psoriasis occurs when skin cells mature too quickly. Skin cells build up on the surface, causing red, scaly patches that often itch or are uncomfortable. Psoriasis flares up because of stress, severe sunburn, irritation, skin creams, antimalarial therapy, or withdrawal from cortisone, or it can be brought on by other triggers. People with psoriasis have an excess of T-helper cell (Th-1) inflammatory cytokines and relatively few Th-2 cytokines. One of the new theories about psoriasis is that superantigens trigger the disease. These prime the T cells to produce high amounts of inflammatory cytokines. These superantigens also contribute to leaky gut, which allows greater exposure to antigens or toxins, including microbial factors. Subsequently these can be deposited along basement membrane in the skin. Immune complexes develop. It's believed that there is a molecular mimicry between H. pylori antigens and keratin 17, which may cause keratin to proliferate. Keratin is the tough, fibrous protein component of skin, hair, and nails. So when we produce a lot more keratin, the skin gets tough and fibrous. If we look at the DIGIN section of the book, all of these factors play a role: leaky gut, dysbiosis, inflammation, and antigens.

Psoriasis can also occur with joint inflammation as psoriatic arthritis (see Chapter 25), and joint inflammation is found in 3 to 7 percent of people with psoriasis. It isn't clear whether psoriasis and psoriatic arthritis are the same disease or two almost identical diseases.

Thirty-six percent of people with psoriasis have one or more family members with psoriasis, which suggests a genetic component. Psoriasis is also influenced by insulin resistance, impaired glucose tolerance, obesity, liver disease, and high cholesterol and/or triglycerides. It's thought to be an indicator of risk for atherosclerosis and may be an early warning sign.

Digestive issues in psoriasis have been found in many cases. There is a clear relationship between celiac, gluten sensitivity, Crohn's disease, and psoriasis. In psoriasis and these other conditions, researchers found increased intestinal permeability and microscopic bowel lesions. Some people with psoriasis also have gastritis, duodenitis, celiac disease, or inflammatory bowel disease. Disturbances in pancreatic function and even acute pancreatitis have been found to be prevalent in people with psoriasis.

Drs. Michael Murray and Joseph Pizzorno note a number of factors that influence the progression of psoriasis, including incomplete digestion of protein, bowel toxemia, food sensitivities, poor liver function, reaction to alcoholic beverages, and eating high amounts of animal fats.

When protein digestion is incomplete or proteins are poorly absorbed, bacteria can break them down and produce toxic substances. One group of these toxins is called polyamines, which have been found to be higher in people with psoriasis than in the average population. Polyamines contribute to psoriasis by blocking production of cyclic AMP. Vitamin A and goldenseal inhibit the formation of polyamines. Because protein digestion begins in the stomach, low levels of hydrochloric acid there can also cause incomplete protein digestion. Digestive enzymes and/or hydrochloric acid supplementation aid protein digestion. (See Chapter 3.)

Poor liver function may contribute to psoriasis as well. Liver function profile tests and the metabolic screening questionnaire can help you determine liver function. Incorporate a detoxification program with an elimination-provocation diet to determine which foods may trigger your psoriasis. (See Chapters 14 and 17.)

Alcohol consumption contributes to psoriasis because alcohol contains many toxic substances, which stress an overburdened liver. Alcohol also increases intestinal permeability.

DYSBIOSIS AND PSORIASIS

Many studies hypothesize that there is a microbe or pathogen that triggers psoriasis. H. pylori has been found in some people with psoriasis. When treated, some people have had large improvements, while there has been no benefit in others. Studies on dysbiosis in psoriasis are lacking. Dr. Zhan Gao and colleagues extracted DNA from skin lesions of six people with psoriasis. He found increased levels of Firmicutes and low levels of Actinobacteria and Propionibacterium species in people with psoriasis compared to controls. Dr. Luciana C. Paulino and colleagues found no significant differences in yeast levels in healthy skin and psoriasis skin.

In a recent study, 21 out of 34 people with psoriasis were found to have *Candida albicans* in the spaces between their fingers or toes, and the majority were also affected by fungi from the tinea family. Other research found a 56 percent increase in nail fungus in people with psoriasis. Another study looked at stool samples of people with psoriasis and other skin disorders. Researchers found a high number of disease-producing microbes, predominantly yeasts, in the colon. This may not be the cause of psoriasis but rather an indication of poor gut ecology. Treatment for yeast infection corresponded with a decrease in skin inflammation.

FOOD AND PSORIASIS

Studies on fasting, vegetarian diets, and diets rich in fish oils have all been shown to produce benefit in people with psoriasis. All of these diets reduce inflammation.

Although I have not seen studies on elimination diets, people with psoriasis have high levels of IgE antibodies, which indicates an allergic component. An elimination diet makes sense to try. Allergy and food sensitivity testing could be helpful in figuring out how someone may benefit the most.

Sixteen percent of people with psoriasis have antibodies to gliadin, the protein found in wheat, rye, and barley. However, when tested for gliadin intolerance, their endomysium antibodies were normal. Nonetheless, a gluten-free diet for three months greatly improved the psoriasis. A follow-up study discovered high levels of tissue transglutaminase antibodies in the skin of people with psoriasis. This decreased by half after a three- to six-month gluten-free trial.

The causes and treatments of psoriasis are complex. Successful treatment must encompass several approaches reflecting its complexity. Look for underlying causes and develop a personal program based on your needs.

Functional Laboratory Testing

- Food and environmental sensitivity testing—IgE and IgG4
- Celiac testing
- Candida testing (either blood or stool)
- Organic acid testing
- Liver function profile
- Intestinal permeability testing
- Blood testing for vitamin and mineral status
- Fatty acid testing

Healing Options

- **Try an elimination-provocation diet.** Explore the relationship between your psoriasis and food and environmental sensitivities through laboratory testing and the elimination-provocation diet. For best results work with a nutritionist or physician who is familiar with food sensitivity protocols.
- **Take a multivitamin with minerals.** Take a good-quality multivitamin with minerals every day. Look for a supplement that contains at least 25,000 IU vitamin A, 400 IU vitamin D, 400 IU vitamin E, 800 mcg folic acid, 200 mcg selenium, 200 mcg chromium, and 25 to 50 mg zinc. Each of these nutrients has been shown to be deficient in people with psoriasis. There are several vitamin A topical creams used by dermatologists for psoriasis. Vitamin A is a critical nutrient for healthy skin.
- **Try antioxidant nutrients.** CoQ10, selenium, and vitamin E supplements have shown benefit. One group reported improvement from use of CoQ10 at 50 mg, vitamin E at 50 mg, and selenium at 48 mcg dissolved in soy lecithin for 30 to 35 days.
- **Increase consumption of beneficial fats and oils.** The research on fish oils is mixed. Eating fish or taking fish oils has been shown to have an anti-inflammatory effect on psoriasis for some people. Fatty acids contribute to healthy skin, hair, and nails, and fish oils promote production of anti-inflammatory prostaglandins. It is also possible that fish oils increase the activity of vitamin D and sunlight. Eat cold-water fish—salmon, halibut, mackerel, sardines, tuna, and herring— two to four times per week or take EPA/DHA capsules along with a balance of omega-6 fatty acids such as evening primrose oil, borage oil, or black currant seed oil.
- **Enjoy some sunlight and get your vitamin D.** Sunlight stimulates our bodies to manufacture vitamin D, which has been shown to be an effective treatment for psoriasis. Ask your doctor to test your vitamin D levels. If low, supplement.

Cod liver oil is a good source of vitamin D because it also contains fish oil and vitamin A, both of benefit in psoriasis. In general, slow tanning improves psoriasis, with sunshine and sunlamps prescribed as part of standard therapy. Normal levels are between 32 and 100 ng/ml. Many integrative clinicians consider levels of 60 to 100 ng/ml to be optimal for people with autoimmune illnesses. Dosage depends on levels. For maintenance, take 2,000 IU of D_3 daily. If deficient, take 5,000 to 10,000 IU of D_3 daily for 8 to 12 weeks, and then retest.

A recent study done in Israel at the Dead Sea, long renowned for its treatment of psoriasis, showed that natural sunlight stimulated significant improvement in disease activity. One group was given just sunlight therapy, and the other received additional therapy in mud packs and sulfur baths. Both groups showed significant improvement in skin symptoms and with psoriatic arthritis, where present. Sunlight and ultraviolet light therapy are common treatments for psoriasis.

- **Take zinc supplements and/or eat zinc-rich foods.** Many studies have determined that people with psoriasis have lower levels of zinc than people in control groups. However, studies using oral zinc supplementation haven't always shown a clear improvement in psoriasis, though such studies have been of short duration—only 6 to 10 weeks. Even though they didn't show improvement in the skin, they did show improvement in immune function and dramatic improvement in joint symptoms. It's possible that either zinc needs to be used along with other nutrients, or the time frame of these studies was too brief to see improvement. Take 50 mg zinc daily.

- **Try chondroitin sulfate.** Several studies have reported improvement in psoriasis in people taking chondroitin sulfate. Take 800 mg daily. Continue for at least two months to see if this is effective for you.

- **Try milk thistle (silymarin).** Extracts of the herb milk thistle have been used since the 15th century for ailments of the liver and gallbladder. Milk thistle, also known as silymarin, contains anti-inflammatory flavonoid complexes that promote the flow of bile and help tone the spleen, gallbladder, and liver. An excellent liver detoxifier, milk thistle has also been shown to have a positive effect on psoriasis. Take three to six capsules of 175 mg standardized 80 percent milk thistle extract daily with water before meals.

- **Try Honduran sarsaparilla.** Sarsaparilla, a flavoring in root beers and confections, has proven to be effective in treating psoriasis, especially the more chronic, large, plaque-forming type. Sarsaparilla binds bacterial endotoxins. Take 2 to 4 teaspoons liquid extract daily, or 250 to 500 mg solid extract daily.

- **Try lecithin and phosphatidylcholine.** Lecithin was used in a 10-year study from 1940 to 1950. People consumed 4 to 8 tablespoons of lecithin daily, along with small amounts of vitamins A, B_1, B_2, B_5, B_6, and D, thyroid and liver preparations, and creams. Out of 155 patients, 118 people responded positively. Lecithin-rich foods include soybeans, wheat germ, nuts, seeds, whole grains, eggs, and oils from soy, nuts, and seeds. Lecithin granules can be purchased in health food stores and added to foods as a cooking ingredient. Lecithin can also be purchased in capsule form, as can the active ingredient in lecithin, phosphatidylcholine. Take 4 to 8 tablespoons of lecithin daily or one to four capsules of phosphatidylcholine daily.

- **Try high-dose folic acid.** There is much research on folate deficiency caused by the drug methotrexate, which is a folate antagonist medication often used for psoriasis. This seems ironic, because folic acid is one of the primary nutrients needed for proper skin formation. Jonathan Wright, MD, recommends extremely high-dose folic acid therapy for psoriasis—50 to 100 mg daily. Alan Gaby, MD, reports on a study of seven people with long-standing psoriasis. They were given 20 mg of folic acid four times daily. Improvements were seen in three to six months of beginning this regimen. Dr. Gaby warns that this is not a good plan for people who have taken methotrexate because it may cause adverse reactions. Be aware that if folic acid is taken by someone with a vitamin B_{12} deficiency, nerve damage can go undetected. If you are going to use high levels of folic acid, have your doctor test your vitamin B_{12} status with serum B_{12}, or more accurately methylmalonic acid testing. I also wonder if the same results could be obtained by using a more absorbable form of folic acid, such as methyltetrahydrofolate at lower doses.

- **Take selenium.** Many studies have shown that people with psoriasis are deficient in selenium. Selenium is part of a molecule called *glutathione peroxidase*, which protects against oxidative damage (free radicals). Giving supplemental selenium to people with psoriasis showed an increase in glutathione peroxidase levels and improvement in immune function, though not an improvement in skin condition. However, these were studies of short duration with selenium as the only supplement. This underscores the concept of patience when using natural therapies and when using more than one nutrient or approach at a time. Take 200 mcg daily, which you can get in a good multivitamin. Selenium can be toxic, so more is not necessarily better. Brazil nuts are an excellent source of selenium. Eat one to two daily to get 200 mcg.

- **Try Saccharomyces boulardii.** Saccharomyces boulardii is a cousin to baker's yeast. It has been shown to raise levels of secretory IgA, which are low in psoriatic arthritis and psoriasis. Take three to six capsules daily.

Topical Treatments to Reduce Skin Inflammation and Symptoms

- **Use aloe vera cream.** A placebo-controlled study of 60 people with psoriasis found that a 0.5 percent aloe vera cream cured 86 percent of the subjects. Each person used the aloe vera cream three times each day for a period of one year, and the researchers concluded that aloe vera cream is a safe and effective cure for psoriasis.

- **Try other topical creams.** Many topical creams, oils, and ointments help psoriasis. Capsaicin, a cayenne pepper cream, helped 66 to 70 percent of the people who used it in a recent trial. The main side effect was that of a burning feeling associated with chili peppers, which quickly subsided. Vitamins A and E have also been used topically with success; one physician alternates them, one each day. Creams containing zinc are also effective, as are salves containing sarsaparilla. Goldenseal ointment or oral supplements can also be helpful.

- **Practice stress-management skills.** Flare-ups of psoriasis often occur after a stressful event. Because stress has to do with our own internalization of an event, even a mildly stressful situation can trigger psoriasis. Learning stress-modification techniques can change your attitude about stressful situations, allowing you to let them roll by more easily. In a recent study, 4 out of 11 people showed significant improvement in psoriatic symptoms with meditation and guided imagery. Hypnotherapy, biofeedback, and walks in nature are other effective tools. Regular aerobic exercise is a powerful stress reducer.

ROSACEA

Rosacea is a chronic inflamed facial condition. It is characterized by redness on the cheeks, nose, chin, and forehead with small bumps or pimples on the face. More rarely it can occur on the scalp, neck, chest, or ears. Over time the redness can become more persistent. You can often also see small blood vessels on the face.

People with rosacea often have watery, bloodshot, or irritated eyes. The condition affects 16 million Americans and is becoming more prevalent. It flares up and goes into remission. Rosacea is a tough illness socially. It affects people's self-esteem, career, and social life.

According to the National Rosacea Society, the most common triggers include sunshine, emotional stress, hot or cold weather, wind, heavy exercise, alcohol consumption, hot baths, spicy foods, indoor heat, and some skin care products.

Research on rosacea and digestion is sparse, yet what is available points to a large component that is digestive in nature. I have seen remarkable improvements in my clients on a gluten-free diet and also with use of betaine HCl to increase stomach acids. Research by Andrea Parodi and colleagues discovered small intestinal bacterial overgrowth (SIBO) in 46 percent of participants (52 out of 113). After treatment with Rifaximin, lesions cleared in 71 percent (20 out of 28) and greatly improved in 21 percent (6 out of 28).

SIBO is associated with lower levels of hydrochloric acid. A few old studies (1920 and 1948) measured hydrochloric acid sufficiency and found rates of insufficiency to be higher in people with rosacea.

There have also been several studies linking *Candida spp.* species with rosacea. *Helicobacteria pylori*, a bacteria most closely connected with stomach ulcers, has also been associated with acne rosacea in studies. If you have rosacea, do explore dysbiosis and infection as an underlying issue.

One researcher reported finding low levels of lipase (fat-splitting enzymes) in people with rosacea. He reported improvements by giving pancreatic enzyme supplements.

Functional Laboratory Testing
- Breath test for small intestinal bacterial overgrowth
- Candida antibodies in serum, or candida in stool analysis
- Organic acid testing
- Stool testing for pancreatic function
- HCl testing
- Food sensitivity testing
- Celiac testing
- Vitamin D levels
- Red blood cell zinc levels
- Vitamin A levels

Healing Options
- **Get tested for SIBO.** Since about 90 percent of people with SIBO and rosacea improved after treatment for SIBO, this is the first place to begin. If discovered, eat a low-carbohydrate diet for several months.
- **Rule out candida.** Take the self-test for candida in Chapter 11. Get tested through organic acid testing, stool, or serum antibodies. If discovered, eat a low-carbohydrate diet and treat the candida with medications and/or natural therapies such as oil of oregano, grapefruit seed extract, garlic, or pau d'arco.
- Rule out *H. pylori*. Any physician can test for *H. pylori* infection. It is strongly associated with acne rosacea.
- **Take digestive enzymes.** One researcher reported finding low levels of lipase (fat-splitting enzymes) in people with rosacea. He reported improvements by

giving pancreatic enzyme supplements. I would probably use lipase-loaded enzymes. Take one with meals.

- **Try an elimination diet.** I have found that this works extremely well for people with rosacea. Gluten and dairy seem to be the biggest culprits, but any food could be inflammatory. See Chapter 14.

- **See if HCl levels are normal.** Take the HCl self-test in Chapter 11.

- **Take probiotics and eat probiotic-rich food.** While there is no research on this, if dysbiosis and gluten sensitivity are main underlying causes of rosacea, it makes sense to protect the gut with probiotics and probiotic-rich foods.

- **Eat brewer's yeast or nutritional yeast.** A study of 96 people with rosacea reported that about 1½ teaspoons daily of brewer's yeast offered great improvement in their rosacea. This was not duplicated by taking synthetic B-complex vitamins.

AFTERWORD

We've covered a lot of ground in *Digestive Wellness*. We've explored how the digestive system works, the DIGIN method for assessing underlying triggers and components of digestive and systemic disease and imbalances, lifestyle and nutritional recommendations, and finally chapters on dozens of specific digestive and systemic disease. Hopefully, you have a deeper understanding of how the digestive system works and what to do when it's out of balance. Most important, I hope that you gained personal insights that will resonate with you over time.

There's so much more that I wanted to include in the book, but it provides an good overview of the topics that are included. Each topic could easily become its own book, but what has been included here gives you plenty to work with. If you are looking for additional resources: books, references, handouts, references for the first through fourth editions, and recommendations for nutritional and herbal supplements, and so on; go to: www.digestivewellnessbook.com.

Thank you for coming with me on this journey.

BIBLIOGRAPHY

The first edition of *Digestive* Wellness was published in 1995. This bibliography includes references that are new to the 5th edition. The full Bibliography to Editions 1-5 can be found online at: www.digestivewellnessbook.com

Author's Preface:

1. Hanaway P. Fire in the Gut Part I: Assessment of Oxidative Stress and Inflammation in Gastrointestinal Dysfunction. Paper presented at: Advanced Practice Module: Restoring Gastrointestinal Equilibrium; July 17–19, 2009; Washington DC.

PART I: Fundamentals

CHAPTER 1   Changing the Way You Feel: When in Doubt, Begin in the Gut

1. Bauer UE, Briss PA, Goodman RA, Bowman BA. Prevention of chronic disease in the 21st century: elimination of the leading preventable causes of premature death and disability in the USA. *Lancet.* 2014;384(9937):45–52.
2. Cordain L, Eaton SB, Sebastian A, et al. Origins and evolution of the Western diet: health implications for the 21st century. *Am J Clin Nutr.* 2005;81(2):341–354.
3. Jones DS HL, Quinn S. *21st Century medicine: A New Model for Medical Education and Practice.* Institute for Functional Medicine;2009.
4. Kidd MR, Saltman DC. Case reports at the vanguard of 21st century medicine. *Journal of medical case reports.* 2012;6:156.
5. Stojanovic D, Markovic D. [Nutrigenomics–the science of the 21st century]. *Vojnosanit Pregl.*68(9):786–791.

CHAPTER 2   A Voyage Through the Digestive System

1. Bourassa MW, Alim I, Bultman SJ, Ratan RR. Butyrate, neuroepigenetics and the gut microbiome: Can a high fiber diet improve brain health? *Neurosci Lett.* 2016;625:56–63.

2. Gutierrez IM, Kang KH, Calvert CE, et al. Risk factors for small bowel bacterial overgrowth and diagnostic yield of duodenal aspirates in children with intestinal failure: a retrospective review. *Journal of pediatric surgery.* 2012;47(6):1150–1154.

3. Miller LS, Vegesna AK, Sampath AM, Prabhu S, Kotapati SK, Makipour K. Ileocecal valve dysfunction in small intestinal bacterial overgrowth: a pilot study. *World J Gastroenterol.* 2012;18(46):6801–6808.

PART II: The DIGIN Model and the 5 Rs

CHAPTER 3   Digestion/Absorption: Replace and Repair

1. Beyer PL, Caviar EM, McCallum RW. Fructose intake at current levels in the United States may cause gastrointestinal distress in normal adults. *J Am Diet Assoc.* 2005;105(10):1559–1566.

2. Ebert K, Witt H. Fructose malabsorption. *Molecular and cellular pediatrics.* 2016;3(1):10.

3. El-Sharkawy AM, Sahota O, Lobo DN. Acute and chronic effects of hydration status on health. *Nutr Rev.* 2015;73 Suppl 2:97–109.

4. Li J, Zhang N, Hu L, et al. Improvement in chewing activity reduces energy intake in one meal and modulates plasma gut hormone concentrations in obese and lean young Chinese men. *Am J Clin Nutr.* 2011;94(3):709–716.

5. Struyvenberg MR, Martin CR, Freedman SD. Practical guide to exocrine pancreatic insufficiency - Breaking the myths. *BMC medicine.* 2017;15(1):29.

CHAPTER 4   Intestinal Permeability/Leaky Membranes

1. Bodammer P, Kerkhoff C, Maletzki C, Lamprecht G. Bovine colostrum increases pore-forming claudin-2 protein expression but paradoxically not ion permeability possibly by a change of the intestinal cytokine milieu. *PLoS One.* 2013;8(5):e64210.

2. Davison G, Marchbank T, March DS, Thatcher R, Playford RJ. Zinc carnosine works with bovine colostrum in truncating heavy exercise-induced increase in gut permeability in healthy volunteers. *Am J Clin Nutr.* 2016;104(2):526–536.

3. Gildea JJ RD, & Bush Z. Protection against Gluten-mediated Tight Junction Injury with a Novel Lignite Extract Supplement. *J of Nutr & Food Sci.* 2016;6(5).

4. Gildea JJ RD, & Bush Z. Protective Effects of Lignite Extract supplement on Intestinal Barrier function in Glyphosate-Mediated Tight junction injury. *J of Clin Nutrition & Dietetics.* 2016;3(1.1).

5. Guerville M, Leroy A, Sinquin A, Laugerette F, Michalski MC, Boudry G. Western-diet consumption induces alteration of barrier function mechanisms in the ileum that correlates with metabolic endotoxemia in rats. *American journal of physiology Endocrinology and metabolism.* 2017;313(2):E107–e120.

6. Halasa M, Maciejewska D, Baskiewicz-Halasa M, Machalinski B, Safranow K, Stachowska E. Oral Supplementation with Bovine Colostrum Decreases Intestinal Permeability and Stool Concentrations of Zonulin in Athletes. *Nutrients.* 2017;9(4).

7. Julio-Pieper M, Bravo JA, Aliaga E, Gotteland M. Review article: intestinal barrier dysfunction and central nervous system disorders—a controversial association. *Aliment Pharmacol Ther.* 2014;40(10):1187–1201.

8. Kamiya S, Nagino M, Kanazawa H, et al. The value of bile replacement during external biliary drainage: an analysis of intestinal permeability, integrity, and microflora. *Ann Surg.* 2004;239(4):510–517.

9. Lin R, Zhou L, Zhang J, Wang B. Abnormal intestinal permeability and microbiota in patients with autoimmune hepatitis. *International journal of clinical and experimental pathology.* 2015;8(5):5153–5160.

10. Marchbank T, Davison G, Oakes JR, et al. The nutriceutical bovine colostrum truncates the increase in gut permeability caused by heavy exercise in athletes. *Am J Physiol Gastrointest Liver Physiol.* 2011;300(3):G477–484.

11. Mu Q, Kirby J, Reilly CM, Luo XM. Leaky Gut As a Danger Signal for Autoimmune Diseases. *Frontiers in immunology.* 2017;8:598.

12. Nouri M, Bredberg A, Westrom B, Lavasani S. Intestinal barrier dysfunction develops at the onset of experimental autoimmune encephalomyelitis, and can be induced by adoptive transfer of auto-reactive T cells. *PLoS One.* 2014;9(9):e106335.

13. Rohr MW, Narasimhulu CA, Rudeski-Rohr TA, Parthasarathy S. Negative Effects of a High-Fat Diet on Intestinal Permeability: A Review. *Adv Nutr.* 2019.

14. Visser J, Rozing J, Sapone A, Lammers K, Fasano A. Tight junctions, intestinal permeability, and autoimmunity: celiac disease and type 1 diabetes paradigms. *Ann N Y Acad Sci.* 2009;1165:195–205.

15. Wang L, Llorente C, Hartmann P, Yang AM, Chen P, Schnabl B. Methods to determine intestinal permeability and bacterial translocation during liver disease. *J Immunol Methods.* 2015;421:44–53.

CHAPTER 5 The GI Microbiome: Our Symbiotic Relationship

1. Aguirre M, Venema K. The art of targeting gut microbiota for tackling human obesity. *Genes Nutr.* 2015;10(4):472.

2. Amato KR, Yeoman CJ, Cerda G, et al. Variable responses of human and non-human primate gut microbiomes to a Western diet. *Microbiome.* 2015;3:53.

3. Barin JG, Tobias LD, Peterson DA. The microbiome and autoimmune disease: Report from a Noel R. Rose Colloquium. *Clin Immunol.* 2015;159(2):183–188.

4. Belizario JE, Napolitano M. Human microbiomes and their roles in dysbiosis, common diseases, and novel therapeutic approaches. *Front Microbiol.* 2015;6:1050.

5. Bengmark S. Nutrition of the critically ill — a 21st-century perspective. *Nutrients.* 2013;5(1):162–207.

6. Birt DF, Phillips GJ. Diet, genes, and microbes: complexities of colon cancer prevention. *Toxicologic pathology.* 2014;42(1):182–188.

7. Byrne CS, Chambers ES, Morrison DJ, Frost G. The role of short chain fatty acids in appetite regulation and energy homeostasis. *International journal of obesity.* 2015; 39(9):1331–1338.

8. Cadwell K. The virome in host health and disease. *Immunity.* 2015;42(5):805–813.

9. Carding S, Verbeke K, Vipond DT, Corfe BM, Owen LJ. Dysbiosis of the gut microbiota in disease. *Microb Ecol Health Dis.* 2015;26:26191.

10. Chassaing B, Koren O, Goodrich JK, et al. Dietary emulsifiers impact the mouse gut microbiota promoting colitis and metabolic syndrome. *Nature.* 2015;519(7541):92–96.

11. Chassaing B, Koren O, Goodrich JK, et al. Corrigendum: Dietary emulsifiers impact the mouse gut microbiota promoting colitis and metabolic syndrome. *Nature.* 2016;536(7615):238.

12. Chen J, He X, Huang J. Diet effects in gut microbiome and obesity. *Journal of food science.* 2014;79(4):R442–451.

13. Conlon MA, Bird AR. The impact of diet and lifestyle on gut microbiota and human health. *Nutrients.* 2014;7(1):17–44.

14. Davis-Richardson AG, Triplett EW. A model for the role of gut bacteria in the development of autoimmunity for type 1 diabetes. *Diabetologia.* 2015;58(7):1386–1393.

15. Donaldson GP, Lee SM, Mazmanian SK. Gut biogeography of the bacterial microbiota. *Nat Rev Microbiol.* 2016;14(1):20–32.

16. Dugas LR, Fuller M, Gilbert J, Layden BT. The obese gut microbiome across the epidemiologic transition. *Emerging themes in epidemiology.* 2016;13:2.

17. Edlund A, Santiago-Rodriguez TM, Boehm TK, Pride DT. Bacteriophage and their potential roles in the human oral cavity. *Journal of oral microbiology.* 2015;7:27423.

18. Fabbiano S, Suarez-Zamorano N, Trajkovski M. Host-Microbiota Mutualism in Metabolic Diseases. *Frontiers in endocrinology.* 2017;8:267.

19. Festi D, Schiumerini R, Eusebi LH, Marasco G, Taddia M, Colecchia A. Gut microbiota and metabolic syndrome. *World J Gastroenterol.* 2014;20(43):16079–16094.

20. Foca A, Liberto MC, Quirino A, Marascio N, Zicca E, Pavia G. Gut inflammation and immunity: what is the role of the human gut virome? *Mediators of inflammation.* 2015;2015:326032.

21. Glendinning L, Free A. Supra-organismal interactions in the human intestine. *Frontiers in cellular and infection microbiology.* 2014;4:47.

22. Jandhyala SM, Talukdar R, Subramanyam C, Vuyyuru H, Sasikala M, Nageshwar Reddy D. Role of the normal gut microbiota. *World J Gastroenterol.* 2015;21(29):8787–8803.

23. Kanai T, Matsuoka K, Naganuma M, Hayashi A, Hisamatsu T. Diet, microbiota, and inflammatory bowel disease: lessons from Japanese foods. *The Korean journal of internal medicine*. 2014;29(4):409–415.

24. Koleva PT, Bridgman SL, Kozyrskyj AL. The infant gut microbiome: evidence for obesity risk and dietary intervention. *Nutrients*. 2015;7(4):2237–2260.

25. Koutsos A, Tuohy KM, Lovegrove JA. Apples and cardiovascular health—is the gut microbiota a core consideration? *Nutrients*. 2015;7(6):3959–3998.

26. Kundu P, Blacher E, Elinav E, Pettersson S. Our Gut Microbiome: The Evolving Inner Self. *Cell*. 2017;171(7):1481–1493.

27. Larmonier CB, Shehab KW, Ghishan FK, Kiela PR. T Lymphocyte Dynamics in Inflammatory Bowel Diseases: Role of the Microbiome. *BioMed research international*. 2015;2015:504638.

28. Lau WL, Vaziri ND. The Leaky Gut and Altered Microbiome in Chronic Kidney Disease. *J Ren Nutr*. 2017;27(6):458–461.

29. Lau WL, Vaziri ND. The Leaky Gut and Altered Microbiome in Chronic Kidney Disease. *J Ren Nutr*. 2017;27(6):458–461.

30. Laursen MF, Zachariassen G, Bahl MI, et al. Having older siblings is associated with gut microbiota development during early childhood. *BMC Microbiol*. 2015;15:154.

31. Li M, Wang M, Donovan SM. Early development of the gut microbiome and immune-mediated childhood disorders. *Seminars in reproductive medicine*. 2014;32(1):74–86.

32. Lloyd-Price J, Abu-Ali G, Huttenhower C. The healthy human microbiome. *Genome medicine*. 2016;8(1):51.

33. Marchesi JR, Adams DH, Fava F, et al. The gut microbiota and host health: a new clinical frontier. *Gut*. 2016;65(2):330–339.

34. Mejia-Leon ME, Barca AM. Diet, Microbiota and Immune System in Type 1 Diabetes Development and Evolution. *Nutrients*. 2015;7(11):9171–9184.

35. Moraes AC, Silva IT, Almeida-Pititto B, Ferreira SR. [Intestinal microbiota and cardiometabolic risk: mechanisms and diet modulation]. *Arq Bras Endocrinol Metabol*. 2014;58(4):317–327.

36. Nardone G, Compare D. The human gastric microbiota: Is it time to rethink the pathogenesis of stomach diseases? *United European Gastroenterol J*. 2015;3(3):255–260.

37. Ni Y, Li J, Panagiotou G. A Molecular-Level Landscape of Diet-Gut Microbiome Interactions: Toward Dietary Interventions Targeting Bacterial Genes. *MBio*. 2015;6(6).

38. Ogilvie LA, Jones BV. The human gut virome: a multifaceted majority. *Front Microbiol*. 2015;6:918.

39. Ou J, Carbonero F, Zoetendal EG, et al. Diet, microbiota, and microbial metabolites in colon cancer risk in rural Africans and African Americans. *Am J Clin Nutr*. 2013;98(1):111–120.

40. Ridaura VK, Faith JJ, Rey FE, et al. Gut microbiota from twins discordant for obesity modulate metabolism in mice. *Science.* 2013;341(6150):1241214.

41. Roberts CL, Keita AV, Duncan SH, et al. Translocation of Crohn's disease Escherichia coli across M-cells: contrasting effects of soluble plant fibres and emulsifiers. *Gut.* 2010;59(10):1331–1339.

42. Savidge TC. Epigenetic Regulation of Enteric Neurotransmission by Gut Bacteria. *Frontiers in cellular neuroscience.* 2015;9:503.

43. Suez J, Korem T, Zilberman-Schapira G, Segal E, Elinav E. Non-caloric artificial sweeteners and the microbiome: findings and challenges. *Gut Microbes.* 2015;6(2):149–155.

44. Tang WH, Hazen SL. The contributory role of gut microbiota in cardiovascular disease. *The Journal of clinical investigation.* 2014;124(10):4204–4211.

45. Versalovic J. The human microbiome and probiotics: implications for pediatrics. *Ann Nutr Metab.* 2013;63 Suppl 2:42–52.

46. Vieira SM, Pagovich OE, Kriegel MA. Diet, microbiota and autoimmune diseases. *Lupus.* 2014;23(6):518–526.

47. Viertel TM, Ritter K, Horz HP. Viruses versus bacteria-novel approaches to phage therapy as a tool against multidrug-resistant pathogens. *The Journal of antimicrobial chemotherapy.* 2014;69(9):2326–2336.

48. Virgin HW. The virome in mammalian physiology and disease. *Cell.* 2014;157(1):142–150.

49. Weaver CM. Diet, gut microbiome, and bone health. *Current osteoporosis reports.* 2015;13(2):125–130.

50. Wong JM. Gut microbiota and cardiometabolic outcomes: influence of dietary patterns and their associated components. *Am J Clin Nutr.* 2014;100 Suppl 1:369s–377s.

51. Woting A, Blaut M. The Intestinal Microbiota in Metabolic Disease. *Nutrients.* 2016;8(4).

52. Xie H, Guo R, Zhong H, et al. Shotgun Metagenomics of 250 Adult Twins Reveals Genetic and Environmental Impacts on the Gut Microbiome. *Cell Syst.* 2016;3(6):572–584.e573.

53. Zhang YJ, Li S, Gan RY, Zhou T, Xu DP, Li HB. Impacts of gut bacteria on human health and diseases. *International journal of molecular sciences.* 2015;16(4):7493–7519.

CHAPTER 6   The GI Microbiome: Prebiotics and Probiotics from Food and Supplements

1. Baothman OA, Zamzami MA, Taher I, Abubaker J, Abu-Farha M. The role of Gut Microbiota in the development of obesity and Diabetes. *Lipids Health Dis.* 2016;15:108.

2. Behera SS, Ray RC, Zdolec N. Lactobacillus plantarum with Functional Properties: An Approach to Increase Safety and Shelf-Life of Fermented Foods. *BioMed research international.* 2018;2018:9361614.

3. Bell V, Ferrao J, Fernandes T. Nutritional Guidelines and Fermented Food Frameworks. *Foods (Basel, Switzerland).* 2017;6(8).

4. Bell V, Ferrao J, Pimentel L, Pintado M, Fernandes T. One Health, Fermented Foods, and Gut Microbiota. *Foods (Basel, Switzerland).* 2018;7(12).

5. Belorkar SA, Gupta AK. Oligosaccharides: a boon from nature's desk. *AMB Express.* 2016;6(1):82.

6. Borchers AT, Selmi C, Meyers FJ, Keen CL, Gershwin ME. Probiotics and immunity. *J Gastroenterol.* 2009;44(1):26–46.

7. Boto-Ordonez M, Urpi-Sarda M, Queipo-Ortuno MI, Tulipani S, Tinahones FJ, Andres-Lacueva C. High levels of Bifidobacteria are associated with increased levels of anthocyanin microbial metabolites: a randomized clinical trial. *Food Funct.* 2014;5(8):1932–1938.

8. Bourrie BC, Willing BP, Cotter PD. The Microbiota and Health Promoting Characteristics of the Fermented Beverage Kefir. *Front Microbiol.* 2016;7:647.

9. Byrne CS, Chambers ES, Morrison DJ, Frost G. The role of short chain fatty acids in appetite regulation and energy homeostasis. *International journal of obesity.* 2015;39(9):1331–1338.

10. Chilton SN, Burton JP, Reid G. Inclusion of fermented foods in food guides around the world. *Nutrients.* 2015;7(1):390–404.

11. Choi IH, Noh JS, Han JS, Kim HJ, Han ES, Song YO. Kimchi, a fermented vegetable, improves serum lipid profiles in healthy young adults: randomized clinical trial. *J Med Food.* 2013;16(3):223–229.

12. Collins S, Reid G. Distant Site Effects of Ingested Prebiotics. *Nutrients.* 2016;8(9).

13. de Oliveira Leite AM, Miguel MA, Peixoto RS, Rosado AS, Silva JT, Paschoalin VM. Microbiological, technological and therapeutic properties of kefir: a natural probiotic beverage. *Brazilian journal of microbiology : [publication of the Brazilian Society for Microbiology].* 2013;44(2):341–349.

14. Dolan KE, Finley HJ, Burns CM, et al. Probiotics and Disease: A Comprehensive Summary-Part 1, Mental and Neurological Health. *Integrative medicine (Encinitas, Calif).* 2016;15(5):46–58.

15. Dolan KE, Pizano JM, Gossard CM, et al. Probiotics and Disease: A Comprehensive Summary-Part 6, Skin Health. *Integrative medicine (Encinitas, Calif).* 2017;16(4):32–41.

16. Du DD, Yoshinaga M, Sonoda M, Kawakubo K, Uehara Y. Blood pressure reduction by Japanese traditional Miso is associated with increased diuresis and natriuresis through dopamine system in Dahl salt-sensitive rats. *Clinical and experimental hypertension (New York, NY : 1993).* 2014;36(5):359–366.

17. Fernandez MA, Marette A. Potential Health Benefits of Combining Yogurt and Fruits Based on Their Probiotic and Prebiotic Properties. *Adv Nutr.* 2017;8(1):155s–164s.

18. Fijan S. Microorganisms with claimed probiotic properties: an overview of recent literature. *International journal of environmental research and public health.* 2014;11(5):4745–4767.

19. Finley HJ, Gasta MG, Dolan KE, et al. Probiotics and Disease: A Comprehensive Summary-Part 8, Gastrointestinal and Genitourinary Disorders. *Integrative medicine (Encinitas, Calif).* 2018;17(1):38–48.

20. Gasta MG, Gossard CM, Williamson CB, et al. Probiotics and Disease: A Comprehensive Summary-Part 5, Respiratory Conditions of the Ears, Nose, and Throat. *Integrative medicine (Encinitas, Calif).* 2017;16(3):28–40.

21. Gasta MG, Williamson CB, Gossard CM, et al. Probiotics and Disease: A Comprehensive Summary-Part 4, Infectious Diseases. *Integrative medicine (Encinitas, Calif).* 2017;16(2):28–38.

22. Gibson GR, Hutkins R, Sanders ME, et al. Expert consensus document: The International Scientific Association for Probiotics and Prebiotics (ISAPP) consensus statement on the definition and scope of prebiotics. *Nat Rev Gastroenterol Hepatol.* 2017;14(8):491–502.

23. Gossard CM, Pizano JM, Burns CM, et al. Probiotics and Disease: A Comprehensive Summary-Part 9, Cancer. *Integrative medicine (Encinitas, Calif).* 2018;17(2):34–46.

24. Hill C, Guarner F, Reid G, et al. Expert consensus document. The International Scientific Association for Probiotics and Prebiotics consensus statement on the scope and appropriate use of the term probiotic. *Nat Rev Gastroenterol Hepatol.* 2014;11(8):506–514.

25. Kasubuchi M, Hasegawa S, Hiramatsu T, Ichimura A, Kimura I. Dietary gut microbial metabolites, short-chain fatty acids, and host metabolic regulation. *Nutrients.* 2015;7(4):2839–2849.

26. Marchesi JR, Adams DH, Fava F, et al. The gut microbiota and host health: a new clinical frontier. *Gut.* 2016;65(2):330–339.

27. Markowiak P, Slizewska K. Effects of Probiotics, Prebiotics, and Synbiotics on Human Health. *Nutrients.* 2017;9(9).

28. Mokoena MP, Mutanda T, Olaniran AO. Perspectives on the probiotic potential of lactic acid bacteria from African traditional fermented foods and beverages. *Food & nutrition research.* 2016;60:29630.

29. Morrison DJ, Preston T. Formation of short chain fatty acids by the gut microbiota and their impact on human metabolism. *Gut Microbes.* 2016;7(3):189–200.

30. Natarajan N, Pluznick JL. From microbe to man: the role of microbial short chain fatty acid metabolites in host cell biology. *American journal of physiology Cell physiology.* 2014;307(11):C979–985.

31. Ostadrahimi A, Taghizadeh A, Mobasseri M, et al. Effect of probiotic fermented milk (kefir) on glycemic control and lipid profile in type 2 diabetic patients: a randomized double-blind placebo-controlled clinical trial. *Iran J Public Health.* 2015;44(2):228–237.

32. Park KY, Jeong JK, Lee YE, Daily JW, 3rd. Health benefits of kimchi (Korean fermented vegetables) as a probiotic food. *J Med Food.* 2014;17(1):6–20.

33. Parker EC, Gossard CM, Dolan KE, et al. Probiotics and Disease: A Comprehensive Summary-Part 2, Commercially Produced Cultured and Fermented Foods Commonly Available in the United States. *Integrative medicine (Encinitas, Calif).* 2016;15(6):22–30.

34. Parker EC, Gossard CM, Dolan KE, et al. Probiotics and Disease: A Comprehensive Summary-Part 2, Commercially Produced Cultured and Fermented Foods Commonly Available in the United States. *Integrative medicine (Encinitas, Calif).* 2016;15(6):22–30.

35. Parvez S, Malik KA, Ah Kang S, Kim HY. Probiotics and their fermented food products are beneficial for health. *J Appl Microbiol.* 2006;100(6):1171–1185.

36. Patra JK, Das G, Paramithiotis S, Shin HS. Kimchi and Other Widely Consumed Traditional Fermented Foods of Korea: A Review. *Front Microbiol.* 2016;7:1493.

37. Pizano JM, Williamson CB, Dolan KE, et al. Probiotics and Disease: A Comprehensive Summary-Part 7, Immune Disorders. *Integrative medicine (Encinitas, Calif).* 2017;16(5):46–57.

38. Shin GH, Kang BC, Jang DJ. Metabolic Pathways Associated with Kimchi, a Traditional Korean Food, Based on In Silico Modeling of Published Data. *Genomics & informatics.* 2016;14(4):222–229.

39. So D, Whelan K, Rossi M, et al. Dietary fiber intervention on gut microbiota composition in healthy adults: a systematic review and meta-analysis. *Am J Clin Nutr.* 2018;107(6):965–983.

40. Swain MR, Anandharaj M, Ray RC, Parveen Rani R. Fermented fruits and vegetables of Asia: a potential source of probiotics. *Biotechnology research international.* 2014;2014:250424.

41. Takagi A, Kano M, Kaga C. Possibility of breast cancer prevention: use of soy isoflavones and fermented soy beverage produced using probiotics. *International journal of molecular sciences.* 2015;16(5):10907–10920.

42. Tamang JP, Watanabe K, Holzapfel WH. Review: Diversity of Microorganisms in Global Fermented Foods and Beverages. *Front Microbiol.* 2016;7:377.

43. Verbeke KA, Boobis AR, Chiodini A, et al. Towards microbial fermentation metabolites as markers for health benefits of prebiotics. *Nutr Res Rev.* 2015;28(1):42–66.

44. Vinolo MA, Rodrigues HG, Nachbar RT, Curi R. Regulation of inflammation by short chain fatty acids. *Nutrients.* 2011;3(10):858–876.

45. Williamson CB, Burns CM, Gossard CM, et al. Probiotics and Disease: A Comprehensive Summary-Part 3, Cardiometabolic Disease and Fatigue Syndromes. *Integrative medicine (Encinitas, Calif).* 2017;16(1):30–41.

46. Zwickey H, Lipski L. Expanding Our View of Herbal Medicine. *J Altern Complement Med.* 2018;24(7):619–620.

CHAPTER 7 The GI Microbiome: Dysbiosis, a Good Neighborhood Gone Bad

1. Banerjee S, Tian T, Wei Z, et al. The ovarian cancer oncobiome. *Oncotarget.* 2017; 8(22):36225–36245.

2. Betrapally NS, Gillevet PM, Bajaj JS. Changes in the Intestinal Microbiome and Alcoholic and Nonalcoholic Liver Diseases: Causes or Effects? *Gastroenterology.* 2016;150(8):1745–1755.e1743.

3. Bull MJ, Plummer NT. Part 2: Treatments for Chronic Gastrointestinal Disease and Gut Dysbiosis. *Integrative medicine (Encinitas, Calif).* 2015;14(1):25–33.

4. Chassaing B, Gewirtz AT. Gut microbiota, low-grade inflammation, and metabolic syndrome. *Toxicologic pathology.* 2014;42(1):49–53.

5. Chen J, Domingue JC, Sears CL. Microbiota dysbiosis in select human cancers: Evidence of association and causality. *Semin Immunol.* 2017;32:25–34.

6. Davis-Richardson AG, Triplett EW. A model for the role of gut bacteria in the development of autoimmunity for type 1 diabetes. *Diabetologia.* 2015;58(7):1386–1393.

7. DeGruttola AK, Low D, Mizoguchi A, Mizoguchi E. Current Understanding of Dysbiosis in Disease in Human and Animal Models. *Inflamm Bowel Dis.* 2016; 22(5):1137–1150.

8. El-Salhy M, Mazzawi T, Hausken T, Hatlebakk JG. Interaction between diet and gastrointestinal endocrine cells. *Biomedical reports.* 2016;4(6):651–656.

9. Everard A, Cani PD. Diabetes, obesity and gut microbiota. *Best Pract Res Clin Gastroenterol.* 2013;27(1):73–83.

10. Gao R, Gao Z, Huang L, Qin H. Gut microbiota and colorectal cancer. *Eur J Clin Microbiol Infect Dis.* 2017;36(5):757–769.

11. Goyal A, Nimmakayala KR, Zonszein J. Is there a paradox in obesity? *Cardiology in review.* 2014;22(4):163–170.

12. Griffin JL, Wang X, Stanley E. Does our gut microbiome predict cardiovascular risk? A review of the evidence from metabolomics. *Circ Cardiovasc Genet.* 2015;8(1):187–191.

13. Hawrelak JA, Cattley T, Myers SP. Essential oils in the treatment of intestinal dysbiosis: A preliminary in vitro study. *Altern Med Rev.* 2009;14(4):380–384.

14. Iliev ID, Leonardi I. Fungal dysbiosis: immunity and interactions at mucosal barriers. *Nat Rev Immunol.* 2017;17(10):635–646.

15. Jayasinghe TN, Chiavaroli V, Holland DJ, Cutfield WS, O'Sullivan JM. The New Era of Treatment for Obesity and Metabolic Disorders: Evidence and Expectations for Gut Microbiome Transplantation. *Frontiers in cellular and infection microbiology.* 2016;6:15.

16. Konrad D, Wueest S. The gut-adipose-liver axis in the metabolic syndrome. *Physiology (Bethesda, Md).* 2014;29(5):304–313.

17. Lau E, Carvalho D, Freitas P. Gut Microbiota: Association with NAFLD and Metabolic Disturbances. *BioMed research international.* 2015;2015:979515.

18. Li J, Zhao F, Wang Y, et al. Gut microbiota dysbiosis contributes to the development of hypertension. *Microbiome.* 2017;5(1):14.

19. Manrique P, Dills M, Young MJ. The Human Gut Phage Community and Its Implications for Health and Disease. *Viruses.* 2017;9(6).

20. McGill AT. Causes of metabolic syndrome and obesity-related co-morbidities Part 1: A composite unifying theory review of human-specific co-adaptations to brain energy consumption. *Archives of public health = Archives belges de sante publique.* 2014;72(1):30.

21. Miyake S, Kim S, Suda W, et al. Dysbiosis in the Gut Microbiota of Patients with Multiple Sclerosis, with a Striking Depletion of Species Belonging to Clostridia XIVa and IV Clusters. *PLoS One.* 2015;10(9):e0137429.

22. Petersen C, Round JL. Defining dysbiosis and its influence on host immunity and disease. *Cellular microbiology.* 2014;16(7):1024–1033.

23. Pope JL, Tomkovich S, Yang Y, Jobin C. Microbiota as a mediator of cancer progression and therapy. *Transl Res.* 2017;179:139–154.

24. Qian LL, Li HT, Zhang L, Fang QC, Jia WP. Effect of the Gut Microbiota on Obesity and Its Underlying Mechanisms: an Update. *Biomed Environ Sci.* 2015;28(11):839–847.

25. Tomasello G, Mazzola M, Leone A, et al. Nutrition, oxidative stress and intestinal dysbiosis: Influence of diet on gut microbiota in inflammatory bowel diseases. *Biomedical papers of the Medical Faculty of the University Palacky, Olomouc, Czechoslovakia.* 2016;160(4):461–466.

26. Upadhyaya S, Banerjee G. Type 2 diabetes and gut microbiome: at the intersection of known and unknown. *Gut Microbes.* 2015;6(2):85–92.

27. Usami M, Miyoshi M, Yamashita H. Gut microbiota and host metabolism in liver cirrhosis. *World J Gastroenterol.* 2015;21(41):11597–11608.

28. Weiss GA, Hennet T. Mechanisms and consequences of intestinal dysbiosis. *Cell Mol Life Sci.* 2017;74(16):2959–2977.

29. Woting A, Blaut M. The Intestinal Microbiota in Metabolic Disease. *Nutrients.* 2016;8(4).

CHAPTER 8 Fire in the Gut: Immunity and Inflammation

1. Donaldson GP, Lee SM, Mazmanian SK. Gut biogeography of the bacterial microbiota. *Nat Rev Microbiol.* 2016;14(1):20–32.

2. Elliott DE, Weinstock JV. Where are we on worms? *Curr Opin Gastroenterol.* 2012;28(6):551–556.

3. Elliott DE, Weinstock JV. Helminth-host immunological interactions: prevention and control of immune-mediated diseases. *Ann N Y Acad Sci.* 2012;1247:83–96.

4. Smyth K, Morton C, Mathew A, et al. Production and Use of Hymenolepis diminuta Cysticercoids as Anti-Inflammatory Therapeutics. *Journal of clinical medicine.* 2017;6(10).

5. Weinstock JV, Elliott DE. Translatability of helminth therapy in inflammatory bowel diseases. *Int J Parasitol.* 2013;43(3–4):245–251.

6. Woolsey ID, Fredensborg BL, Jensen PM, Kapel CM, Meyling NV. An insect-tapeworm model as a proxy for anthelminthic effects in the mammalian host. *Parasitol Res.* 2015;114(7):2777–2780.

CHAPTER 9 Reactions: Food Sensitivities, Intolerances, and Allergies

1. Arnold LE, Lofthouse N, Hurt E. Artificial food colors and attention-deficit/hyperactivity symptoms: conclusions to dye for. *Neurotherapeutics : the journal of the American Society for Experimental NeuroTherapeutics.* 2012;9(3):599–609.

2. Barrett JS, Irving PM, Shepherd SJ, Muir JG, Gibson PR. Comparison of the prevalence of fructose and lactose malabsorption across chronic intestinal disorders. *Aliment Pharmacol Ther.* 2009;30(2):165–174.

3. Bunyavanich S, Rifas-Shiman SL, Platts-Mills TA, et al. Peanut allergy prevalence among school-age children in a US cohort not selected for any disease. *J Allergy Clin Immunol.* 2014;134(3):753–755.

4. Catassi C, Alaedini A, Bojarski C, et al. The Overlapping Area of Non-Celiac Gluten Sensitivity (NCGS) and Wheat-Sensitive Irritable Bowel Syndrome (IBS): An Update. *Nutrients.* 2017;9(11).

5. Catassi C, Elli L, Bonaz B, et al. Diagnosis of Non-Celiac Gluten Sensitivity (NCGS): The Salerno Experts' Criteria. *Nutrients.* 2015;7(6):4966–4977.

6. Cuomo R, Andreozzi P, Zito FP, Passananti V, De Carlo G, Sarnelli G. Irritable bowel syndrome and food interaction. *World J Gastroenterol.* 2014;20(27):8837–8845.

7. Di Stefano M, Pesatori EV, Manfredi GF, et al. Non-Celiac Gluten Sensitivity in patients with severe abdominal pain and bloating: The accuracy of ALCAT 5. *Clinical nutrition ESPEN.* 2018;28:127–131.

8. Du Toit G, Roberts G, Sayre PH, et al. Randomized trial of peanut consumption in infants at risk for peanut allergy. *N Engl J Med.* 2015;372(9):803–813.

9. Du Toit G, Sayre PH, Roberts G, et al. Effect of Avoidance on Peanut Allergy after Early Peanut Consumption. *N Engl J Med.* 2016;374(15):1435–1443.

10. Figueiredo L, Régis WCBJN. Medicinal mushrooms in adjuvant cancer therapies: an approach to anticancer effects and presumed mechanisms of action. 2017;42(1):28.

11. Hertzler SR, Savaiano DA. Colonic adaptation to daily lactose feeding in lactose maldigesters reduces lactose intolerance. *Am J Clin Nutr.* 1996;64(2):232–236.

12. Lennerz BS, Vafai SB, Delaney NF, et al. Effects of sodium benzoate, a widely used food preservative, on glucose homeostasis and metabolic profiles in humans. *Mol Genet Metab.* 2015;114(1):73–79.

13. Makharia A, Catassi C, Makharia GK. The Overlap between Irritable Bowel Syndrome and Non-Celiac Gluten Sensitivity: A Clinical Dilemma. *Nutrients.* 2015;7(12):10417–10426.

14. Nigg JT, Lewis K, Edinger T, Falk M. Meta-analysis of attention-deficit/hyperactivity disorder or attention-deficit/hyperactivity disorder symptoms, restriction diet, and synthetic food color additives. *J Am Acad Child Adolesc Psychiatry.* 2012;51(1):86–97.e88.

15. Pan L, Qin G, Zhao Y, Wang J, Liu F, Che D. Effects of soybean agglutinin on mechanical barrier function and tight junction protein expression in intestinal epithelial cells from piglets. *International journal of molecular sciences.* 2013;14(11):21689–21704.

16. Pitt TJ, Becker AB, Chan-Yeung M, et al. Reduced risk of peanut sensitization following exposure through breast-feeding and early peanut introduction. *J Allergy Clin Immunol.* 2018;141(2):620–625.e621.

17. Shakoor Z, AlFaifi A, AlAmro B, AlTawil LN, AlOhaly RY. Prevalence of IgG-mediated food intolerance among patients with allergic symptoms. *Annals of Saudi medicine.* 2016;36(6):386–390.

18. Skypala IJ, Williams M, Reeves L, Meyer R, Venter C. Sensitivity to food additives, vaso-active amines and salicylates: a review of the evidence. *Clinical and translational allergy.* 2015;5:34.

19. Tang ML, Ponsonby AL, Orsini F, et al. Administration of a probiotic with peanut oral immunotherapy: A randomized trial. *J Allergy Clin Immunol.* 2015;135(3):737–744.e738.

20. Teuri U, Vapaatalo H, Korpela R. Fructooligosaccharides and lactulose cause more symptoms in lactose maldigesters and subjects with pseudohypolactasia than in control lactose digesters. *Am J Clin Nutr.* 1999;69(5):973–979.

21. Vesa TH, Korpela RA, Sahi T. Tolerance to small amounts of lactose in lactose maldigesters. *Am J Clin Nutr.* 1996;64(2):197–201.

22. Vojdani A, Vojdani C. Immune reactivity to food coloring. *Altern Ther Health Med.* 2015;21 Suppl 1:52–62.

23. Yasuoka T, Sasaki M, Fukunaga T, et al. The effects of lectins on indomethacin-induced small intestinal ulceration. *International journal of experimental pathology.* 2003;84(5):231–237.

24. Yu CJ, Du JC, Chiou HC, et al. Sugar-Sweetened Beverage Consumption Is Adversely Associated with Childhood Attention Deficit/Hyperactivity Disorder. *International journal of environmental research and public health.* 2016;13(7).

CHAPTER 10   The Enteric Nervous System: The Gut–Brain Connection

1. Barrett E, Ross RP, O'Toole PW, Fitzgerald GF, Stanton C. gamma-Aminobutyric acid production by culturable bacteria from the human intestine. *J Appl Microbiol.* 2012;113(2):411–417.

2. Breit S, Kupferberg A, Rogler G, Hasler G. Vagus Nerve as Modulator of the Brain-Gut Axis in Psychiatric and Inflammatory Disorders. *Frontiers in psychiatry.* 2018;9:44.

3. Cenit MC, Sanz Y, Codoner-Franch P. Influence of gut microbiota on neuropsychiatric disorders. *World J Gastroenterol.* 2017;23(30):5486–5498.

4. de Lartigue G. Role of the vagus nerve in the development and treatment of diet-induced obesity. *The Journal of physiology.* 2016;594(20):5791–5815.

5. Dhakal R, Bajpai VK, Baek KH. Production of gaba (gamma - Aminobutyric acid) by microorganisms: a review. *Brazilian journal of microbiology : [publication of the Brazilian Society for Microbiology].* 2012;43(4):1230–1241.

6. Dinan TG, Cryan JF. Melancholic microbes: a link between gut microbiota and depression? *Neurogastroenterol Motil.* 2013;25(9):713–719.

7. Dinan TG, Stanton C, Cryan JF. Psychobiotics: a novel class of psychotropic. *Biol Psychiatry.* 2013;74(10):720–726.

8. Huang R, Wang K, Hu J. Effect of Probiotics on Depression: A Systematic Review and Meta-Analysis of Randomized Controlled Trials. *Nutrients.* 2016;8(8).

9. Koopman FA, Chavan SS, Miljko S, et al. Vagus nerve stimulation inhibits cytokine production and attenuates disease severity in rheumatoid arthritis. *Proc Natl Acad Sci U S A.* 2016;113(29):8284–8289.

10. Maiese K. Neurotransmission. Merck Manual Professional Version. https://www.merckmanuals.com/professional/neurologic-disorders/neurotransmission/neurotransmission. Published n.d. Accessed 7–31, 2019.

11. Mittal R, Debs LH, Patel AP, et al. Neurotransmitters: The Critical Modulators Regulating Gut-Brain Axis. *J Cell Physiol.* 2017;232(9):2359–2372.

12. Pessione E, Cirrincione S. Bioactive Molecules Released in Food by Lactic Acid Bacteria: Encrypted Peptides and Biogenic Amines. *Front Microbiol.* 2016;7:876.

13. Pokusaeva K, Johnson C, Luk B, et al. GABA-producing Bifidobacterium dentium modulates visceral sensitivity in the intestine. *Neurogastroenterol Motil.* 2017;29(1).

14. Slykerman RF, Hood F, Wickens K, et al. Effect of Lactobacillus rhamnosus HN001 in Pregnancy on Postpartum Symptoms of Depression and Anxiety: A Randomised Double-blind Placebo-controlled Trial. *EBioMedicine.* 2017;24:159–165.

15. Smythies LE, Smythies JR. Microbiota, the immune system, black moods and the brain-melancholia updated. *Front Hum Neurosci.* 2014;8:720.

16. Tan DX, Zheng X, Kong J, et al. Fundamental issues related to the origin of melatonin and melatonin isomers during evolution: relation to their biological functions. *International journal of molecular sciences.* 2014;15(9):15858–15890.

17. Tang F, Reddy BL, Saier MH, Jr. Psychobiotics and their involvement in mental health. *J Mol Microbiol Biotechnol.* 2014;24(4):211–214.

18. Thomas LV, Suzuki K, Zhao J. Probiotics: a proactive approach to health. A symposium report. *Br J Nutr.* 2015;114 Suppl 1:S1–s15.

19. Zhou L, Foster JA. Psychobiotics and the gut-brain axis: in the pursuit of happiness. *Neuropsychiatr Dis Treat.* 2015;11:715–723.

CHAPTER 11   Functional Medicine Testing and Questionnaires

1. Al-Abri SA, Olson KR. Baking soda can settle the stomach but upset the heart: case files of the Medical Toxicology Fellowship at the University of California, San Francisco. *J Med Toxicol.* 2013;9(3):255–258.

2. Barrett JS, Irving PM, Shepherd SJ, Muir JG, Gibson PR. Comparison of the prevalence of fructose and lactose malabsorption across chronic intestinal disorders. *Aliment Pharmacol Ther.* 2009;30(2):165–174.

3. Beyer PL, Caviar EM, McCallum RW. Fructose intake at current levels in the United States may cause gastrointestinal distress in normal adults. *J Am Diet Assoc.* 2005;105(10):1559–1566.

4. Cutler P. Food sensitivities. *Can Fam Physician.* 1984;30:133–136.

5. Ebert K, Witt H. Fructose malabsorption. *Molecular and cellular pediatrics.* 2016;3(1):10.

6. Elwyn G, Taubert M, Davies S, Brown G, Allison M, Phillips C. Which test is best for Helicobacter pylori? A cost-effectiveness model using decision analysis. *Br J Gen Pract.* 2007;57(538):401–403.

7. GAtkinson W, Sheldon TA, Shaath N, Whorwell PJ. Food elimination based on IgG antibodies in irritable bowel syndrome: a randomised controlled trial. *Gut.* 2004;53(10):1459–1464.

8. Gene E, Sanchez-Delgado J, Calvet X, Gisbert JP, Azagra R. What is the best strategy for diagnosis and treatment of Helicobacter pylori in the prevention of recurrent peptic ulcer bleeding? A cost-effectiveness analysis. *Value in health : the journal of the International Society for Pharmacoeconomics and Outcomes Research.* 2009;12(5):759–762.

9. Hollon J, Puppa EL, Greenwald B, Goldberg E, Guerrerio A, Fasano A. Effect of gliadin on permeability of intestinal biopsy explants from celiac disease patients and patients with non-celiac gluten sensitivity. *Nutrients.* 2015;7(3):1565–1576.

10. Karakula-Juchnowicz H, Szachta P, Opolska A, et al. The role of IgG hypersensitivity in the pathogenesis and therapy of depressive disorders. *Nutr Neurosci.* 2014.

11. Mullin GE, Swift KM, Lipski L, Turnbull LK, Rampertab SD. Testing for food reactions: the good, the bad, and the ugly. *Nutr Clin Pract.* 2010;25(2):192–198.

12. Solutions M. Sucrose Breath Test. 2014. https://www.metsol.com/assets/sites/3/Sucrose-Breath-Test.pdf

13. Vojdani A, Lambert J. The onset of enhanced intestinal permeability and food sensitivity triggered by medication used in dental procedures: a case report. *Case reports in gastrointestinal medicine.* 2012;2012:265052.

PART III: Coming Back into Balance

CHAPTER 13 Food Is Your Best Medicine

1. Buckland G, Travier N, Cottet V, et al. Adherence to the mediterranean diet and risk of breast cancer in the European prospective investigation into cancer and nutrition cohort study. *Int J Cancer.* 2013;132(12):2918–2927.

2. Caracciolo B, Xu W, Collins S, Fratiglioni L. Cognitive decline, dietary factors and gut-brain interactions. *Mech Ageing Dev.* 2014;136–137:59–69.

3. Casas R, Sacanella E, Estruch R. The immune protective effect of the Mediterranean diet against chronic low-grade inflammatory diseases. *Endocrine, metabolic & immune disorders drug targets.* 2014;14(4):245–254.

4. Dernini S, Berry EM, Serra-Majem L, et al. Med Diet 4.0: the Mediterranean diet with four sustainable benefits. *Public Health Nutr.* 2017;20(7):1322–1330.

5. Donovan MG, Selmin OI, Doetschman TC, Romagnolo DF. Mediterranean Diet: Prevention of Colorectal Cancer. *Frontiers in nutrition.* 2017;4:59.

6. Dussaillant C, Echeverria G, Urquiaga I, Velasco N, Rigotti A. [Current evidence on health benefits of the mediterranean diet]. *Revista medica de Chile.* 2016;144(8):1044–1052.

7. Farsinejad-Marj M, Talebi S, Ghiyasvand R, Miraghajani M. Adherence to Mediterranean diet and risk of breast cancer in premenopausal and postmenopausal women. *Archives of Iranian medicine.* 2015;18(11):786–792.

8. Mancini JG, Filion KB, Atallah R, Eisenberg MJ. Systematic Review of the Mediterranean Diet for Long-Term Weight Loss. *Am J Med.* 2016;129(4):407–415.e404.

9. Martinez-Gonzalez MA, Martin-Calvo N. Mediterranean diet and life expectancy; beyond olive oil, fruits, and vegetables. *Curr Opin Clin Nutr Metab Care.* 2016;19(6):401–407.

10. Martinez-Gonzalez MA, Salas-Salvado J, Estruch R, Corella D, Fito M, Ros E. Benefits of the Mediterranean Diet: Insights From the PREDIMED Study. *Prog Cardiovasc Dis.* 2015;58(1):50–60.

11. Potentas E, Witkowska AM, Zujko ME. Mediterranean diet for breast cancer prevention and treatment in postmenopausal women. *Prz Menopauzalny.* 2015;14(4):247–253.

12. Schwingshackl L, Hoffmann G. Adherence to Mediterranean diet and risk of cancer: an updated systematic review and meta-analysis of observational studies. *Cancer medicine.* 2015.

13. Singh B, Parsaik AK, Mielke MM, et al. Association of mediterranean diet with mild cognitive impairment and Alzheimer's disease: a systematic review and meta-analysis. *J Alzheimers Dis.* 2014;39(2):271–282.

14. Sivamaruthi BS, Kesika P, Prasanth MI, Chaiyasut C. A Mini Review on Antidiabetic Properties of Fermented Foods. *Nutrients.* 2018;10(12).

15. Sofi F, Casini A. Mediterranean diet and non-alcoholic fatty liver disease: new therapeutic option around the corner? *World J Gastroenterol.* 2014;20(23):7339–7346.

16. Toledo E, Salas-Salvado J, Donat-Vargas C, et al. Mediterranean Diet and Invasive Breast Cancer Risk Among Women at High Cardiovascular Risk in the PREDIMED Trial: A Randomized Clinical Trial. *JAMA Intern Med.* 2015;175(11):1752–1760.

17. Tseng M, Sellers TA, Vierkant RA, Kushi LH, Vachon CM. Mediterranean diet and breast density in the Minnesota Breast Cancer Family Study. *Nutr Cancer.* 2008;60(6):703–709.

18. Zinocker MK, Lindseth IA. The Western Diet-Microbiome-Host Interaction and Its Role in Metabolic Disease. *Nutrients.* 2018;10(3).

CHAPTER 14 Therapeutic Elimination Diets for GI Healing

1. Alexander DD, Bylsma LC, Elkayam L, Nguyen DL. Nutritional and health benefits of semi-elemental diets: A comprehensive summary of the literature. *World journal of gastrointestinal pharmacology and therapeutics.* 2016;7(2):306–319.

2. Altobelli E, Del Negro V, Angeletti PM, Latella G. Low-FODMAP Diet Improves Irritable Bowel Syndrome Symptoms: A Meta-Analysis. *Nutrients.* 2017;9(9).

3. Berni Canani R, Pezzella V, Amoroso A, Cozzolino T, Di Scala C, Passariello A. Diagnosing and Treating Intolerance to Carbohydrates in Children. *Nutrients.* 2016;8(3):157.

4. Bisht B, Darling WG, Grossmann RE, et al. A multimodal intervention for patients with secondary progressive multiple sclerosis: feasibility and effect on fatigue. *J Altern Complement Med.* 2014;20(5):347–355.

5. Bisht B, Darling WG, White EC, et al. Effects of a multimodal intervention on gait and balance of subjects with progressive multiple sclerosis: a prospective longitudinal pilot study. *Degenerative neurological and neuromuscular disease.* 2017;7:79–93.

6. Britto S, Kellermayer R. Carbohydrate Monotony as Protection and Treatment for Inflammatory Bowel Disease. *J Crohns Colitis.* 2019.

7. Catassi G, Lionetti E, Gatti S, Catassi C. The Low FODMAP Diet: Many Question Marks for a Catchy Acronym. *Nutrients.* 2017;9(3).

8. Chumpitazi BP, Cope JL, Hollister EB, et al. Randomised clinical trial: gut microbiome biomarkers are associated with clinical response to a low FODMAP diet in children with the irritable bowel syndrome. *Aliment Pharmacol Ther.* 2015;42(4):418–427.

9. Ciampa BP, Reyes Ramos E, Borum M, Doman DB. The Emerging Therapeutic Role of Medical Foods for Gastrointestinal Disorders. *Gastroenterol Hepatol (N Y)*. 2017;13(2):104–115.

10. Cozma-Petrut A, Loghin F, Miere D, Dumitrascu DL. Diet in irritable bowel syndrome: What to recommend, not what to forbid to patients! *World J Gastroenterol*. 2017;23(21):3771–3783.

11. Cozma-Petrut A, Loghin F, Miere D, Dumitrascu DL. Diet in irritable bowel syndrome: What to recommend, not what to forbid to patients! *World J Gastroenterol*. 2017;23(21):3771–3783.

12. Dugum M, Barco K, Garg S. Managing irritable bowel syndrome: The low-FODMAP diet. *Cleve Clin J Med*. 2016;83(9):655–662.

13. Durchschein F, Petritsch W, Hammer HF. Diet therapy for inflammatory bowel diseases: The established and the new. *World J Gastroenterol*. 2016;22(7):2179–2194.

14. Egger J, Carter CM, Soothill JF, Wilson J. Oligoantigenic diet treatment of children with epilepsy and migraine. *J Pediatr*. 1989;114(1):51–58.

15. Enko D, Meinitzer A, Mangge H, et al. Concomitant Prevalence of Low Serum Diamine Oxidase Activity and Carbohydrate Malabsorption. *Canadian journal of gastroenterology & hepatology*. 2016;2016:4893501.

16. Esposito T, Lobaccaro JM, Esposito MG, et al. Effects of low-carbohydrate diet therapy in overweight subjects with autoimmune thyroiditis: possible synergism with ChREBP. *Drug Des Devel Ther*. 2016;10:2939–2946.

17. Hackett C, Kolber MR. Low FODMAP diet. *Can Fam Physician*. 2015;61(8):691.

18. Harvie RM, Chisholm AW, Bisanz JE, et al. Long-term irritable bowel syndrome symptom control with reintroduction of selected FODMAPs. *World J Gastroenterol*. 2017;23(25):4632–4643.

19. Hill P, Muir JG, Gibson PR. Controversies and Recent Developments of the Low-FODMAP Diet. *Gastroenterol Hepatol (N Y)*. 2017;13(1):36–45.

20. Hou JK, Lee D, Lewis J. Diet and inflammatory bowel disease: review of patient-targeted recommendations. *Clin Gastroenterol Hepatol*. 2014;12(10):1592–1600.

21. Irish AK, Erickson CM, Wahls TL, Snetselaar LG, Darling WG. Randomized control trial evaluation of a modified Paleolithic dietary intervention in the treatment of relapsing-remitting multiple sclerosis: a pilot study. *Degenerative neurological and neuromuscular disease*. 2017;7:1–18.

22. Kakodkar S, Mutlu EA. Diet as a Therapeutic Option for Adult Inflammatory Bowel Disease. *Gastroenterology clinics of North America*. 2017;46(4):745–767.

23. Knight-Sepulveda K, Kais S, Santaolalla R, Abreu MT. Diet and Inflammatory Bowel Disease. *Gastroenterol Hepatol (N Y)*. 2015;11(8):511–520.

24. Konijeti GG, Kim N, Lewis JD, et al. Efficacy of the Autoimmune Protocol Diet for Inflammatory Bowel Disease. *Inflamm Bowel Dis.* 2017;23(11):2054–2060.

25. Krogsgaard LR, Lyngesen M, Bytzer P. Systematic review: quality of trials on the symptomatic effects of the low FODMAP diet for irritable bowel syndrome. *Aliment Pharmacol Ther.* 2017;45(12):1506–1513.

26. Lee JE, Bisht B, Hall MJ, et al. A Multimodal, Nonpharmacologic Intervention Improves Mood and Cognitive Function in People with Multiple Sclerosis. *J Am Coll Nutr.* 2017;36(3):150–168.

27. Lucendo AJ, Arias A. Treatment of adult eosinophilic esophagitis with diet. *Dig Dis.* 2014;32(1-2):120–125.

28. Ly V, Bottelier M, Hoekstra PJ, Arias Vasquez A, Buitelaar JK, Rommelse NN. Elimination diets' efficacy and mechanisms in attention deficit hyperactivity disorder and autism spectrum disorder. *European child & adolescent psychiatry.* 2017;26(9):1067–1079.

29. Manzotti G, Breda D, Di Gioacchino M, Burastero SE. Serum diamine oxidase activity in patients with histamine intolerance. *International journal of immunopathology and pharmacology.* 2016;29(1):105–111.

30. Nanayakkara WS, Skidmore PM, O'Brien L, Wilkinson TJ, Gearry RB. Efficacy of the low FODMAP diet for treating irritable bowel syndrome: the evidence to date. *Clinical and experimental gastroenterology.* 2016;9:131–142.

31. Ohkura Y, Haruta S, Tanaka T, Ueno M, Udagawa H. Effectiveness of postoperative elemental diet (Elental(R)) in elderly patients after gastrectomy. *World journal of surgical oncology.* 2016;14(1):268.

32. Okada T, Nakajima Y, Nishikage T, et al. A prospective study of nutritional supplementation for preventing oral mucositis in cancer patients receiving chemotherapy. *Asia Pac J Clin Nutr.* 2017;26(1):42–48.

33. Olendzki BC, Silverstein TD, Persuitte GM, Ma Y, Baldwin KR, Cave D. An anti-inflammatory diet as treatment for inflammatory bowel disease: a case series report. *Nutr J.* 2014;13:5.

34. Otten J, Stomby A, Waling M, et al. A heterogeneous response of liver and skeletal muscle fat to the combination of a Paleolithic diet and exercise in obese individuals with type 2 diabetes: a randomised controlled trial. *Diabetologia.* 2018;61(7):1548–1559.

35. Otten J, Stomby A, Waling M, et al. Benefits of a Paleolithic diet with and without supervised exercise on fat mass, insulin sensitivity, and glycemic control: a randomized controlled trial in individuals with type 2 diabetes. *Diabetes Metab Res Rev.* 2017;33(1).

36. Pedersen N, Ankersen DV, Felding M, et al. Low-FODMAP diet reduces irritable bowel symptoms in patients with inflammatory bowel disease. *World J Gastroenterol.* 2017;23(18):3356–3366.

37. Peters SL, Yao CK, Philpott H, Yelland GW, Muir JG, Gibson PR. Randomised clinical trial: the efficacy of gut-directed hypnotherapy is similar to that of the low FODMAP diet for the treatment of irritable bowel syndrome. *Aliment Pharmacol Ther.* 2016;44(5):447–459.

38. Philpott H, Nandurkar S, Royce SG, Thien F, Gibson PR. Allergy tests do not predict food triggers in adult patients with eosinophilic oesophagitis. A comprehensive prospective study using five modalities. *Aliment Pharmacol Ther.* 2016;44(3):223–233.

39. Quigley EMM. Editorial: food for thought-the low-FODMAP diet and IBS in perspective. *Aliment Pharmacol Ther.* 2017;46(2):206–207.

40. Rao SS, Yu S, Fedewa A. Systematic review: dietary fibre and FODMAP-restricted diet in the management of constipation and irritable bowel syndrome. *Aliment Pharmacol Ther.* 2015;41(12):1256–1270.

41. Rosell-Camps A, Zibetti S, Perez-Esteban G, Vila-Vidal M, Ferres-Ramis L, Garcia-Teresa-Garcia E. Histamine intolerance as a cause of chronic digestive complaints in pediatric patients. *Rev Esp Enferm Dig.* 2013;105(4):201–206.

42. Rostami K, Al Dulaimi D. Elemental diets role in treatment of high ileostomy output and other gastrointestinal disorders. *Gastroenterology and hepatology from bed to bench.* 2015;8(1):71–76.

43. Ruemmele FM. Role of Diet in Inflammatory Bowel Disease. *Ann Nutr Metab.* 2016;68 Suppl 1:33–41.

44. Schumann D, Langhorst J, Dobos G, Cramer H. Randomised clinical trial: yoga vs a low-FODMAP diet in patients with irritable bowel syndrome. *Aliment Pharmacol Ther.* 2018;47(2):203–211.

45. Soriano RA, Ramos-Soriano AG. Clinical and Pathologic Remission of Pediatric Ulcerative Colitis with Serum-Derived Bovine Immunoglobulin Added to the Standard Treatment Regimen. *Case reports in gastroenterology.* 2017;11(2):335–343.

46. Suskind DL, Wahbeh G, Cohen SA, et al. Patients Perceive Clinical Benefit with the Specific Carbohydrate Diet for Inflammatory Bowel Disease. *Dig Dis Sci.* 2016;61(11):3255–3260.

47. Uno Y, van Velkinburgh JC. Logical hypothesis: Low FODMAP diet to prevent diverticulitis. *World journal of gastrointestinal pharmacology and therapeutics.* 2016;7(4):503–512.

48. Uy N, Graf L, Lemley KV, Kaskel F. Effects of gluten-free, dairy-free diet on childhood nephrotic syndrome and gut microbiota. *Pediatr Res.* 2015;77(1–2):252–255.

49. Vandenplas Y, Plaskie K, Hauser B. Safety and adequacy of a semi-elemental formula for children with gastro-intestinal disease. *Amino acids.* 2010;38(3):909–914.

50. Varju P, Farkas N, Hegyi P, et al. Low fermentable oligosaccharides, disaccharides, monosaccharides and polyols (FODMAP) diet improves symptoms in adults suffering from irritable bowel syndrome (IBS) compared to standard IBS diet: A meta-analysis of clinical studies. *PLoS One.* 2017;12(8):e0182942.

51. Vincenzi M, Del Ciondolo I, Pasquini E, Gennai K, Paolini B. Effects of a Low FOD-MAP Diet and Specific Carbohydrate Diet on Symptoms and Nutritional Adequacy of Patients with Irritable Bowel Syndrome: Preliminary Results of a Single-blinded Randomized Trial. *Journal of translational internal medicine.* 2017;5(2):120–126.

52. Wahls T, Scott MO, Alshare Z, et al. Dietary approaches to treat MS-related fatigue: comparing the modified Paleolithic (Wahls Elimination) and low saturated fat (Swank) diets on perceived fatigue in persons with relapsing-remitting multiple sclerosis: study protocol for a randomized controlled trial. *Trials.* 2018;19(1):309.

53. Wahls TL. The seventy percent solution. *Journal of general internal medicine.* 2011;26(10):1215–1216.

54. Wahls TL, Chenard CA, Snetselaar LG. Review of Two Popular Eating Plans within the Multiple Sclerosis Community: Low Saturated Fat and Modified Paleolithic. *Nutrients.* 2019;11(2).

55. Whalen KA, Judd S, McCullough ML, Flanders WD, Hartman TJ, Bostick RM. Paleolithic and Mediterranean Diet Pattern Scores Are Inversely Associated with All-Cause and Cause-Specific Mortality in Adults. *J Nutr.* 2017;147(4):612–620.

56. Wilder-Smith CH, Olesen SS, Materna A, Drewes AM. Predictors of response to a low-FODMAP diet in patients with functional gastrointestinal disorders and lactose or fructose intolerance. *Aliment Pharmacol Ther.* 2017;45(8):1094–1106.

57. Zhou SY, Gillilland M, 3rd, Wu X, et al. FODMAP diet modulates visceral nociception by lipopolysaccharide-mediated intestinal inflammation and barrier dysfunction. *The Journal of clinical investigation.* 2018;128(1):267–280.

CHAPTER 16 Balancing Stress on All Levels

1. Flowers NT. EV, Anda RF, Felitti VJ. Adverse Childhood Experiences and Gastrointestinal Symptoms in Adulthood. *AGA Abstracts.* n.d. Accessed 1-5-19.

2. Langgartner D, Lowry CA, Reber SO. Old Friends, immunoregulation, and stress resilience. *Pflugers Arch.* 2018.

3. Park SH, Videlock EJ, Shih W, Presson AP, Mayer EA, Chang L. Adverse childhood experiences are associated with irritable bowel syndrome and gastrointestinal symptom severity. *Neurogastroenterol Motil.* 2016;28(8):1252–1260.

4. Oh B, Lee KJ, Zaslawski C, et al. Health and well-being benefits of spending time in forests: systematic review. *Environmental health and preventive medicine.* 2017;22(1):71.

CHAPTER 17 Cleansing and Detoxification

1. Beever R. Far-infrared saunas for treatment of cardiovascular risk factors: summary of published evidence. *Can Fam Physician.* 2009;55(7):691–696.

2. Brunt VE, Howard MJ, Francisco MA, Ely BR, Minson CT. Passive heat therapy improves endothelial function, arterial stiffness and blood pressure in sedentary humans. *The Journal of physiology*. 2016;594(18):5329–5342.

3. Cheng CW, Villani V, Buono R, et al. Fasting-Mimicking Diet Promotes Ngn3-Driven beta-Cell Regeneration to Reverse Diabetes. *Cell*. 2017;168(5):775–788.e712.

4. Choi IY, Lee C, Longo VD. Nutrition and fasting mimicking diets in the prevention and treatment of autoimmune diseases and immunosenescence. *Molecular and cellular endocrinology*. 2017;455:4–12.

5. Choi IY, Piccio L, Childress P, et al. A Diet Mimicking Fasting Promotes Regeneration and Reduces Autoimmunity and Multiple Sclerosis Symptoms. *Cell reports*. 2016;15(10):2136–2146.

6. Crinnion W. Components of practical clinical detox programs--sauna as a therapeutic tool. *Altern Ther Health Med*. 2007;13(2):S154–156.

7. Crinnion WJ. Sauna as a valuable clinical tool for cardiovascular, autoimmune, toxicant- induced and other chronic health problems. *Altern Med Rev*. 2011;16(3):215–225.

8. Genuis SJ, Birkholz D, Ralitsch M, Thibault N. Human detoxification of perfluorinated compounds. *Public Health*. 2010;124(7):367–375.

9. Hannuksela ML, Ellahham S. Benefits and risks of sauna bathing. *Am J Med*. 2001;110(2):118–126.

10. Hussain J, Cohen M. Clinical Effects of Regular Dry Sauna Bathing: A Systematic Review. *Evid Based Complement Alternat Med*. 2018;2018:1857413.

11. Hyland C, Bradman A, Gerona R, et al. Organic diet intervention significantly reduces urinary pesticide levels in U.S. children and adults. *Environ Res*. 2019;171:568–575.

12. Khamwong P, Paungmali A, Pirunsan U, Joseph L. Prophylactic Effects of Sauna on Delayed-Onset Muscle Soreness of the Wrist Extensors. *Asian journal of sports medicine*. 2015;6(2):e25549.

13. Kilburn KH, Warsaw RH, Shields MG. Neurobehavioral dysfunction in firemen exposed to polycholorinated biphenyls (PCBs): possible improvement after detoxification. *Arch Environ Health*. 1989;44(6):345–350.

14. Kukkonen-Harjula K, Kauppinen K. How the sauna affects the endocrine system. *Annals of clinical research*. 1988;20(4):262–266.

15. Laukkanen JA, Laukkanen T, Kunutsor SK. Cardiovascular and Other Health Benefits of Sauna Bathing: A Review of the Evidence. *Mayo Clin Proc*. 2018;93(8):1111–1121.

16. Laukkanen T, Kunutsor S, Kauhanen J, Laukkanen JA. Sauna bathing is inversely associated with dementia and Alzheimer's disease in middle-aged Finnish men. *Age Ageing*. 2017;46(2):245–249.

17. Longo VD, Antebi A, Bartke A, et al. Interventions to Slow Aging in Humans: Are We Ready? *Aging cell*. 2015;14(4):497–510.

18. Longo VD, Panda S. Fasting, Circadian Rhythms, and Time-Restricted Feeding in Healthy Lifespan. *Cell metabolism.* 2016;23(6):1048–1059.

19. Mattson MP, Longo VD, Harvie M. Impact of intermittent fasting on health and disease processes. *Ageing Res Rev.* 2017;39:46–58.

20. Oosterveld FG, Rasker JJ, Floors M, et al. Infrared sauna in patients with rheumatoid arthritis and ankylosing spondylitis. A pilot study showing good tolerance, short-term improvement of pain and stiffness, and a trend towards long-term beneficial effects. *Clin Rheumatol.* 2009;28(1):29–34.

21. Ross GH, Sternquist MC. Methamphetamine exposure and chronic illness in police officers: significant improvement with sauna-based detoxification therapy. *Toxicol Ind Health.* 2012;28(8):758–768.

22. Sears ME, Kerr KJ, Bray RI. Arsenic, cadmium, lead, and mercury in sweat: a systematic review. *Journal of environmental and public health.* 2012;2012:184745.

23. Vatansever F, Hamblin MR. Far infrared radiation (FIR): its biological effects and medical applications. *Photonics & lasers in medicine.* 2012;4:255–266.

24. Zaccardi F, Laukkanen T, Willeit P, Kunutsor SK, Kauhanen J, Laukkanen JA. Sauna Bathing and Incident Hypertension: A Prospective Cohort Study. *American journal of hypertension.* 2017;30(11):1120–1125.

PART IV: Natural Therapies for Common Digestive Problems

CHAPTER 18 The Mouth: Bad Breath/Halitosis, Cheilosis, Gingivitis and Periodontal Disease, Nutrients and Teeth, Mouth Ulcers/Canker Sores, Thrush, Tongue Problems, and Burning Tongue

1. Bale BF, Doneen AL, Vigerust DJ. High-risk periodontal pathogens contribute to the pathogenesis of atherosclerosis. *Postgrad Med J.* 2017;93(1098):215–220.

2. Dursun E, Akalin FA, Genc T, Cinar N, Erel O, Yildiz BO. Oxidative Stress and Periodontal Disease in Obesity. *Medicine.* 2016;95(12):e3136.

3. Grubbs V, Vittinghoff E, Beck JD, et al. Association Between Periodontal Disease and Kidney Function Decline in African Americans: The Jackson Heart Study. *J Periodontol.* 2015;86(10):1126–1132.

4. Jenzsch A, Eick S, Rassoul F, Purschwitz R, Jentsch H. Nutritional intervention in patients with periodontal disease: clinical, immunological and microbiological variables during 12 months. *Br J Nutr.* 2009;101(6):879–885.

5. Kaye EK, Chen N, Cabral HJ, Vokonas P, Garcia RI. Metabolic Syndrome and Periodontal Disease Progression in Men. *Journal of dental research.* 2016;95(7):822–828.

6. Kim YJ, Moura LM, Caldas CP, Perozini C, Ruivo GF, Pallos D. Evaluation of periodontal condition and risk in patients with chronic kidney disease on hemodialysis. *Einstein (Sao Paulo, Brazil).* 2017;15(2):173–177.

7. Martinez-Herrera M, Silvestre-Rangil J, Silvestre FJ. Association between obesity and periodontal disease. A systematic review of epidemiological studies and controlled clinical trials. *Medicina oral, patologia oral y cirugia bucal.* 2017;22(6):e708–e715.

8. Michaud DS, Kelsey KT, Papathanasiou E, Genco CA, Giovannucci E. Periodontal disease and risk of all cancers among male never smokers: an updated analysis of the Health Professionals Follow-up Study. *Annals of oncology : official journal of the European Society for Medical Oncology.* 2016;27(5):941–947.

9. Momen-Heravi F, Babic A, Tworoger SS, et al. Periodontal disease, tooth loss and colorectal cancer risk: Results from the Nurses' Health Study. *Int J Cancer.* 2017;140(3):646–652.

10. Najeeb S, Zafar MS, Khurshid Z, Zohaib S, Almas K. The Role of Nutrition in Periodontal Health: An Update. *Nutrients.* 2016;8(9).

11. Nwizu NN, Marshall JR, Moysich K, et al. Periodontal Disease and Incident Cancer Risk among Postmenopausal Women: Results from the Women's Health Initiative Observational Cohort. *Cancer Epidemiol Biomarkers Prev.* 2017;26(8):1255–1265.

12. Papageorgiou SN, Hagner M, Nogueira AV, Franke A, Jager A, Deschner J. Inflammatory bowel disease and oral health: systematic review and a meta-analysis. *Journal of clinical periodontology.* 2017;44(4):382–393.

13. Teshome A, Yitayeh A. Relationship between periodontal disease and preterm low birth weight: systematic review. *The Pan African medical journal.* 2016;24:215.

14. Xu S, Song M, Xiong Y, Liu X, He Y, Qin Z. The association between periodontal disease and the risk of myocardial infarction: a pooled analysis of observational studies. *BMC cardiovascular disorders.* 2017;17(1):50.

15. Yu YH, Chasman DI, Buring JE, Rose L, Ridker PM. Cardiovascular risks associated with incident and prevalent periodontal disease. *Journal of clinical periodontology.* 2015;42(1):21–28.

16. Zhang J, Jiang H, Sun M, Chen J. Association between periodontal disease and mortality in people with CKD: a meta-analysis of cohort studies. *BMC nephrology.* 2017;18(1):269.

CHAPTER 19   The Esophagus and Stomach: Belching, Barrett's Esophagus, Eosinophilic Esophagitis, Dyspepsia, Gastritis, and Gastroparesis

1. Akhondi-Meybodi M, Aghaei, M. A., & Hashemian, Z. The role of diet in the management of non-ulcer dyspepsia. *Middle East journal of digestive diseases.* 2015;7(1):19–24.

2. Carlson DA, Hirano I, Zalewski A, Gonsalves N, Lin Z, Pandolfino JE. Improvement in Esophageal Distensibility in Response to Medical and Diet Therapy in Eosinophilic Esophagitis. *Clinical and translational gastroenterology.* 2017;8(10):e119.

3. Cotton CC, Erim D, Eluri S, et al. Cost Utility Analysis of Topical Steroids Compared With Dietary Elimination for Treatment of Eosinophilic Esophagitis. *Clin Gastroenterol Hepatol.* 2017;15(6):841–849.e841.

4. Erwin EA, Kruszewski PG, Russo JM, Schuyler AJ, Platts-Mills TA. IgE antibodies and response to cow's milk elimination diet in pediatric eosinophilic esophagitis. *J Allergy Clin Immunol.* 2016;138(2):625–628.e622.

5. Gonsalves N, Hirano I. Editorial: long-term effectiveness of elimination diet therapy for eosinophilic oesophagitis-is the glass half full or half empty? *Aliment Pharmacol Ther.* 2018;47(1):135–136.

6. Groetch M, Venter C, Skypala I, et al. Dietary Therapy and Nutrition Management of Eosinophilic Esophagitis: A Work Group Report of the American Academy of Allergy, Asthma, and Immunology. *The journal of allergy and clinical immunology In practice.* 2017;5(2):312–324.e329.

7. Information DoD. How to Request Domperidone for Expanded Access Use. 2018. https://www.fda.gov/drugs/developmentapprovalprocess/howdrugsaredevelopedandapproved/approvalapplications/investigationalnewdrugindapplication/ucm368736.htm.

8. Kliewer KL, Venter C, Cassin AM, et al. Should wheat, barley, rye, and/or gluten be avoided in a 6-food elimination diet? *J Allergy Clin Immunol.* 2016;137(4):1011–1014.

9. Levine ME, Koch SY, & Koch KL. Lipase Supplementation before a High-Fat Meal Reduces Perceptions of Fullness in Healthy Subjects. *Gut and liver.* 2014;9(4):464–469.

10. Lucendo AJ. Eosinophilic esophagitis: current evidence-based diagnosis and treatment in children and adults. *Minerva gastroenterologica e dietologica.* 2018;64(1):62–74.

11. Lucendo AJ, Arias A, Gonzalez-Cervera J, et al. Empiric 6-food elimination diet induced and maintained prolonged remission in patients with adult eosinophilic esophagitis: a prospective study on the food cause of the disease. *J Allergy Clin Immunol.* 2013;131(3):797–804.

12. Madisch A, Andresen V, Enck P, Labenz J, Frieling T, & Schemann, M. The Diagnosis and Treatment of Functional Dyspepsia. *Deutsches Arzteblatt international.* 2018; 115(13):222–232.

13. Majeed M MS, Nagabhushanam K, Arumugam S, Pande A, Paschapur M, Ali F. Evaluation of the Safety and Efficacy of a Multienzyme Complex in Patients with Functional Dyspepsia: A Randomized, Double-Blind, Placebo-Controlled Study. *J Med Food.* 2018;21(11):1120–1128.

14. McGowan EC, Platts-Mills TA. Eosinophilic Esophagitis From an Allergy Perspective: How to Optimally Pursue Allergy Testing & Dietary Modification in the Adult Population. *Curr Gastroenterol Rep.* 2016;18(11):58.

15. Philpott H, Nandurkar S, Royce SG, Thien F, Gibson PR. Allergy tests do not predict food triggers in adult patients with eosinophilic oesophagitis. A comprehensive prospective study using five modalities. *Aliment Pharmacol Ther.* 2016;44(3):223–233.

16. Philpott H, Nandurkar S, Royce SG, Thien F, Gibson PR. A prospective open clinical trial of a proton pump inhibitor, elimination diet and/or budesonide for eosinophilic oesophagitis. *Aliment Pharmacol Ther.* 2016;43(9):985–993.

17. Runge TM, Abrams JA, Shaheen NJ. Epidemiology of Barrett's Esophagus and Esophageal Adenocarcinoma. *Gastroenterology clinics of North America.* 2015;44(2):203–231.

18. Snider EJ, Freedberg DE, Abrams JA. Potential Role of the Microbiome in Barrett's Esophagus and Esophageal Adenocarcinoma. *Dig Dis Sci.* 2016;61(8):2217–2225.

19. Tan VP. The low-FODMAP diet in the management of functional dyspepsia in East and Southeast Asia. Journal of Gastroenterology and Hepatology. *Journal of Gastroenterology and Hepatology.* 2017;32:46–52.

20. Tatsuta M, Iishi H. Effect of treatment with liu-jun-zi-tang (TJ-43) on gastric emptying and gastrointestinal symptoms in dyspeptic patients. *Aliment Pharmacol Ther.* 1993;7(4):459–462.

21. Wytiaz V, Homko C, Duffy F, Schey R, Parkman HP. Foods provoking and alleviating symptoms in gastroparesis: patient experiences. *Dig Dis Sci.* 2015;60(4):1052–1058.

22. Zito FP, Polese B, Vozzella L, Gala A, Genovese D, Verlezza V, Medugno F, Santini A, Barrea L, Cargiolli M, Andreozzi P, Sarnelli G, … Cuomo R. Good adherence to Mediterranean diet can prevent gastrointestinal symptoms: A survey from Southern Italy. *World journal of gastrointestinal pharmacology and therapeutics.* 2016;7(4):564–571.

CHAPTER 20   The Liver: Fatty Liver Disease, Hepatitis, and Cirrhosis

1. Federico A, Dallio M, Loguercio C. Silymarin/Silybin and Chronic Liver Disease: A Marriage of Many Years. *Molecules (Basel, Switzerland).* 2017;22(2).

2. Horvath A, Leber B, Schmerboeck B, et al. Randomised clinical trial: the effects of a multispecies probiotic vs. placebo on innate immune function, bacterial translocation and gut permeability in patients with cirrhosis. *Aliment Pharmacol Ther.* 2016;44(9):926–935.

3. Nakanishi H, Kurosaki M, Tsuchiya K, et al. L-carnitine Reduces Muscle Cramps in Patients With Cirrhosis. *Clin Gastroenterol Hepatol.* 2015;13(8):1540–1543.

4. Nishikawa H, Osaki Y. Liver Cirrhosis: Evaluation, Nutritional Status, and Prognosis. *Mediators of inflammation.* 2015;2015:872152.

5. Shiraki M, Shimizu M, Moriwaki H, Okita K, Koike K. Carnitine dynamics and their effects on hyperammonemia in cirrhotic Japanese patients. *Hepatology research : the official journal of the Japan Society of Hepatology.* 2017;47(4):321–327.

6. Usami M, Miyoshi M, Yamashita H. Gut microbiota and host metabolism in liver cirrhosis. *World J Gastroenterol.* 2015;21(41):11597–11608.

7. Vajravelu ME, Keren R, Weber DR, Verma R, De Leon DD, Denburg MR. Incidence and risk of celiac disease after type 1 diabetes: A population-based cohort study using the health improvement network database. *Pediatr Diabetes.* 2018;19(8):1422–1428.

8. Yang Z, Zhuang L, Lu Y, Xu Q, Chen X. Effects and tolerance of silymarin (milk thistle) in chronic hepatitis C virus infection patients: a meta-analysis of randomized controlled trials. *BioMed research international.* 2014;2014:941085.

CHAPTER 21 The Pancreas: Pancreatic Insufficiency, Pancreatitis, and Diabetes

1. Betrapally NS, Gillevet PM, Bajaj JS. Changes in the Intestinal Microbiome and Alcoholic and Nonalcoholic Liver Diseases: Causes or Effects? *Gastroenterology.* 2016;150(8):1745–1755.e1743.

2. Craig ME, Prinz N, Boyle CT, et al. Prevalence of Celiac Disease in 52,721 Youth With Type 1 Diabetes: International Comparison Across Three Continents. *Diabetes Care.* 2017;40(8):1034–1040.

3. Davis-Richardson AG, Triplett EW. A model for the role of gut bacteria in the development of autoimmunity for type 1 diabetes. *Diabetologia.* 2015;58(7):1386–1393.

4. El-Salhy M, Mazzawi T, Hausken T, Hatlebakk JG. Interaction between diet and gastrointestinal endocrine cells. *Biomedical reports.* 2016;4(6):651–656.

5. Everard A, Cani PD. Diabetes, obesity and gut microbiota. *Best Pract Res Clin Gastroenterol.* 2013;27(1):73–83.

6. Griffin JL, Wang X, Stanley E. Does our gut microbiome predict cardiovascular risk? A review of the evidence from metabolomics. *Circ Cardiovasc Genet.* 2015;8(1):187–191.

7. Gulden E, Wong FS, Wen L. The gut microbiota and Type 1 Diabetes. *Clin Immunol.* 2015;159(2):143–153.

8. Hagopian W, Lee HS, Liu E, et al. Co-occurrence of Type 1 Diabetes and Celiac Disease Autoimmunity. *Pediatrics.* 2017;140(5).

9. John GK, Mullin GE. The Gut Microbiome and Obesity. *Current oncology reports.* 2016;18(7):45.

10. Kallio KA, Hatonen KA, Lehto M, Salomaa V, Mannisto S, Pussinen PJ. Endotoxemia, nutrition, and cardiometabolic disorders. *Acta diabetologica.* 2015;52(2):395–404.

11. Kaur N, Bhadada SK, Minz RW, Dayal D, Kochhar R. Interplay between Type 1 Diabetes Mellitus and Celiac Disease: Implications in Treatment. *Dig Dis.* 2018;36(6):399–408.

12. McGill AT. Causes of metabolic syndrome and obesity-related co-morbidities Part 1: A composite unifying theory review of human-specific co-adaptations to brain energy consumption. *Archives of public health = Archives belges de sante publique.* 2014;72(1):30.

13. Qian LL, Li HT, Zhang L, Fang QC, Jia WP. Effect of the Gut Microbiota on Obesity and Its Underlying Mechanisms: an Update. *Biomed Environ Sci.* 2015;28(11):839–847.

14. Sabico S, Al-Mashharawi A, Al-Daghri NM, et al. Effects of a multi-strain probiotic supplement for 12 weeks in circulating endotoxin levels and cardiometabolic profiles of medication naive T2DM patients: a randomized clinical trial. *J Transl Med.* 2017;15(1):249.

15. Upadhyaya S, Banerjee G. Type 2 diabetes and gut microbiome: at the intersection of known and unknown. *Gut Microbes.* 2015;6(2):85–92.

16. Wickens KL, Barthow CA, Murphy R, et al. Early pregnancy probiotic supplementation with Lactobacillus rhamnosus HN001 may reduce the prevalence of gestational diabetes mellitus: a randomised controlled trial. *Br J Nutr.* 2017;117(6):804–813.

17. Woting A, Blaut M. The Intestinal Microbiota in Metabolic Disease. *Nutrients.* 2016;8(4).

CHAPTER 22 The Gallbladder: Gallstones and Cholecystectomy

1. Bakke AM, Chikwati EM, Venold FF, et al. Bile enhances glucose uptake, reduces permeability, and modulates effects of lectins, trypsin inhibitors and saponins on intestinal tissue. *Comparative biochemistry and physiology Part A, Molecular & integrative physiology.* 2014;168:96–109.

2. Breneman JC. Allergy elimination diet as the most effective gallbladder diet. *Ann Allergy.* 1968;26(2):83–87.

3. Jones BV, Begley M, Hill C, Gahan CG, Marchesi JR. Functional and comparative metagenomic analysis of bile salt hydrolase activity in the human gut microbiome. *Proc Natl Acad Sci U S A.* 2008;105(36):13580–13585.

4. Kamiya S, Nagino M, Kanazawa H, et al. The value of bile replacement during external biliary drainage: an analysis of intestinal permeability, integrity, and microflora. *Ann Surg.* 2004;239(4):510–517.

5. Laukkarinen J, Sand J, Nordback I. The underlying mechanisms: how hypothyroidism affects the formation of common bile duct stones-a review. *HPB surgery : a world journal of hepatic, pancreatic and biliary surgery.* 2012;2012:102825.

6. Pavlidis P, Powell N, Vincent RP, Ehrlich D, Bjarnason I, Hayee B. Systematic review: bile acids and intestinal inflammation-luminal aggressors or regulators of mucosal defence? *Aliment Pharmacol Ther.* 2015;42(7):802–817.

7. Ridlon JM, Bajaj JS. The human gut sterolbiome: bile acid-microbiome endocrine aspects and therapeutics. *Acta pharmaceutica Sinica B.* 2015;5(2):99–105.

8. Ridlon JM, Kang DJ, Hylemon PB, Bajaj JS. Bile acids and the gut microbiome. *Curr Opin Gastroenterol.* 2014;30(3):332–338.

9. Werner A, Minich DM, Havinga R, et al. Fat malabsorption in essential fatty acid-deficient mice is not due to impaired bile formation. *Am J Physiol Gastrointest Liver Physiol.* 2002;283(4):G900–908.

CHAPTER 23 The Small Intestine: Flatulence/Gas, Celiac Disease, and Nonceliac Gluten Sensitivity

1. Alaedini A, Lebwohl B, Wormser GP, Green PH, Ludvigsson JFJBM. Borrelia infection and risk of celiac disease. 2017;15(1):169.
2. Camilleri M. Management Options for Irritable Bowel Syndrome. *Mayo Clin Proc.* 2018;93(12):1858–1872.
3. Catassi C. Gluten Sensitivity. *Ann Nutr Metab.* 2015;67 Suppl 2:16–26.
4. Catassi C, Alaedini A, Bojarski C, et al. The Overlapping Area of Non-Celiac Gluten Sensitivity (NCGS) and Wheat-Sensitive Irritable Bowel Syndrome (IBS): An Update. *Nutrients.* 2017;9(11).
5. Chmielewska A, Piescik-Lech M, Szajewska H, Shamir R. Primary Prevention of Celiac Disease: Environmental Factors with a Focus on Early Nutrition. *Ann Nutr Metab.* 2015;67 Suppl 2:43–50.
6. Czaja-Bulsa G. Non coeliac gluten sensitivity - A new disease with gluten intolerance. *Clin Nutr.* 2015;34(2):189–194.
7. Elli L, Branchi F, Tomba C, et al. Diagnosis of gluten related disorders: Celiac disease, wheat allergy and non-celiac gluten sensitivity. *World J Gastroenterol.* 2015;21(23):7110–7119.
8. Elli L, Roncoroni L, Bardella MT. Non-celiac gluten sensitivity: Time for sifting the grain. *World J Gastroenterol.* 2015;21(27):8221–8226.
9. Hogg-Kollars S, Al Dulaimi D, Tait K, Rostami K. Type 1 diabetes mellitus and gluten induced disorders. *Gastroenterology and hepatology from bed to bench.* 2014;7(4):189–197.
10. Igbinedion SO, Ansari J, Vasikaran A, et al. Non-celiac gluten sensitivity: All wheat attack is not celiac. *World J Gastroenterol.* 2017;23(40):7201–7210.
11. Isasi C, Tejerina E, Moran LM. Non-celiac gluten sensitivity and rheumatic diseases. *Reumatologia clinica.* 2016;12(1):4–10.
12. Jimenez Ortega AI, Martinez Garcia RM, Quiles Blanco MJ, Majid Abu Naji JA, Gonzalez Iglesias MJ. Celiac disease and new diseases related to gluten. *Nutr Hosp.* 2016;33(Suppl 4):345.
13. Joseph J, Depp C, Shih PB, Cadenhead KS, Schmid-Schonbein G. Modified Mediterranean Diet for Enrichment of Short Chain Fatty Acids: Potential Adjunctive Therapeutic to Target Immune and Metabolic Dysfunction in Schizophrenia? *Front Neurosci.* 2017;11:155.

14. Lernmark A. Environmental factors in the etiology of type 1 diabetes, celiac disease, and narcolepsy. *Pediatr Diabetes*. 2016;17 Suppl 22:65–72.

15. Mahmud FH, De Melo EN, Noordin K, et al. The Celiac Disease and Diabetes-Dietary Intervention and Evaluation Trial (CD-DIET) protocol: a randomised controlled study to evaluate treatment of asymptomatic coeliac disease in type 1 diabetes. *BMJ open*. 2015;5(5):e008097.

16. Makharia A, Catassi C, Makharia GK. The Overlap between Irritable Bowel Syndrome and Non-Celiac Gluten Sensitivity: A Clinical Dilemma. *Nutrients*. 2015;7(12):10417–10426.

17. Mesnage R, Antoniou MN. Facts and Fallacies in the Debate on Glyphosate Toxicity. *Frontiers in public health*. 2017;5:316.

18. Ortiz C, Valenzuela R, Lucero AY. [Celiac disease, non celiac gluten sensitivity and wheat allergy: comparison of 3 different diseases triggered by the same food]. *Revista chilena de pediatria*. 2017;88(3):417–423.

19. Parra-Medina R, Molano-Gonzalez N, Rojas-Villarraga A, et al. Prevalence of celiac disease in latin america: a systematic review and meta-regression. *PLoS One*. 2015;10(5):e0124040.

20. Pham-Short A, Donaghue KC, Ambler G, Phelan H, Twigg S, Craig ME. Screening for Celiac Disease in Type 1 Diabetes: A Systematic Review. *Pediatrics*. 2015;136(1):e170–176.

21. Pruimboom L, de Punder K. The opioid effects of gluten exorphins: asymptomatic celiac disease. *Journal of health, population, and nutrition*. 2015;33:24.

22. Pynnonen PA, Isometsa ET, Aronen ET, Verkasalo MA, Savilahti E, Aalberg VA. Mental disorders in adolescents with celiac disease. *Psychosomatics*. 2004;45(4):325–335.

23. Riddle MS, Murray JA, Cash BD, Pimentel M, Porter CK. Pathogen-specific risk of celiac disease following bacterial causes of foodborne illness: a retrospective cohort study. *Dig Dis Sci*. 2013;58(11):3242–3245.

24. Samsel A, Seneff S. Glyphosate, pathways to modern diseases II: Celiac sprue and gluten intolerance. *Interdisciplinary toxicology*. 2013;6(4):159–184.

25. Samsel A, Seneff S. Glyphosate, pathways to modern diseases III: Manganese, neurological diseases, and associated pathologies. *Surg Neurol Int*. 2015;6:45.

26. Schnedl WJ, Lackner S, Enko D, Schenk M, Mangge H, Holasek SJ. Non-celiac gluten sensitivity: people without celiac disease avoiding gluten-is it due to histamine intolerance? *Inflamm Res*. 2018;67(4):279–284.

27. Sharma A, Liu X, Hadley D, et al. Identification of Non-HLA Genes Associated with Celiac Disease and Country-Specific Differences in a Large, International Pediatric Cohort. *PLoS One*. 2016;11(3):e0152476.

28. Silano M, Agostoni C, Sanz Y, Guandalini S. Infant feeding and risk of developing celiac disease: a systematic review. *BMJ open*. 2016;6(1):e009163.

29. Skodje GI, Sarna VK, Minelle IH, et al. Fructan, Rather Than Gluten, Induces Symptoms in Patients With Self-Reported Non-Celiac Gluten Sensitivity. *Gastroenterology.* 2018;154(3):529–539.e522.

30. Szajewska H, Shamir R, Chmielewska A, et al. Systematic review with meta-analysis: early infant feeding and coeliac disease—update 2015. *Aliment Pharmacol Ther.* 2015; 41(11):1038–1054.

31. Troncone R, Jabri B. Coeliac disease and gluten sensitivity. *J Intern Med.* 2011;269(6):582–590.

32. Vasagar B, Cox J, Herion JT, Ivanoff E. World epidemiology of non-celiac gluten sensitivity. *Minerva gastroenterologica e dietologica.* 2017;63(1):5–15.

33. Volta U, Bardella MT, Calabro A, Troncone R, Corazza GR. An Italian prospective multicenter survey on patients suspected of having non-celiac gluten sensitivity. *BMC medicine.* 2014;12:85.

CHAPTER 24 The Colon or Large Intestine: Constipation, Diarrhea, Diverticular Disease, Irritable Bowel Syndrome, Inflammatory Bowel Disease, and Hemorrhoids

1. Alexander DD, Bylsma LC, Elkayam L, Nguyen DL. Nutritional and health benefits of semi-elemental diets: A comprehensive summary of the literature. *World journal of gastrointestinal pharmacology and therapeutics.* 2016;7(2):306–319.

2. Balemans D, Mondelaers SU, Cibert-Goton V, et al. Evidence for long-term sensitization of the bowel in patients with post-infectious-IBS. *Sci Rep.* 2017;7(1):13606.

3. Basson A, Trotter A, Rodriguez-Palacios A, Cominelli F. Mucosal Interactions between Genetics, Diet, and Microbiome in Inflammatory Bowel Disease. *Frontiers in immunology.* 2016;7(290).

4. Burgis JC, Nguyen K, Park KT, Cox K. Response to strict and liberalized specific carbohydrate diet in pediatric Crohn's disease. *World J Gastroenterol.* 2016;22(6):2111–2117.

5. Card T, Enck P, Barbara G, et al. Post-infectious IBS: Defining its clinical features and prognosis using an internet-based survey. *United European Gastroenterol J.* 2018;6(8):1245–1253.

6. Chang J, Leong RW, Wasinger VC, Ip M, Yang M, Phan TG. Impaired Intestinal Permeability Contributes to Ongoing Bowel Symptoms in Patients With Inflammatory Bowel Disease and Mucosal Healing. *Gastroenterology.* 2017;153(3):723–731.e721.

7. Chen SJ, Liu XW, Liu JP, Yang XY, Lu FG. Ulcerative colitis as a polymicrobial infection characterized by sustained broken mucus barrier. *World J Gastroenterol.* 2014;20(28):9468–9475.

8. Ciampa BP, Reyes Ramos E, Borum M, Doman DB. The Emerging Therapeutic Role of Medical Foods for Gastrointestinal Disorders. *Gastroenterol Hepatol (N Y).* 2017;13(2):104–115.

9. Cuomo R, Cargiolli M, Cassarano S, Carabotti M, Annibale B. Treatment of diverticular disease, targeting symptoms or underlying mechanisms. *Curr Opin Pharmacol.* 2018;43:124–131.

10. Dahl C, Crichton M, Jenkins J, et al. Evidence for Dietary Fibre Modification in the Recovery and Prevention of Reoccurrence of Acute, Uncomplicated Diverticulitis: A Systematic Literature Review. *Nutrients.* 2018;10(2).

11. DiNicolantonio JJ, Lucan SC. Is fructose malabsorption a cause of irritable bowel syndrome? *Med Hypotheses.* 2015;85(3):295–297.

12. Durchschein F, Petritsch W, Hammer HF. Diet therapy for inflammatory bowel diseases: The established and the new. *World J Gastroenterol.* 2016;22(7):2179–2194.

13. Gibson PR. Use of the low-FODMAP diet in inflammatory bowel disease. *J Gastroenterol Hepatol.* 2017;32 Suppl 1:40–42.

14. Hou JK, Lee D, Lewis J. Diet and inflammatory bowel disease: review of patient-targeted recommendations. *Clin Gastroenterol Hepatol.* 2014;12(10):1592–1600.

15. Jones BJ, Lees R, Andrews J, Frost P, Silk DB. Comparison of an elemental and polymeric enteral diet in patients with normal gastrointestinal function. *Gut.* 1983;24(1):78–84.

16. Jung KW, Seo M, Cho YH, et al. Prevalence of Fructose Malabsorption in Patients With Irritable Bowel Syndrome After Excluding Small Intestinal Bacterial Overgrowth. *Journal of neurogastroenterology and motility.* 2018;24(2):307–316.

17. Kakodkar S, Farooqui AJ, Mikolaitis SL, Mutlu EA. The Specific Carbohydrate Diet for Inflammatory Bowel Disease: A Case Series. *J Acad Nutr Diet.* 2015;115(8):1226–1232.

18. Kakodkar S, Mutlu EA. Diet as a Therapeutic Option for Adult Inflammatory Bowel Disease. *Gastroenterology clinics of North America.* 2017;46(4):745–767.

19. Khandalavala BN, Nirmalraj MC. Resolution of Severe Ulcerative Colitis with the Specific Carbohydrate Diet. *Case reports in gastroenterology.* 2015;9(2):291–295.

20. Klem F, Wadhwa A, Prokop LJ, et al. Prevalence, Risk Factors, and Outcomes of Irritable Bowel Syndrome After Infectious Enteritis: A Systematic Review and Meta-analysis. *Gastroenterology.* 2017;152(5):1042–1054.e1041.

21. Krokowicz L, Stojcev Z, Kaczmarek BF, et al. Microencapsulated sodium butyrate administered to patients with diverticulosis decreases incidence of diverticulitis—a prospective randomized study. *Int J Colorectal Dis.* 2014;29(3):387–393.

22. Legaki E, Gazouli M. Influence of environmental factors in the development of inflammatory bowel diseases. *World journal of gastrointestinal pharmacology and therapeutics.* 2016;7(1):112–125.

23. Lira-Junior R, Figueredo CM. Periodontal and inflammatory bowel diseases: Is there evidence of complex pathogenic interactions? *World J Gastroenterol.* 2016;22(35):7963–7972.

24. Maguire LH, Song M, Strate LE, Giovannucci EL, Chan AT. Higher serum levels of vitamin D are associated with a reduced risk of diverticulitis. *Clin Gastroenterol Hepatol.* 2013;11(12):1631–1635.

25. Malhotra R, Turner K, Sonnenberg A, Genta RM. High prevalence of inflammatory bowel disease in United States residents of Indian ancestry. *Clin Gastroenterol Hepatol.* 2015;13(4):683–689.

26. McIlroy J, Ianiro G, Mukhopadhya I, Hansen R, Hold GL. Review article: the gut microbiome in inflammatory bowel disease-avenues for microbial management. *Aliment Pharmacol Ther.* 2018;47(1):26–42.

27. Melchior C, Gourcerol G, Dechelotte P, Leroi AM, Ducrotte P. Symptomatic fructose malabsorption in irritable bowel syndrome: A prospective study. *United European Gastroenterol J.* 2014;2(2):131–137.

28. Michielan A, D'Inca R. Intestinal Permeability in Inflammatory Bowel Disease: Pathogenesis, Clinical Evaluation, and Therapy of Leaky Gut. *Mediators of inflammation.* 2015;2015:628157.

29. Muhvic-Urek M, Tomac-Stojmenovic M, Mijandrusic-Sincic B. Oral pathology in inflammatory bowel disease. *World J Gastroenterol.* 2016;22(25):5655–5667.

30. Nishida A, Inoue R, Inatomi O, Bamba S, Naito Y, Andoh A. Gut microbiota in the pathogenesis of inflammatory bowel disease. *Clinical journal of gastroenterology.* 2018;11(1):1–10.

31. Obih C, Wahbeh G, Lee D, et al. Specific carbohydrate diet for pediatric inflammatory bowel disease in clinical practice within an academic IBD center. *Nutrition.* 2016;32(4):418–425.

32. Owczarek D, Rodacki T, Domagala-Rodacka R, Cibor D, Mach T. Diet and nutritional factors in inflammatory bowel diseases. *World J Gastroenterol.* 2016;22(3): 895–905.

33. Papageorgiou SN, Hagner M, Nogueira AV, Franke A, Jager A, Deschner J. Inflammatory bowel disease and oral health: systematic review and a meta-analysis. *Journal of clinical periodontology.* 2017;44(4):382–393.

34. Penagini F, Dilillo D, Borsani B, et al. Nutrition in Pediatric Inflammatory Bowel Disease: From Etiology to Treatment. A Systematic Review. *Nutrients.* 2016;8(6).

35. Rapozo DC, Bernardazzi C, de Souza HS. Diet and microbiota in inflammatory bowel disease: The gut in disharmony. *World J Gastroenterol.* 2017;23(12):2124–2140.

36. Rashvand S, Somi MH, Rashidkhani B, Hekmatdoost A. Dietary protein intakes and risk of ulcerative colitis. *Medical journal of the Islamic Republic of Iran.* 2015;29:253.

37. Rezapour M, Ali S, Stollman N. Diverticular Disease: An Update on Pathogenesis and Management. *Gut and liver.* 2018;12(2):125–132.

38. Rostami K, Al Dulaimi D. Elemental diets role in treatment of high ileostomy output and other gastrointestinal disorders. *Gastroenterology and hepatology from bed to bench.* 2015;8(1):71–76.

39. Severi C, Carabotti M, Cicenia A, Pallotta L, Annibale B. Recent advances in understanding and managing diverticulitis. *F1000Research.* 2018;7.

40. Siah KT, Wong RK, Ho KY. Melatonin for the treatment of irritable bowel syndrome. *World J Gastroenterol.* 2014;20(10):2492–2498.

41. Suskind DL, Wahbeh G, Gregory N, Vendettuoli H, Christie D. Nutritional therapy in pediatric Crohn disease: the specific carbohydrate diet. *J Pediatr Gastroenterol Nutr.* 2014;58(1):87–91.

42. Tanaka M, Kawakami A, Iwao Y, Fukushima T, Yamamoto-Mitani N. Coping Strategies for Possible Flare-Ups and Their Perceived Effectiveness in Patients With Inflammatory Bowel Disease. *Gastroenterol Nurs.* 2016;39(1):42–47.

43. Theochari NA, Stefanopoulos A, Mylonas KS, Economopoulos KP. Antibiotics exposure and risk of inflammatory bowel disease: a systematic review. *Scand J Gastroenterol.* 2018;53(1):1–7.

44. Yang CM, Li YQ. [The therapeutic effects of eliminating allergic foods according to food-specific IgG antibodies in irritable bowel syndrome]. *Zhonghua Nei Ke Za Zhi.* 2007;46(8):641–643.

PART V: Natural Therapies for the Diverse Consequences of Faulty Digestion

CHAPTER 25   Arthritis and Other Connective Tissue Disorders: Osteoarthritis, Rheumatoid Arthritis, Psoriatic Arthritis, Ankylosing Spondylitis, Scleroderma, and Sjögren's Syndrome

1. Andreasson K, Alrawi Z, Persson A, Jonsson G, Marsal J. Intestinal dysbiosis is common in systemic sclerosis and associated with gastrointestinal and extraintestinal features of disease. *Arthritis research & therapy.* 2016;18(1):278.

2. Asquith M, Elewaut D, Lin P, Rosenbaum JT. The role of the gut and microbes in the pathogenesis of spondyloarthritis. *Best practice & research Clinical rheumatology.* 2014;28(5):687–702.

3. Conti V, Leone MC, Casato M, Nicoli M, Granata G, Carlesimo M. High prevalence of gluten sensitivity in a cohort of patients with undifferentiated connective tissue disease. *Eur Ann Allergy Clin Immunol.* 2015;47(2):54–57.

4. Costello ME, Elewaut D, Kenna TJ, Brown MA. Microbes, the gut and ankylosing spondylitis. *Arthritis research & therapy.* 2013;15(3):214.

5. Dahan S, Segal Y, Shoenfeld Y. Dietary factors in rheumatic autoimmune diseases: a recipe for therapy? *Nature Reviews Rheumatology.* 2017;13:348.

6. Denton C. The elimination/challenge diet. *Minnesota medicine.* 2012;95(12):43–44.

7. Ebringer A, Wilson C. HLA molecules, bacteria and autoimmunity. *J Med Microbiol.* 2000;49(4):305–311.

8. El-Sohemy A. Nutrigenetics. *Forum Nutr.* 2007;60:25–30.

9. Feuerstein J. Reversal of premature ovarian failure in a patient with Sjogren syndrome using an elimination diet protocol. *J Altern Complement Med.* 2010;16(7):807–809.

10. Gamlin L, Brostoff J. Food sensitivity and rheumatoid arthritis. *Environmental toxicology and pharmacology.* 1997;4(1–2):43–49.

11. Glenska-Olender J, Durlik K, Konieczna I, Kowalska P, Gaweda J, Kaca W. Detection of human antibodies binding with smooth and rough LPSs from Proteus mirabilis O3 strains S1959, R110, R45. *Antonie Van Leeuwenhoek.* 2017;110(11):1435–1443.

12. Jonas WB, Rapoza CP, Blair WF. The effect of niacinamide on osteoarthritis: a pilot study. *Inflamm Res.* 1996;45(7):330–334.

13. Karatay S, Erdem T, Yildirim K, et al. The effect of individualized diet challenges consisting of allergenic foods on TNF-alpha and IL-1beta levels in patients with rheumatoid arthritis. *Rheumatology (Oxford).* 2004;43(11):1429–1433.

14. Kim-Lee C, Suresh L, Ambrus JL, Jr. Gastrointestinal disease in Sjogren's syndrome: related to food hypersensitivities. *Springerplus.* 2015;4:766.

15. Martin RH. The role of nutrition and diet in rheumatoid arthritis. *Proc Nutr Soc.* 1998;57(2):231–234.

16. Mehta H, Goulet PO, Mashiko S, et al. Early-Life Antibiotic Exposure Causes Intestinal Dysbiosis and Exacerbates Skin and Lung Pathology in Experimental Systemic Sclerosis. *J Invest Dermatol.* 2017;137(11):2316–2325.

17. Miggiano GA, Gagliardi L. [Diet, nutrition and rheumatoid arthritis]. *La Clinica terapeutica.* 2005;156(3):115–123.

18. Prousky JE. The use of Niacinamide and Solanaceae (Nightshade) Elimination in the Treatment of Osteoarthritis. *J of Orthomolecular Medicine.* 2015;30(1):13–21.

19. Rashid T, Ebringer A, Wilson C. The link between Proteus mirabilis, environmental factors and autoantibodies in rheumatoid arthritis. *Clin Exp Rheumatol.* 2017;35(5):865–871.

20. Rashid T, Wilson C, Ebringer A. The link between ankylosing spondylitis, Crohn's disease, Klebsiella, and starch consumption. *Clinical & developmental immunology.* 2013;2013:872632.

21. Rashid T, Wilson C, Ebringer A. Raised incidence of ankylosing spondylitis among Inuit populations could be due to high HLA-B27 association and starch consumption. *Rheumatology international.* 2015;35(6):945–951.

22. Schrander JJ, Marcelis C, de Vries MP, van Santen-Hoeufft HM. Does food intolerance play a role in juvenile chronic arthritis? *Br J Rheumatol.* 1997;36(8):905–908.

23. Vojdani A. A Potential Link between Environmental Triggers and Autoimmunity. *Autoimmune Dis.* 2014;2014:437231.

24. Volkmann ER, Chang YL, Barroso N, et al. Association of Systemic Sclerosis With a Unique Colonic Microbial Consortium. *Arthritis & rheumatology (Hoboken, NJ).* 2016;68(6):1483–1492.

CHAPTER 26 Autoimmune Diseases Overview

1. Abe K, Takahashi A, Fujita M, et al. Dysbiosis of oral microbiota and its association with salivary immunological biomarkers in autoimmune liver disease. *PLoS One.* 2018;13(7):e0198757.

2. Choi IY, Piccio L, Childress P, et al. A Diet Mimicking Fasting Promotes Regeneration and Reduces Autoimmunity and Multiple Sclerosis Symptoms. *Cell reports.* 2016;15(10):2136–2146.

3. de Oliveira GLV, Leite AZ, Higuchi BS, Gonzaga MI, Mariano VS. Intestinal dysbiosis and probiotic applications in autoimmune diseases. *Immunology.* 2017;152(1):1–12.

4. Ho JT, Chan GC, Li JC. Systemic effects of gut microbiota and its relationship with disease and modulation. *BMC immunology.* 2015;16:21.

5. Horta-Baas G, Romero-Figueroa MDS, Montiel-Jarquin AJ, Pizano-Zarate ML, Garcia-Mena J, Ramirez-Duran N. Intestinal Dysbiosis and Rheumatoid Arthritis: A Link between Gut Microbiota and the Pathogenesis of Rheumatoid Arthritis. *J Immunol Res.* 2017;2017:4835189.

6. Jahromi SR, Sahraian MA, Ashtari F, et al. Islamic fasting and multiple sclerosis. *BMC neurology.* 2014;14:56.

7. Kohling HL, Plummer SF, Marchesi JR, Davidge KS, Ludgate M. The microbiota and autoimmunity: Their role in thyroid autoimmune diseases. *Clin Immunol.* 2017;183:63–74.

8. Lin L, Zhang J. Role of intestinal microbiota and metabolites on gut homeostasis and human diseases. *BMC immunology.* 2017;18(1):2.

9. Mandl T, Marsal J, Olsson P, Ohlsson B, Andreasson K. Severe intestinal dysbiosis is prevalent in primary Sjogren's syndrome and is associated with systemic disease activity. *Arthritis research & therapy.* 2017;19(1):237.

10. Yadav SK, Boppana S, Ito N, et al. Gut dysbiosis breaks immunological tolerance toward the central nervous system during young adulthood. *Proc Natl Acad Sci U S A.* 2017;114(44):E9318–e9327.

CHAPTER 27 Behcet's Disease

1. Chen Y, Luo D, Cai JF, et al. Effectiveness and safety of Glycyrrhizae Decoction for Purging Stomach-Fire in Behcet disease patients: Study protocol for a randomized controlled and double-blinding trail. *Medicine.* 2018;97(13):e0265.

2. Jun JH, Choi TY, Zhang J, Ko MM, Lee MS. Herbal medicine for Behcet's disease: A protocol for a systematic review and meta-analysis. *Medicine.* 2018;97(13):e0165.

3. Kavandi H, Hajialilo M, Khabbazi A. Efficacy of Nigella sativa seeds oil in patients with Behcet's disease: a double-blind randomized controlled trial. *Avicenna J Phytomed.* 2018;8(6):498–503.

4. Kim MS, Kim SO, Lim WK, et al. Novel effects of On-Chung-Eum, the traditional plant medicine, on cytokine production in human mononuclear cells from Behcet's. *Immunopharmacol Immunotoxicol.* 2003;25(1):65–72.

5. Pronai L, Arimori S. BG-104 enhances the decreased plasma superoxide scavenging activity in patients with Behcet's disease, Sjogren's syndrome or hematological malignancy. *Biotherapy (Dordrecht, Netherlands).* 1991;3(4):365–371.

6. Thorat JD, Ng I. Acute dural sinus thrombosis following ingestion of an herbal tonic: case report. *Journal of stroke and cerebrovascular diseases : the official journal of National Stroke Association.* 2007;16(5):232–235.

7. Wu D, Lin W, Wong KW. Herbal medicine (Gancao Xiexin decoction) for Behcet disease: A systematic review protocol. *Medicine.* 2018;97(37):e12324.

8. Wu ZW, Yang CY, Bian TY. Behcet's disease: clinical report of 88 cases treated with herbal decoctions. *Journal of traditional Chinese medicine = Chung i tsa chih ying wen pan.* 1983;3(3):223–226.

9. Zhou WY, Zhang H, Zhuang ZY. Chinese medicine in the treatment of Behcet's disease's uveitis: a case report. *Chin J Integr Med.* 2012;18(3):219–221.

CHAPTER 28   Cardiometabolic Health

1. Boulangé CL, Neves AL, Chilloux J, Nicholson JK, Dumas M-EJGM. Impact of the gut microbiota on inflammation, obesity, and metabolic disease. 2016;8(1):42.

2. Bull MJ, Plummer NT. Part 2: Treatments for Chronic Gastrointestinal Disease and Gut Dysbiosis. *Integrative medicine (Encinitas, Calif).* 2015;14(1):25–33.

3. Cani PD, Osto M, Geurts L, Everard A. Involvement of gut microbiota in the development of low-grade inflammation and type 2 diabetes associated with obesity. *Gut Microbes.* 2012;3(4):279–288.

4. Cerdo T, Garcia-Santos JA, M GB, Campoy C. The Role of Probiotics and Prebiotics in the Prevention and Treatment of Obesity. *Nutrients.* 2019;11(3).

5. Cox LM, Blaser MJ. Antibiotics in early life and obesity. *Nature reviews Endocrinology.* 2015;11(3):182–190.

6. Davis-Richardson AG, Triplett EW. A model for the role of gut bacteria in the development of autoimmunity for type 1 diabetes. *Diabetologia.* 2015;58(7):1386–1393.

7. Devaraj S, Hemarajata P, Versalovic J. The human gut microbiome and body metabolism: implications for obesity and diabetes. *Clinical chemistry.* 2013;59(4):617–628.

8. Kasai C, Sugimoto K, Moritani I, et al. Comparison of the gut microbiota composition between obese and non-obese individuals in a Japanese population, as analyzed by terminal restriction fragment length polymorphism and next-generation sequencing. *BMC Gastroenterol.* 2015;15:100.

9. Liu R, Zhang C, Shi Y, et al. Dysbiosis of Gut Microbiota Associated with Clinical Parameters in Polycystic Ovary Syndrome. *Front Microbiol.* 2017;8:324.

10. Mar Rodriguez M, Perez D, Javier Chaves F, et al. Obesity changes the human gut mycobiome. *Sci Rep.* 2015;5:14600.

11. Million M, Lagier JC, Yahav D, Paul M. Gut bacterial microbiota and obesity. *Clinical microbiology and infection : the official publication of the European Society of Clinical Microbiology and Infectious Diseases.* 2013;19(4):305–313.

12. Nagata S, Chiba Y, Wang C, Yamashiro Y. The effects of the Lactobacillus casei strain on obesity in children: a pilot study. *Beneficial microbes.* 2017;8(4):535–543.

13. Nagpal R, Kumar M, Yadav AK, et al. Gut microbiota in health and disease: an overview focused on metabolic inflammation. *Beneficial microbes.* 2016;7(2):181–194.

14. Neuman H, Forsythe P, Uzan A, Avni O, Koren O. Antibiotics in early life: dysbiosis and the damage done. *FEMS microbiology reviews.* 2018;42(4):489–499.

15. Rasmussen SH, Shrestha S, Bjerregaard LG, et al. Antibiotic exposure in early life and childhood overweight and obesity: A systematic review and meta-analysis. *Diabetes Obes Metab.* 2018;20(6):1508–1514.

16. Rial SA, Karelis AD, Bergeron KF, Mounier C. Gut Microbiota and Metabolic Health: The Potential Beneficial Effects of a Medium Chain Triglyceride Diet in Obese Individuals. *Nutrients.* 2016;8(5).

17. Shao X, Ding X, Wang B, et al. Antibiotic Exposure in Early Life Increases Risk of Childhood Obesity: A Systematic Review and Meta-Analysis. *Frontiers in endocrinology.* 2017;8:170.

18. Williamson CB, Burns CM, Gossard CM, et al. Probiotics and Disease: A Comprehensive Summary-Part 3, Cardiometabolic Disease and Fatigue Syndromes. *Integrative medicine (Encinitas, Calif).* 2017;16(1):30–41.

19. Woting A, Blaut M. The Intestinal Microbiota in Metabolic Disease. *Nutrients.* 2016;8(4).

CHAPTER 29   Myalgic Encephalomyelitis/Chronic Fatigue Syndrome

1. Giloteaux L, Goodrich JK, Walters WA, Levine SM, Ley RE, Hanson MR. Reduced diversity and altered composition of the gut microbiome in individuals with myalgic encephalomyelitis/chronic fatigue syndrome. *Microbiome.* 2016;4(1):30.

2. Godas Sieso T, Gomez Gil E, Salamero Baro M, Fernandez-Huerta JM, Fernandez-Sola J. [Relationship between chronic fatigue syndrome and type A behaviour]. *Med Clin (Barc).* 2009;133(14):539–541.

3. Logan AC, Venket Rao A, Irani D. Chronic fatigue syndrome: lactic acid bacteria may be of therapeutic value. *Med Hypotheses.* 2003;60.

4. Logan AC, Wong C. Chronic fatigue syndrome: oxidative stress and dietary modifications. *Altern Med Rev.* 2001;6(5):450–459.

5. Maes M, Mihaylova I, Leunis JC. Increased serum IgA and IgM against LPS of enterobacteria in chronic fatigue syndrome (CFS): indication for the involvement of gram-negative enterobacteria in the etiology of CFS and for the presence of an increased gut-intestinal permeability. *J Affect Disord.* 2007;99(1–3):237–240.

6. Morris G, Berk M, Carvalho AF, Caso JR, Sanz Y, Maes M. The Role of Microbiota and Intestinal Permeability in the Pathophysiology of Autoimmune and Neuroimmune Processes with an Emphasis on Inflammatory Bowel Disease Type 1 Diabetes and Chronic Fatigue Syndrome. *Curr Pharm Des.* 2016;22(40):6058–6075.

7. Nagy-Szakal D, Williams BL, Mishra N, et al. Fecal metagenomic profiles in subgroups of patients with myalgic encephalomyelitis/chronic fatigue syndrome. *Microbiome.* 2017; 5(1):44.

8. Wallis A, Ball M, McKechnie S, Butt H, Lewis DP, Bruck D. Examining clinical similarities between myalgic encephalomyelitis/chronic fatigue syndrome and D-lactic acidosis: a systematic review. *J Transl Med.* 2017;15(1):129.

CHAPTER 30   Fibromyalgia

1. Cole JA, Rothman KJ, Cabral HJ, Zhang Y, Farraye FA. Migraine, fibromyalgia, and depression among people with IBS: a prevalence study. *BMC Gastroenterol.* 2006;6:26.

2. Goebel A, Buhner S, Schedel R, Lochs H, Sprotte G. Altered intestinal permeability in patients with primary fibromyalgia and in patients with complex regional pain syndrome. *Rheumatology (Oxford).* 2008;47(8):1223–1227.

3. Lamb JJ, Konda VR, Quig DW, et al. A program consisting of a phytonutrient-rich medical food and an elimination diet ameliorated fibromyalgia symptoms and promoted toxic-element detoxification in a pilot trial. *Altern Ther Health Med.* 2011;17(2):36–44.

4. Pimentel M, Wallace D, Hallegua D, et al. A link between irritable bowel syndrome and fibromyalgia may be related to findings on lactulose breath testing. *Ann Rheum Dis.* 2004;63(4):450–452.

5. Regland B, Forsmark S, Halaouate L, et al. Response to vitamin B12 and folic acid in myalgic encephalomyelitis and fibromyalgia. *PLoS One.* 2015;10(4):e0124648.

6. Rodrigo L, Blanco I, Bobes J, de Serres FJ. Clinical impact of a gluten-free diet on health-related quality of life in seven fibromyalgia syndrome patients with associated celiac disease. *BMC Gastroenterol.* 2013;13:157.

7. Rossi A, Di Lollo AC, Guzzo MP, et al. Fibromyalgia and nutrition: what news? *Clin Exp Rheumatol.* 2015;33(1 Suppl 88):S117–125.

8. Slim M, Calandre EP, Rico-Villademoros F. An insight into the gastrointestinal component of fibromyalgia: clinical manifestations and potential underlying mechanisms. *Rheumatology international.* 2015;35(3):433–444.

9. Sturgeon JA, Darnall BD, Zwickey HL, et al. Proinflammatory cytokines and DHEA-S in women with fibromyalgia: impact of psychological distress and menopausal status. *Journal of pain research.* 2014;7:707–716.

CHAPTER 31   Migraine Headaches

1. Alpay K, Ertas M, Orhan EK, Ustay DK, Lieners C, Baykan B. Diet restriction in migraine, based on IgG against foods: a clinical double-blind, randomised, cross-over trial. *Cephalalgia : an international journal of headache.* 2010;30(7):829–837.
2. Aydinlar EI, Dikmen PY, Tiftikci A, et al. IgG-based elimination diet in migraine plus irritable bowel syndrome. *Headache.* 2013;53(3):514–525.
3. Bunner AE, Agarwal U, Gonzales JF, Valente F, Barnard ND. Nutrition intervention for migraine: a randomized crossover trial. *The journal of headache and pain.* 2014;15:69.
4. Cole JA, Rothman KJ, Cabral HJ, Zhang Y, Farraye FA. Migraine, fibromyalgia, and depression among people with IBS: a prevalence study. *BMC Gastroenterol.* 2006;6:26.
5. Egger J, Carter CM, Soothill JF, Wilson J. Oligoantigenic diet treatment of children with epilepsy and migraine. *J Pediatr.* 1989;114(1):51–58.
6. Mitchell N, Hewitt CE, Jayakody S, et al. Randomised controlled trial of food elimination diet based on IgG antibodies for the prevention of migraine like headaches. *Nutr J.* 2011;10:85.
7. Pelsser LM, Frankena K, Buitelaar JK, Rommelse NN. Effects of food on physical and sleep complaints in children with ADHD: a randomised controlled pilot study. *European journal of pediatrics.* 2010;169(9):1129–1138.
8. Stuart S, Cox HC, Lea RA, Griffiths LR. The role of the MTHFR gene in migraine. *Headache.* 2012;52(3):515–520.
9. van Hemert S, Breedveld AC, Rovers JM, et al. Migraine associated with gastrointestinal disorders: review of the literature and clinical implications. *Frontiers in neurology.* 2014;5:241.

CHAPTER 32   Mental Health: Depression, Anxiety, and Schizophrenia

1. Boyle NB, Lawton C, Dye L. The Effects of Magnesium Supplementation on Subjective Anxiety and Stress-A Systematic Review. *Nutrients.* 2017;9(5).
2. Byrne G, Rosenfeld G, Leung Y, et al. Prevalence of Anxiety and Depression in Patients with Inflammatory Bowel Disease. *Canadian journal of gastroenterology & hepatology.* 2017;2017:6496727.
3. Campagna G, Pesce M, Tatangelo R, Rizzuto A, La Fratta I, Grilli A. The progression of coeliac disease: its neurological and psychiatric implications. *Nutr Res Rev.* 2017;30(1):25–35.

4. Caso JR, Balanza-Martinez V, Palomo T, Garcia-Bueno B. The Microbiota and Gut-Brain Axis: Contributions to the Immunopathogenesis of Schizophrenia. *Curr Pharm Des.* 2016;22(40):6122–6133.

5. Chan W, Shim HH, Lim MS, et al. Symptoms of anxiety and depression are independently associated with inflammatory bowel disease-related disability. *Dig Liver Dis.* 2017;49(12):1314–1319.

6. Ergun C, Urhan M, Ayer A. A review on the relationship between gluten and schizophrenia: Is gluten the cause? *Nutr Neurosci.* 2018;21(7):455–466.

7. Esenyel S, Unal F, Vural P. Depression and anxiety in child and adolescents with follow-up celiac disease and in their families. *Turk J Gastroenterol.* 2014;25(4):381–385.

8. Garakani A, Win T, Virk S, Gupta S, Kaplan D, Masand PS. Comorbidity of irritable bowel syndrome in psychiatric patients: a review. *Am J Ther.* 2003;10(1):61–67.

9. Hadjivassiliou M, Duker AP, Sanders DS. Gluten-related neurologic dysfunction. *Handb Clin Neurol.* 2014;120:607–619.

10. Hauser W, Janke KH, Klump B, Gregor M, Hinz A. Anxiety and depression in adult patients with celiac disease on a gluten-free diet. *World J Gastroenterol.* 2010;16(22):2780–2787.

11. Hausteiner-Wiehle C, Henningsen P. Irritable bowel syndrome: relations with functional, mental, and somatoform disorders. *World J Gastroenterol.* 2014;20(20):6024–6030.

12. Huang R, Wang K, Hu J. Effect of Probiotics on Depression: A Systematic Review and Meta-Analysis of Randomized Controlled Trials. *Nutrients.* 2016;8(8).

13. Jackson J, Eaton W, Cascella N, et al. Gluten sensitivity and relationship to psychiatric symptoms in people with schizophrenia. *Schizophrenia research.* 2014;159(2–3):539–542.

14. Jackson J, Eaton W, Cascella N, et al. A gluten-free diet in people with schizophrenia and anti-tissue transglutaminase or anti-gliadin antibodies. *Schizophrenia research.* 2012;140(1-3):262–263.

15. Karadag E, Samancioglu S, Ozden D, Bakir E. Effects of aromatherapy on sleep quality and anxiety of patients. *Nursing in critical care.* 2017;22(2):105–112.

16. Kasper S, Muller WE, Volz HP, Moller HJ, Koch E, Dienel A. Silexan in anxiety disorders: Clinical data and pharmacological background. *The world journal of biological psychiatry : the official journal of the World Federation of Societies of Biological Psychiatry.* 2018;19(6):412–420.

17. Kyrou I, Christou A, Panagiotakos D, et al. Effects of a hops (Humulus lupulus L.) dry extract supplement on self-reported depression, anxiety and stress levels in apparently healthy young adults: a randomized, placebo-controlled, double-blind, crossover pilot study. *Hormones (Athens, Greece).* 2017;16(2):171–180.

18. Lach G, Schellekens H, Dinan TG, Cryan JF. Anxiety, Depression, and the Microbiome: A Role for Gut Peptides. *Neurotherapeutics : the journal of the American Society for Experimental NeuroTherapeutics.* 2018;15(1):36–59.

19. Lakhan SE, Vieira KF. Nutritional and herbal supplements for anxiety and anxiety-related disorders: systematic review. *Nutr J.* 2010;9:42.

20. Malan-Muller S, Valles-Colomer M, Raes J, Lowry CA, Seedat S, Hemmings SMJ. The Gut Microbiome and Mental Health: Implications for Anxiety- and Trauma-Related Disorders. *Omics.* 2018;22(2):90–107.

21. Moos WH, Faller DV, Harpp DN, et al. Microbiota and Neurological Disorders: A Gut Feeling. *BioResearch open access.* 2016;5(1):137–145.

22. Neuendorf R, Harding A, Stello N, Hanes D, Wahbeh H. Depression and anxiety in patients with Inflammatory Bowel Disease: A systematic review. *J Psychosom Res.* 2016;87:70–80.

23. Pirbaglou M, Katz J, de Souza RJ, Stearns JC, Motamed M, Ritvo P. Probiotic supplementation can positively affect anxiety and depressive symptoms: a systematic review of randomized controlled trials. *Nutrition research (New York, NY).* 2016;36(9):889–898.

24. Porcelli B, Verdino V, Bossini L, Terzuoli L, Fagiolini A. Celiac and non-celiac gluten sensitivity: a review on the association with schizophrenia and mood disorders. *Auto Immun Highlights.* 2014;5(2):55–61.

25. Pratte MA, Nanavati KB, Young V, Morley CP. An alternative treatment for anxiety: a systematic review of human trial results reported for the Ayurvedic herb ashwagandha (Withania somnifera). *J Altern Complement Med.* 2014;20(12):901–908.

26. Samaroo D, Dickerson F, Kasarda DD, et al. Novel immune response to gluten in individuals with schizophrenia. *Schizophrenia research.* 2010;118(1-3):248–255.

27. Severance EG, Prandovszky E, Castiglione J, Yolken RH. Gastroenterology issues in schizophrenia: why the gut matters. *Current psychiatry reports.* 2015;17(5):27.

28. Smith LB, Lynch KF, Kurppa K, et al. Psychological Manifestations of Celiac Disease Autoimmunity in Young Children. *Pediatrics.* 2017;139(3).

29. Stevens BR, Goel R, Seungbum K, et al. Increased human intestinal barrier permeability plasma biomarkers zonulin and FABP2 correlated with plasma LPS and altered gut microbiome in anxiety or depression. *Gut.* 2018;67(8):1555–1557.

30. Tseng PT, Zeng BS, Chen YW, Wu MK, Wu CK, Lin PY. A meta-analysis and systematic review of the comorbidity between irritable bowel syndrome and bipolar disorder. *Medicine.* 2016;95(33):e4617.

CHAPTER 33   Osteoporosis: The GI Connection

1. Chen YC, Greenbaum J, Shen H, Deng HW. Association Between Gut Microbiota and Bone Health: Potential Mechanisms and Prospective. *J Clin Endocrinol Metab.* 2017;102(10):3635–3646.

2. Di Stefano M, Veneto G, Malservisi S, Corazza GR. Small intestine bacterial overgrowth and metabolic bone disease. *Dig Dis Sci.* 2001;46(5):1077–1082.

3. Hernandez CJ, Guss JD, Luna M, Goldring SR. Links Between the Microbiome and Bone. *Journal of bone and mineral research : the official journal of the American Society for Bone and Mineral Research.* 2016;31(9):1638–1646.

4. Iqbal J, Yuen T, Sun L, Zaidi M. From the gut to the strut: where inflammation reigns, bone abstains. *The Journal of clinical investigation.* 2016;126(6):2045–2048.

5. Irwin R, Raehtz S, Parameswaran N, McCabe LR. Intestinal inflammation without weight loss decreases bone density and growth. *American journal of physiology Regulatory, integrative and comparative physiology.* 2016;311(6):R1149–r1157.

6. Li JY, Chassaing B, Tyagi AM, et al. Sex steroid deficiency-associated bone loss is microbiota dependent and prevented by probiotics. *The Journal of clinical investigation.* 2016;126(6):2049–2063.

7. McCabe LR, Parameswaran N. Advances in Probiotic Regulation of Bone and Mineral Metabolism. *Calcif Tissue Int.* 2018;102(4):480–488.

8. Narva M, Nevala R, Poussa T, Korpela R. The effect of Lactobacillus helveticus fermented milk on acute changes in calcium metabolism in postmenopausal women. *Eur J Nutr.* 2004;43(2):61–68.

9. Shimizu Y. Gut microbiota in common elderly diseases affecting activities of daily living. *World J Gastroenterol.* 2018;24(42):4750–4758.

10. Wang J, Wang Y, Gao W, et al. Diversity analysis of gut microbiota in osteoporosis and osteopenia patients. *PeerJ.* 2017;5:e3450.

CHAPTER 34   Skin Conditions

1. Afifi L, Danesh MJ, Lee KM, et al. Dietary Behaviors in Psoriasis: Patient-Reported Outcomes from a U.S. National Survey. *Dermatology and therapy.* 2017;7(2):227–242.

2. Coondoo A, Phiske M, Verma S, Lahiri K. Side-effects of topical steroids: A long overdue revisit. *Indian dermatology online journal.* 2014;5(4):416–425.

3. Egeberg A, Hansen PR, Gislason GH, Thyssen JP. Clustering of autoimmune diseases in patients with rosacea. *J Am Acad Dermatol.* 2016;74(4):667–672.e661.

4. Gravina A, Federico A, Ruocco E, et al. Helicobacter pylori infection but not small intestinal bacterial overgrowth may play a pathogenic role in rosacea. *United European Gastroenterol J.* 2015;3(1):17–24.

5. Guarneri C, Lotti J, Fioranelli M, Roccia MG, Lotti T, Guarneri F. Possible role of Helicobacter pylori in diseases of dermatological interest. *Journal of biological regulators and homeostatic agents.* 2017;31(2 Suppl. 2):57–77.

6. Lazaridou E, Korfitis C, Kemanetzi C, et al. Rosacea and Helicobacter pylori: links and risks. *Clinical, cosmetic and investigational dermatology.* 2017;10:305–310.

7. Saleh P, Naghavi-Behzad M, Herizchi H, Mokhtari F, Mirza-Aghazadeh-Attari M, Piri R. Effects of Helicobacter pylori treatment on rosacea: A single-arm clinical trial study. *J Dermatol.* 2017;44(9):1033–1037.

8. Triantafillidis JK, Mantzaris G, Stamataki A, Asvestis K, Malgarinos G, Gikas A. Complete remission of severe scleritis and psoriasis in a patient with active Crohn's disease using Modulen IBD as an exclusive immunomodulating diet. *J Clin Gastroenterol.* 2008;42(5):550–551.

9. Yang X. Relationship between Helicobacter pylori and Rosacea: review and discussion. *BMC Infect Dis.* 2018;18(1):318.

INDEX

Page numbers in italics refer to figures or tables.

ABOUT THE AUTHOR

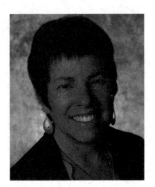

Liz Lipski, PhD, CNS, BCHN, FACN, IFMCP, LDN. After having been in clinical practice for 35 years, Dr. Lipski now devotes her time to teaching, training, consulting, and writing. Liz Lipski is currently a Professor and the Director of the Academic Development for the Nutrition programs in Clinical Nutrition at Maryland University of Integrative Health. She is the architect of the Doctor of Clinical Nutrition program, the first integrative program of its type in the United States.

Dr. Lipski holds a PhD in Clinical Nutrition, is a Fellow of the American College of Nutrition, and holds two board certifications in clinical nutrition and one in functional medicine. She is a faculty educator for The Institute for Functional Medicine and the Metabolic Medicine Institute fellowship program. She currently sits on the board for the Accreditation Council for Professional Nutrition Education, the Certified International Health Coaches, and the Autism Hope Alliance. She is a consultant for Conversion Labs.

Dr. Lipski has coauthored many peer reviewed papers and written textbook chapters. Her other books include: *Digestive Wellness for Children*, and *Leaky Gut Syndrome*.

She is the founder of InnovativeHealing.com, where she offers webinar-based Mentoring Programs and Advanced Nutrition Forums for nutritionists, dietitians, and other clinicians.

She lives in Oregon with her husband, and spends her free time gardening, camping, and spending as much time as possible with her adult children and grandchildren.

Websites

Book:

www.digestivewellnessbook.com

Course:

www.artofdigestivewelless.com

Main Website:

www.innovativehealing.com

University Website:

www.muih.edu

Supplement Store:

https://us.fullscript.com/welcome/lizlipski